GW01375358

Assessing Grammar

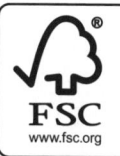

COMMUNICATION DISORDERS ACROSS LANGUAGES

Series Editors: Dr Nicole Müller and Dr Martin Ball, *University of Louisiana at Lafayette, USA*

While the majority of work in communication disorders has focused on English, there has been a growing trend in recent years for the publication of information on languages other than English. However, much of this is scattered through a large number of journals in the field of speech pathology/communication disorders, and therefore, not always readily available to the practitioner, researcher and student. It is the aim of this series to bring together into book form surveys of existing studies on specifi c languages, together with new materials for the language(s) in question. We also have launched a series of companion volumes dedicated to issues related to the cross-linguistic study of communication disorders. The series does not include English (as so much work is readily available), but covers a wide number of other languages (usually separately, though sometimes two or more similar languages may be grouped together where warranted by the amount of published work currently available). We have been able to publish volumes on Finnish, Spanish, Chinese and Turkish, and books on multilingual aspects of stuttering, aphasia, and speech disorders, with several others in preparation.

Full details of all the books in this series and of all our other publications can be found on http://www.multilingual-matters.com, or by writing to Multilingual Matters, St Nicholas House, 31-34 High Street, Bristol BS1 2AW, UK.

Assessing Grammar
The Languages of LARSP

Edited by
Martin J. Ball, David Crystal and Paul Fletcher

MULTILINGUAL MATTERS
Bristol • Buffalo • Toronto

Library of Congress Cataloging in Publication Data
A catalog record for this book is available from the Library of Congress.
Assessing Grammar: The Languages of LARSP/Edited by Martin J. Ball, David Crystal and Paul Fletcher.
Communication Disorders Across Languages: 7
Includes bibliographical references and index.
I. Ball, Martin J. (Martin John) II. Crystal, David, 1941- III. Fletcher, Paul, 1943- IV. Series: Communication disorders across languages ; 7.
[DNLM: 1. Language Tests. 2. Child. 3. Language Development Disorders--diagnosis. 4. Language Development. 5. Speech-Language Pathology--methods. WM 475]
LC classification not assigned
618.92'855–dc23 2011048970

British Library Cataloguing in Publication Data
A catalogue entry for this book is available from the British Library.

ISBN-13: 978-1-84769-638-0 (hbk)
ISBN-13: 978-1-84769-637-3 (pbk)

Multilingual Matters
UK: St Nicholas House, 31-34 High Street, Bristol BS1 2AW, UK.
USA: UTP, 2250 Military Road, Tonawanda, NY 14150, USA.
Canada: UTP, 5201 Dufferin Street, North York, Ontario M3H 5T8, Canada.

Copyright © 2012 Martin J. Ball, David Crystal, Paul Fletcher and the authors of individual chapters.

All rights reserved. No part of this work may be reproduced in any form or by any means without permission in writing from the publisher.

The policy of Multilingual Matters/Channel View Publications is to use papers that are natural, renewable and recyclable products, made from wood grown in sustainable forests. In the manufacturing process of our books, and to further support our policy, preference is given to printers that have FSC and PEFC Chain of Custody certification. The FSC and/or PEFC logos will appear on those books where full certification has been granted to the printer concerned.

Typeset by The Charlesworth Group.
Printed and bound in Great Britain by Short Run Press Ltd.

Contents

Contributors		vii
Introduction *Martin J. Ball*		1
1	On the Origin of LARSPecies *David Crystal*	4
2	LARSP Thirty Years On *Paul Fletcher, Thomas Klee and William Gavin*	12
3	'Computerized Profiling' of Clinical Language Samples and the Issue of Time *Steven Long*	29
4	HARSP: A Developmental Language Profile for Hebrew *Ruth A. Berman and Lyle Lustigman*	43
5	Profiling Linguistic Disability in German-Speaking Children *Harald Clahsen and Detlef Hansen*	77
6	GRAMAT: A Dutch Adaptation of LARSP *Gerard W. Bol*	92
7	LLARSP: A Grammatical Profile for Welsh *Martin J. Ball and Enlli Môn Thomas*	110
8	An Investigation of Syntax in Children of Bengali (Sylheti)-Speaking Families *Jane Stokes*	139
9	ILARSP: A Grammatical Profile of Irish *Tina Hickey*	149

10	Persian: Devising the P-LARSP *Habibeh Samadi and Mick Perkins*	167
11	Frisian TARSP. Based on the methodology of Dutch TARSP *Jelske Dijkstra and Liesbeth Schlichting*	189
12	C-LARSP: Developing a Chinese Grammatical Profile *Lixian Jin, with Bee Lim Oh and Rogayah A. Razak*	208
13	F-LARSP: A Computerized Tool for Measuring Morphosyntactic Abilities in French *Christophe Parisse, Christelle Maillart and Jodi Tommerdahl*	230
14	Spanish Acquisition and the Development of PERSL *Ana Isabel Codesido-García, Carmen Julia Coloma, Elena Garayzábal-Heinze, Victoria Marrero, Elvira Mendoza and Mª Mercedes Pavez*	245
15	LARSP for Turkish (TR-LARSP) *Seyhun Topbaş, Özlem Cangökçe-Yaşar and Martin J. Ball*	282
	Subject Index	306
	Author Index	315

Contributors

Martin J. Ball is Hawthorne-BoRSF Endowed Professor at the University of Louisiana at Lafayette. He is co-editor of the journal Clinical Linguistics and Phonetics (Taylor & Francis), and the book series Communication Disorders Across Languages (Multilingual Matters). His main research interests include sociolinguistics, clinical phonetics and phonology, and the linguistics of Welsh. He is an honorary Fellow of the Royal College of Speech and Language Therapists, and a Fellow of the Royal Society of Arts. Among his recent books are *Handbook of Clinical Linguistics* (co-edited with M. Perkins, N. Müller and S. Howard, Blackwell, 2008), and *Phonology for Communication Disorders* (co-authored with N. Müller and B. Rutter, Psychology Press, 2010).

Gerard Bol has worked at the University of Groningen since 1993. His research topic is developmental language disorders. This includes not only Specific Language Impairment, but also language disorders as a result of hearing impairment and cognitive problems. With that, methodology and quantification in child language research are issues he has published on. Gerard Bol is coauthor of the Dutch adaptation of the LARSP method by Crystal, Fletcher and Garman, called GRAMAT. Recent publications have concentrated on morphosyntax in typically developing Dutch children and those with SLI, including chapters in edited collections and papers in major peer-reviewed journals.

Ruth Berman, née Aronson, Professor Emeritus in linguistics, Tel Aviv University, with chair in Language across the Life Span, BA University of Cape Town, MA Columbia University, PhD Hebrew University (1973). Main research domains: Modern Hebrew grammar and lexicon; cross-linguistic first language acquisition, later language development, and text production from childhood to adolescence. Publications include: *Modern Hebrew Structure,* 1978; *Acquisition of Hebrew,* 1985; *Relating Events in Narrative,* 1994 with Dan I. Slobin; *Language Development across Childhood and Adolescence* (edited, 2004), and a special issue of *Journal of Pragmatics* (2005) on developing discourse stance. Former president of the International Association for the Study of Child Language [IASCL], and an honorary member of the Linguistic Society of America and the Spanish Language Acquisition Association.

Özlem Cangökçe-Yaşar has a bachelor's degree in Linguistics and has been awarded her Master's degree in Speech and Language Therapy. Currently she is employed as a research assistant at the Education, Research and Training Centre for Speech and Language Pathology (DİLKOM) as well as a PhD student in the Department of Speech & Language Pathology at Anadolu University, Eskişehir, Turkey.

Harald Clahsen is Alexander-von-Humboldt Professor at the University of Potsdam (Germany) and director of the new Potsdam Research Institute for Multilingualism. He is also a Fellow of the British Academy. He has published eight books and more than 100 research articles on first and second language acquisition, developmental and acquired language disorders and language processing. He has been the coordinator of several large research projects, and he co-edits Benjamins' book series on Language Development and Language Disorders. He received the Gerhard-Hess Award from the German Research Council for his work on language acquisition and an award from the University of Düsseldorf for his book on child language disorders.

Ana Isabel Codesido-García is full-time Associate Professor of Linguistics at the University of Santiago de Compostela (Galicia-Spain). Her main research interests include clinical linguistics, educational linguistics and forensic linguistics. Her doctoral dissertation (2003) dealt with qualitative assessment and evaluation of SLI in Spain. She has been recently incorporated to a research group focused on the early speech development in Spanish learning cochlear implant users, directed by Professor Ignacio Moreno-Torres (University of Málaga-Spain).

Carmen Julia Coloma is a linguist and holds a Master's degree in special education, and a PhD in health psychology. She was formerly the Principal of the School of Language and Speech, at the University of Chile, and is now an Associate Professor at that University. Her areas of research are related to phonology, grammar and narrative discourse of language impaired children. She has also developed studies related to oral language and its influences on learning to read. She has published many scientific articles; *Narrative Discourse in Children* is her most recent book.

David Crystal is honorary professor of linguistics at the University of Bangor, Wales, UK. He was formerly professor of linguistic science at the University of Reading, where he was responsible for developing undergraduate and advanced courses in linguistics and language pathology, and where the early research into linguistic profiling took place. Since leaving Reading in 1984, he has worked from his home in Holyhead, North Wales, as a writer, editor, lecturer, and broadcaster on linguistics, applied linguistics, and English language studies. His books include *The Cambridge Encyclopedia of Language*, *The Stories of English* and *Internet Linguistics*.

Jelske Dijkstra is working as a PhD-student at the Fryske Akademy in Leeuwarden, the Netherlands. Her study focuses on the early bilingual (Frisian/Dutch) language development of young children living in the province of Fryslân. Her research interests include speech and language development of young children, multilingualism and speech technology. One of her recent publications is a book about the language instrument

F-TARSP, *F-TARSP: Fryske Taal Analyze Remediearring en Screening Proseduere. In Fryske bewurking fan 'e TARSP* (Fryske Akademy/Afûk, 2008).

Paul Fletcher is Emeritus Professor, Speech and Hearing Sciences, University College Cork. Since the 1970s he has published widely on language development and language impairment in children speaking English, and more recently on those speaking Cantonese and Mandarin. His research focus, initially primarily on syntax, has broadened to include vocabulary, and the interaction between vocabulary and syntax in language development. He is a past president of the International Association for the Study of Child Language, and an honorary member of the Irish Association of Speech and Language Therapists.

Elena Garayzábal-Heinze is an Associate Professor of Linguistics at the Universidad Autónoma of Madrid (Spain); she is also a speech therapist and takes an active part as therapist and counselor in the Spanish Williams Syndrome Association and the Spanish Smith-Magenis Syndrome Association. She is a member of the editorial board of the electronic journal *Revista de Logopedia*. Her main research interests include clinical linguistics and forensic linguistics. She is a research member in different national and international research projects related to rare diseases and cochlear implant users. Among her recent books are *Lingüística Clínica y Logopedia* (Antonio Machado, 2006) and *Guía de Intervención Logopédica en el Síndrome de Williams* (co-authored with M. Fernández and E. Diez-Itza, Síntesis, 2010).

William Gavin serves as the Director of the Brainwaves Research Laboratory and is Associate Professor in the Department of Human Development and Family Studies at Colorado State University. Since receiving his doctorate degree in Experimental Psychology at the University of Miami (Coral Gables, Florida), he has been conducting research on a variety of topics related to child development. His early research focused primarily on speech and language development in infants and toddlers. His current research investigates the neurophysiological mechanisms that underlie the relationship of perception of sensory stimuli with the development of language and cognition in children with and without disabilities using electroencephalography (EEG) and event-related potentials (ERPs).

Detlef M. Hansen is Full Professor at the University of Wuerzburg (Germany) and Head of Department of Special Education – Speech and Language Pathology. His main research work and publications are in the field of Specific Language Impairment, speech and language assessment and therapy. For his research work on speech therapy with SLI-children he received the Gustav-Otto-Kanter-Award from the University of Cologne (Germany).

Tina Hickey lectures in the School of Psychology, UCD Dublin, and her publications include articles and books on the acquisition of Irish as L1, early immersion education, bilingualism, and second-language reading. In recent years she has been a Government of Ireland Fellow, and a Visiting

Scholar at the ESRC Centre for Research on Bilingualism in Bangor. She has served as Convenor of the AILA Child Language Commission, as Treasurer of IASCL, and is a member of the editorial board of the International Journal of Bilingual Education and Bilingualism. She is a former President of the Irish Association for Applied Linguistics and the Reading Association of Ireland. A recent book *Multilingual Europe: Diversity and Learning* (Trentham) was co-edited with Charmian Kenner.

Lixian Jin is Professor of Linguistics and Intercultural Learning at De Montfort University, UK, has been conducting research into bilingual clinical assessments and learners of English for over twenty years. Her research interests, with over 100 publications, include grammatical assessments of bilingual children for speech and language therapy (SLT), cultures of learning and intercultural and health communication, using innovative research methods of narrative and metaphor analysis to lead internationally funded research projects in Malaysia, Singapore and China for SLT clients and dyslexia learners. She is an editorial member for a number of international SLT and ELT journals.

Thomas Klee is Professor in the Department of Communication Disorders at University of Canterbury and Deputy Director of the New Zealand Institute of Language, Brain and Behaviour. He was twice Associate Editor of the *Journal of Speech, Language, and Hearing Research* and currently serves on the editorial boards of *Evidence-Based Communication Assessment and Intervention* and *Child Language Teaching and Therapy*. He led the development of a new MSc in Evidence-Based Practice in Communication Disorders at Newcastle University (UK) and has held research funding from the UK's Economic and Social Research Council, the Nuffield Foundation and the Hong Kong Research Grants Council. His research is currently funded by the Marsden Fund of the Royal Society of New Zealand and focuses on improving the way in which children with language difficulties are identified.

Steven Long is Associate Professor and Director of the Graduate Program in Speech Pathology and Audiology at Marquette University, Milwaukee, Wisconsin. His interests are centered around clinical linguistics and child therapy. He is the author (with M. Fey and R. Channell) of Computerized Profiling, a collection of computer programs for doing linguistic analyses of speech samples.

Lyle Lustigman, MA in linguistics, Tel Aviv University, doctoral student in the Cognitive Studies program on interfaces in early language development. Rottenstreich Fellowship, the Council for Higher Education, Israel (2010–2013), senior research assistant on Advanced Language Learners project (German-Israel Foundation, 2005-2008), project coordinator, Development of Complex Syntax in Hebrew (Israel Science Foundation, 2010–2013), directed by Ruth Berman. Publications include: Berman, R.A., Lustigman, L., & Nir-Sagiv, B. (2008) 'Discourse analysis as a window on later language development', *Israel Studies in Language and Society,* 1, 10–47 (in Hebrew); Lustigman, L. (in press), 'Developing structural specification: Productivity in early Hebrew verb usage', *First Language*; Lustigman, L. (in press), 'Non-finiteness in early Hebrew verbs', *Brill's Annual of Afroasiatic Languages and Linguistics (BAALL).*

Christelle Maillart is lecturer at the University of Liège in Belgium. She is speech and language therapist. Her teaching expertise and research interests include language acquisition, preschool and school age developmental language disorders and specific language impairment.

Victoria Marrero, holds a PhD in Linguistics from the *Complutense University of Madrid*, and is Professor of Linguistics and Spanish Language at the *National Distance Education University* (UNED) in Spain. Her main areas of interest are Phonetics, Speech Perception, Clinical Linguistics, Language Acquisition and Spanish as a Second Language for Immigrants. She has participated in research projects funded by the European Union, and by the Spanish Ministry of Science. Her latest book is entitled *El Lenguaje Humano* and *Invitación a la Lingüística* (coord V. Escandell, ed. UNED-CEURA). She has co-edited the Proceedings of the II International Conference on Clinical Linguistics, and authored/co-authored 10 other books, as well as numerous articles in journals such as *Speech Communication, Revista de Filología Española, Revista de Logopedia,* and *Foniatría y Audiología.*

Elvira Mendoza is Professor of Psychology and Logopedics in the Department of Personality, Assessment and Psychological Treatment at the University of Granada, Spain. She has published widely in areas such as language comprehension, Specific Language Impairment and language development. Her most recent works deal with Language Assessment (Revista de Logopedia, Foniatría y Audiología, 2010, 2011) and Grammatical Comprehension (CEG. TEA, 2005) and Specific Language Impairment. Currently she is vice president of the Spanish Association of Logopedics, Phoniatrics and Audiology.

Bee Lim Oh is a qualified speech and language therapist in Malaysia, graduated from the Universiti Kebangsaan Malaysia in 2010. She was one of the student research assistants who participated in the research project on the language development of Chinese-speaking children in Malaysia. She developed her research skills by collecting and analysing data and was a team member to carry out research at De Montfort University, UK during the project period.

Christophe Parisse is a full-time researcher at Modyco (Modèles, Dynamiques, Corpus), INSERM, University of Paris Ouest Nanterre La Défense, France. His main research interests include language development and developmental language disorders, from a cognitive linguistics perspective. He has contributed widely to the development of corpus analysis of child language and his work includes theoretical research about French language characteristics and psycholinguistic processes, as well as applied research such as computer tools for corpus processing. He has published widely in these areas in peer-reviewed journals in both French and English.

María Mercedes Pavez is a linguist and Associate Professor in the School of Language and Speech at the University of Chile. Her research topics are applied linguistics in language impairment and language development. She has researched on phonological disorders, and grammatical and narrative development in children with language problems. She has published tests for phonological and grammatical evaluation in Spanish speaking children and many scientific papers. *Narrative development in children* is her latest book.

Mick Perkins is Emeritus Professor of Clinical Linguistics in the Department of Human Communication Sciences at the University of Sheffield, UK. He has published widely both in his specialism of clinical linguistics and also in areas such as pragmatics, semantics and language development. His most recent books are *Pragmatic Impairment* (2007, CUP) and the *Handbook of Clinical Linguistics* (2008, Blackwell – co-edited with Martin Ball, Nicole Müller and Sara Howard). He was a founder member of the International Clinical Phonetics and Linguistics Association (ICPLA) and was its Vice-President from 2000 to 2006.

Rogayah A Razak, PhD is an associate professor in clinical linguistics at Universiti Kebangsaan Malaysia. She pioneered the clinical linguistic field in Malaysia by introducing a postgraduate programme in 2007. Her current research interests include child language development, construction of indigenous tools and linguistic analysis of disordered clinical data. Her publications include *The Syntax and Semantics of Quantification in Malay* (2003), numerous articles on developmental language, test adaptations such as the *Malay Boston NamingTest* (2007) and has constructed the Malay Syntactic Test prototype (2011) and is currently standardizing the *Malay Preschool Language Assessment Tool* (2010).

Habibeh Samadi is an honorary fellow of the University of Sheffield, Department of Human Communication Sciences and formerly an assistant professor at Kerman University of Medical Sciences, Medical School, Iran. Her main research interests are Persian (Farsi) language acquisition, child language acquisition and clinical syntax and morphology.

J. Liesbeth Schlichting is a voluntary researcher at the University of Groningen, Department of Special education, formerly a research fellow at the Academic Hospital of Utrecht University. Her main interests are language testing, language therapy and teaching reading to deaf students. Her main research interests include early vocabularies, the syntactic development of Dutch children, and nonword repetition. Recent language tests are the Schlichting Test voor Taalbegrip (Schlichting Test of Language Comprehension, Bohn Stafleu van Loghum, 2010, 2011) and the Schlichting Test voor Taalproductie (Schlichting Test of Language Production) Bohn Stafleu van Loghum, 2010, 2011), both with co-author H.C. lutje Spelberg.

Jane Stokes is a senior lecturer in speech and language therapy at the University of Greenwich in the UK. She has worked as a speech and language therapist in London and Hong Kong. She has always enjoyed clinical work with children and adults with communication difficulties and managing teams in linguistically and culturally diverse communities. Recently she has been involved in developing the curriculum for a new postgraduate diploma in speech and language therapy run as a collaboration between University of Greenwich and Canterbury Christ Church University. In this role she has drawn on her experience in the National Health Service to prepare student practitioners for the challenges of working in health, education and social care settings in the UK. Throughout her career she has been committed to joint work with people who share her enthusiasm for continuous improvement of the services provided to children and families who speak languages other than English.

Enlli Môn Thomas is currently a Lecturer in Education at Bangor University, and a core member of the executive of the ESRC Centre for Research on Bilingualism in Theory and Practice. She graduated with a degree in Psychology, but went on to pursue her interests in language, gaining a PhD looking at children's acquisition of grammatical gender in Welsh. Her research interests include Welsh language acquisition, bilingual acquisition, minority language acquisition, bilingual and minority language assessment, and approaches to language teaching in education. She has authored journal articles and book chapters on theoretical and practice aspects to bilingualism and acquisition.

Jodi Tommerdahl is an Associate Professor at the University of Texas at Arlington. She received her PhD from la Sorbonne (Paris IV) and is on the editorial board of Child Language Teaching and Therapy. Her main research interests lie in clinical linguistics, reasoning, and the interface of thought and language. She is currently setting up a neurophysiology laboratory to examine language and reasoning in relation to learning and education.

Seyhun Topbaş is Professor of Speech and Language Pathology at Anadolu University, Eskişehir, Turkey. She is one of the pioneers of the Speech & Language Pathology profession in Turkey, the founder of the graduate programs in Speech and Language Therapy and DİLKOM (Education, Research and Training Centre for Speech and Language Pathology) at Anadolu University. Dr Topbas has developed a standardized Turkish Articulation and Phonology Test and has authored many articles and chapters in international and national journals. She has written and been the editor of three books in speech and language disorders. The most recent was published internationally by Multilingual Matters titled *Communication Disorders in Turkish* (co-authored by Dr Mehmet Yavaş). She is currently a member of ASHA, and elected committee member of *International Issues Board*, and a member of IALP, ICPLA, and on the editorial board of *Clinical Linguistics and Phonetics*.

Introduction
Martin J. Ball

The publication of *The grammatical analysis of language disability* (Crystal *et al.*, 1976) came as a most welcome boon for teachers of English grammatical structure to speech/language pathology students. At last we had a principled approach to clients' language data that allowed a comprehensive analysis together with a metric based on developmental norms.

So widely used was this approach at the time that a new verb was born: *to larsp*, and we all became expert *larspers*. Indeed, the profile approach to language data was soon recognized internationally, and only a few years later versions of LARSP appeared designed for other languages (Hebrew was the first in 1982, see Chapter 4). Over the three-plus decades since its first appearance, versions of LARSP have been designed for numerous languages, and one of the purposes of this book was to collect as many of these together as possible, to act as a source book for clinicians working with different languages. However, it was clear also that there were several lacunae in the provision of profiles, in that some major languages had had no profiles designed for them. Therefore, a second purpose of this collection was to provide a place where new versions of LARSP could be introduced (albeit some of these are still works in progress).

The editors of this collection provided guidelines to the contributors about how to structure chapters. We felt that readers would welcome a grammatical sketch of the language concerned; information, where available, on normal patterns of grammatical acquisition; details on the database used to draw up these patterns; and the design of the chart itself. However, different teams of authors are at different stages in the development of their profiles. Some are reporting on versions that were designed quite some time ago, whereas others are still in the process of finalizing their designs. This results, of course, in chapters that display quite some variation in content and approach. So, while some profiles are ready for clinical application (and indeed have been so applied), others are only at the trial stage and may lack details of grammatical patterns in the final developmental stages. This is unavoidable in a collection that includes both mature and new profiles.

There are also other differences between chapters. While authors have for the most part adhered to grammatical analyses along the lines described in Crystal *et al.* (1976; see also Chapter 2), there are some departures from this in certain chapters. Partly this is to do with the requirements of the individual languages, or to the preferred analyses of authors or author teams.

Some interesting similarities and differences emerge from comparing the different profiles described in these chapters. Most authors have kept to the same sections and subsections in the profile charts as are used in LARSP. On the other hand, while most have kept to single-page charts, some authors have felt that multi-page charts are easier. For example, both Welsh and Irish display initial consonant mutation and more word-level morphology than is found in English. Ball and Thomas (Chapter 7) use three charts to cover syntax, mutations and morphology respectively, while Hickey (Chapter 9) uses only one. Indeed, it is the morphologically rich languages that display most differences in chart design as shown, for example, in Turkish, where again a separate morphology chart is needed. Another point concerns the developmental metric used in LARSP. This is copied in several of the charts described in this collection, but for those languages where developmental norms have not been fully established, a simple stage-by-stage approach has been used; further research will show whether these stages do coincide with developmental milestones.

The editors have chosen to order the chapters in the collection in a quasi-chronological manner, that is, in the order in which the original profiles were first developed. So, after David Crystal's description of the origin of LARSPecies in Chapter 1, we place Fletcher, Klee and Gavin's re-assessment of the English LARSP. This is followed (out of chronological sequence) by Steven Long's examination of computerized profiling (as it deals mainly with the English LARSP). The first non-English profile was designed for Hebrew and so Berman and Lustigman's description of HARSP is Chapter 4. Next in chronological order come German (Clahsen & Hansen), Dutch (Bol) and Welsh (Ball & Thomas). Stokes's description of work on the Sylheti dialect of Bengali is Chapter 8, Hickey on Irish is Chapter 9, and Chapter 10 deals with Persian (Samadi & Perkins). Dijkstra and Schlichting's chapter on Frisian completes the set of chapters based on established profiles, though interestingly her work is based on an earlier Dutch version of LARSP, which was an alternative to Bol's work (Schlichting, 1987). The final four chapters contain the profiles developed especially for this volume and are arranged alphabetically by the name of the language in English. They are Chinese (Jin and colleagues), French (Parisse and colleagues), Spanish (with teams from Madrid, Santiago de Compostela, and Chile), and Turkish (Seyhun Topbaş and her colleagues).

Naturally, in any such endeavour, there are always some that 'got away'. We had information that suggested that unpublished versions of LARSP had been created for certain Scandinavian languages (Danish and Norwegian); for Japanese; and that preliminary work had been done on versions for French, Hungarian, and Giriama (a Bantu language of East Africa). None of these proved traceable. There were also those that we thought we had got, and that 'got away' during the preparation of the collection. Authors had agreed to produce a new chapter on Hungarian, and revise a dissertation version for Panjabi. Unfortunately, despite being signed up to the project, neither set of authors was able to complete their contributions and withdrew fairly late in the process. Nevertheless, we feel we have a good balance between major and lesser-used languages, between Indo-European languages and those of other families, and a good geographical spread. Indeed, as we have profiles for both English and Chinese, one could claim we cover the great majority of speakers in the world!

This brings us to future developments: new languages of LARSP. There are currently two doctoral students in the Department of Communicative Disorders at the University of Louisiana at Lafayette working on preliminary stages of LARSP-like profiles: one for Greek and the other for Russian. A new team of researchers has expressed an interest in developing a Hungarian version (but was unable to meet the deadline for this book). We know also that a version for Malay is currently being worked on.

In any future new collection of languages of LARSP one would clearly like to see versions for languages where speech/language pathology provision is available. This would imply languages such as Portuguese (Brazil and Portugal), Italian, other eastern European languages, more languages of India, Japanese, Korean, Cantonese and some of the major languages of South Africa. Clearly, we have scope here for future collections of the languages of LARSP!

Please note, that copyright in all the Charts appearing in this book rests with the respective authors, and in the case of the F-TARSP chart, with the Fryske Akademy.

References

Crystal, D., Fletcher, P. and Garman, M. (1976) *The Grammatical Analysis of Language Disability*. London: Edward Arnold.

Schlichting, L. (1987) *TARSP: Taal Analyse Remediëring en Screening Procedure, Taalontwikkelingsschaal van Nederlandse Kinderen van 1-4 Jaar*. Amsterdam: Pearson.

1 On the Origin of LARSPecies
David Crystal

The origins of LARSP lie in a serendipitous encounter with a language-delayed child, at a time when a linguistically informed analysis of language was not a routine weapon in the speech pathologist's armoury. In Britain, it was not until 1972 that a government report on speech therapy services (the Quirk Report) made a statement that now seems blindingly obvious, but which at the time indicated the distance still to be travelled in clinical training and practice[1]:

> the would-be practitioner of therapy ... must in future regard language as the central core of his basic discipline.

The consequence was an immediate raising of the profile for linguistics, as the relevant science of language. A new climate formed and a clinical linguistic perspective became routine. LARSP, expounded in 1976 in the book *The grammatical analysis of language disability*,[2] was part of that climate. But its origins lie a decade before, in that chance encounter.

The Department of Linguistic Science at the University of Reading was established in 1965. One of my roles was to teach courses in the structure of English and child language acquisition, and so, when a phone call came through from the Royal Berkshire Hospital, just down the road, it was put through to me. It was from the audiologist, Dr Kevin Murphy, who was hoping that there was someone who could visit his department to advise on the assessment of a 3-year-old child whose speech was puzzling them. There were no hearing problems, it seems, and intelligence and social skills were normal, but she wasn't saying very much, and when she did speak her utterances evidently sounded immature.

I spent an afternoon observing a session with her therapist. It was the first language-delayed child I had ever seen, but her language output was immediately recognizable to anyone familiar with the limited but growing literature on language development in children. Asked for my opinion about what was going on, I gave a report which (if I were giving it today) would say that this child was making slow progress at Stage II, with several isolated phrases, verb-related gaps in clause structure, no clause element expansion in the direction of Stage III and a worryingly high proportion of minor sentences at Stage I. But this was not today: it was 1968. And as I continued with my description of the child's grammatical difficulties and her developmental level, it was evident that my listeners had no idea what I was talking about.

We took time out to discuss the problem. Grammatical analysis, it appeared, had not been part of the training of any of the professionals in the room. They had a vague memory of 'doing grammar' in their school days, but that had not been a particularly pleasant experience; they had forgotten most of it, and in any case it didn't seem to relate to the practical demands of the clinic. Nor had they ever been given a course on child language development. That was hardly surprising. Child language studies were in their infancy in the 1960s. There was no journal of child language (that did not begin until 1975), no child language association (that was 1970), and the major books that would one day define the subject were yet to be written (Roger Brown's *A First Language*, for example, wasn't published until 1973). I well recall the difficulty of finding material for students to read, in those days, and – in a pre-CHILDES era[3] – getting hold of audio examples of real children to demonstrate developmental reality. I spent many hours recording my young children, as a consequence, and I know several other linguists who were doing the same.

LARSP, I can see now, was born on that afternoon. I was asked to write up my observations in a report, and present it to a group at the hospital. I did so, giving them a handout which had primitive levels of development (what would later be Stages I to V) illustrated by a few types of construction. The child was evidently about two years grammatically delayed. My session included a basic grammar tutorial about clause and phrase structure. The data from the child was analysed and located at the appropriate points. It was possible to see a pattern: where she was. It was also possible to see the deficit: where she ought to be (for her age). And because the material was organized into developmental stages, it was possible to address the question that was foremost in everyone's mind: how do we get her from where she was to where she ought to be? The principle of following normal development was already well established in paediatric circles, so it was possible to suggest to the speech therapist that the next session should focus on structures which would first consolidate the stage where the child was (introducing verbs, in particular), and then integrating phrase structure within clause elements. A remedial programme was agreed, and therapy began. It is no surprise today, several thousand interventions later, to know that it worked. But at the time, the fact that the therapy was principled, that the child made progress, and that the procedure was generalizable to other patients with language disability (adults as well as children), produced reactions of genuine surprise, delight and relief.

It was grammar that had to be the primary focus of attention, and rightly so. Although the child I had seen evidently had an immature vocabulary and pronunciation, it was her grammatical difficulties which needed the most urgent treatment. This is because grammar is the key to understanding language disability. Vocabulary, because of its huge scope (tens of thousands of words to be learned) is sometimes said to be the primary goal of therapy, and it has certainly taken up a huge amount of testing time. But vocabulary without grammar is a dead end. Without a command of sentence structure, it is not possible to make sense of words. Words by themselves are entities with uncertain meaning. A one-word sentence has many possible interpretations. A word such as *apple* has several competing meanings ('fruit, computer, Beatles...'). Only by putting words into sentences is it possible to say which meaning we wish to convey. All the structures of grammar, from the largest clauses to the smallest word-endings, are there to help make sense of our words. Procedures for other aspects of language are important, of course, but grammar remains at the centre of clinical enquiry, as the dimension within which semantic and phonological observations need to be integrated. That is why LARSP was the first kind of procedure to be developed.[4]

As a young linguist, interested in the potential of linguistics to be useful as well as fascinating, I found the clinical domain enthralling and enticing. A two-track process of development followed: on the one hand, it was crucial to gain as much clinical experience as possible, to test the hypotheses about grammatical delay, and here the hospital and local speech therapy clinics played a critical role; and it was essential to consolidate the analysis, filling it out on the basis of contemporary research findings, establishing norms and integrating it into a single procedure. This second task took much longer than I was expecting, because in the early 1970s child language research was a rapidly expanding field, and many new developmental findings had to be incorporated into the procedure. At the same time, it was evident that there were huge gaps – areas of grammatical development where little or no empirical research had been done. I initially supplemented the research literature with data taken from samples of my own children, who had by this time (a boy born in 1964, a girl born in 1966) gone through all the relevant grammatical stages without incident. But a more systematic approach was needed. The principle of many heads making light work obtained. The cavalry had arrived in the department, in the form of Michael Garman and Paul Fletcher, and with their overlapping interests and expertise a fuller picture of grammatical development to age three soon emerged. The later stages of acquisition were less well studied, and our Stage VII is really no more than a placeholder, reminding people that there is grammar still to be learned after age five, but this didn't bother us. Most patients were going to be at a much earlier stage, and if any of them managed to reach Stage VII they would hardly need the help provided by a LARSP. The same point applied when using the chart to work with adult aphasics.

By early 1974 we had an account that we felt was developmentally robust. We took it out on the road, giving in-service courses to groups of speech therapists in various parts of the UK, all of whom were very keen to take on board this early encounter with a linguistic perspective. The benefit for us was that many in our audiences were highly experienced clinicians, and their comments helped us shape the final version of the chart as well as giving us confidence about our judgements.

Just as important as the developmental side of the project was its practical purpose. There was no point in working up a procedure that clinicians and remedial teachers would find unusable. The mid-1970s was a period when formal language teaching had disappeared from British schools (it had gone from most school syllabuses by the mid-1960s)[5] and well before the recommendations of the Quirk report had been implemented in speech therapy training courses. There was a limit to the amount of grammatical apparatus that professionals would be able to assimilate, and real constraints on the amount of clinical time it would take to use a new procedure. The shortage of speech therapists meant that most patients were being seen for perhaps half an hour a week, with heavy caseloads leaving little time for analytical reflection. Feedback from clinicians made it clear that they wanted a procedure which would fit on one side of a sheet of paper.

As linguists, we had two choices to make. Which grammatical model to choose? And how much grammatical detail to introduce? After much debate, we used a model in which a clear distinction is made between sentence structure (syntax) and word structure (morphology) – a highly relevant clinical distinction. Complex sentences are analysed into sequences of clauses; clauses are analysed into a series of elements (Subject, Verb, Object, Complement, Adverbial); and clause elements are represented by phrases (such as noun phrase, verb phrase, prepositional phrase).[6] We reduced the amount of grammatical detail by focusing on a small number of developmentally salient constructions and making a copious use of the category 'Other'. We experimented with several designs before settling on the final version, which did, happily, fit on to a single page.

What kind of procedure had emerged? We had spent some time looking at the tests and procedures that were already being used in relation to other areas of child development. It was immediately obvious that grammatical development was unlike anything else: for a start there were too many variables operating simultaneously – formal choices in clause and phrase structure (SV, DN, etc), sentence functions (statement, question, etc), morphology *(-ing, -ed*, etc) and patterns of interaction (especially questions and responses). It would never be possible to reduce these to a single 'test' score. The notion of a *profile* of performance, already used in linguistics (in such areas as stylistics), seemed the only sensible way to proceed. And it was evidently going to be desirable to bring together the four chief clinical desiderata: screening, assessment, diagnosis and therapy. Bearing in mind, also, the fact that many children with language problems were being managed in school (rather than, or as well as, in a clinic), it was important to introduce an educational perspective. How were all these variables to be combined?

Diagnosis seemed a distant goal, given the lack of clinical case studies. In any case, the broad diagnostic categories already being used ('language delay', 'language disorder') were enough to be getting on with. It was likely that it would eventually be possible to establish a more refined set of diagnostic categories, identified by their grammatical symptomatology, but this was not going to be possible until a large number of individual patients had been thoroughly investigated using a standard sampling procedure – and, moreover, over a period of time. Assessment, and its first cousin, screening, seemed more realistic immediate goals, along with the notion of remediation (a term that seemed to straddle clinic and classroom), so these three elements influenced our choice of the name for the procedure.

A good acronym was evidently critical. Acronyms were everywhere in the clinical domain (WISC, PPVT, RDLS...), and we appreciated the value of a succinct label in everyday discourse. Fortunately, the initial letters of Assessment, Screening, and Remediation, along with P for Procedure, formed a pronounceable unit, ARSP. That was the easy bit. The more intriguing question was which letter to use to introduce the acronym. G for Grammar was the obvious choice, but GARSP (pronounced 'gasp' in Received Pronunciation) had the wrong connotations and elicited hilarity from anyone we mentioned it to – as did GRARSP. It is always wise to try out acronyms in real sentences before choosing them, and it seemed somewhat inelegant to talk of a patient having been GRARSPed. We settled for LARSP, where L stood for Language. Today, with several other profiles and procedures around focusing on other aspects of language (semantics, phonology, etc), that choice feels too general. LARSP does not deal with all aspects of language. But in the mid-1970s, it seemed a reasonable decision. Grammar was virtually synonymous with the notion of language in the minds of therapists, and the change of direction from 'speech' to 'language' (which eventually became formally incorporated into the official nomenclature of the profession in the UK) was chiefly associated with a move from pronunciation to grammar. (In the event, the application of LARSP to other languages led to the some authors replacing the initial letter, as several chapters in this book illustrate.)

The structure of the chart reflected its utilitarian purpose (see Figure 1.1). The main types of organization in sentence structure and function are represented under various headings laid out horizontally on the chart. The main stages of grammatical acquisition are laid out vertically on the chart, beneath the thick black line. The main patterns of grammatical interaction between therapist/teacher and patient/pupil are summarized above the thick black line, in Sections B, C and D. The bottom line of the chart contains certain kinds of summarizing information, and Section A is included primarily as a time-saving device in using the procedure. We quickly learned that an awful lot of time was being wasted by clinicians struggling to analyse utterances that any experienced grammarian would see straight

Section A Time-saving section
Sections B C D Information about interaction
Types of sentence structure and function Stages of grammatical acquisition I–VII
Summarizing line

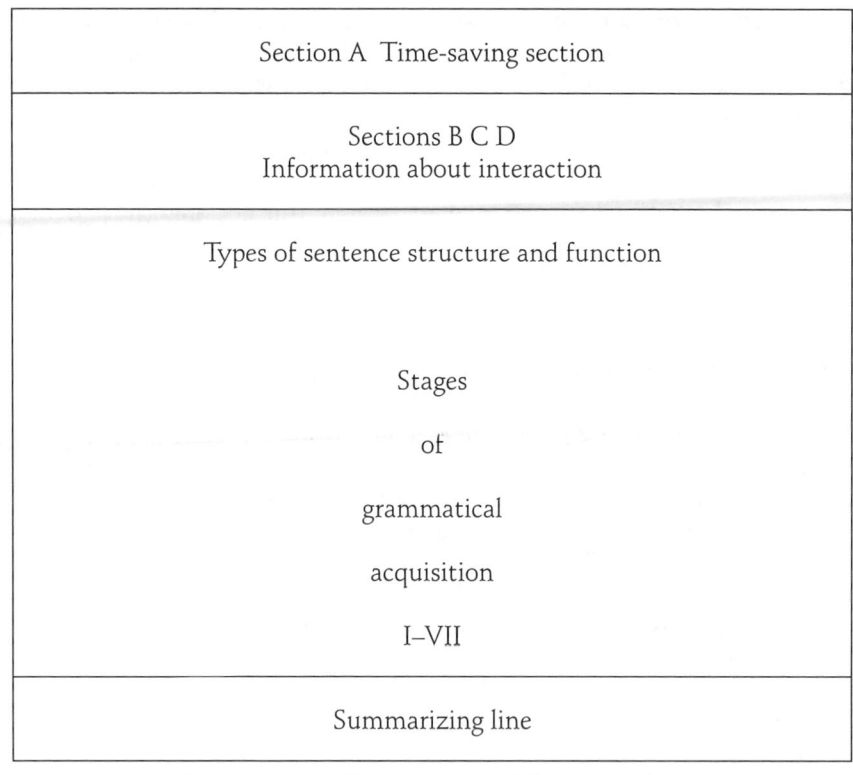

Figure 1.1 Outline structure of the LARSP chart

away were not worth the effort because they were incomplete, ambiguous or whatever. There was a natural tendency to want to analyse everything, and it's an important moment when one realizes that a significant feature of an assessment is the proportion of utterances that *cannot* be given a sensible grammatical analysis. Section A, with its categories of Unanalysed and Problematic, and their five subdivisions, was partly intended to take the worry out of the situation, as well as being clinically informative in its own right.

Sections B and C reflected our sense that it was crucial to alert clinicians to the importance of the way they talked to their patients. An early observation had been that two of the most popular question stimuli were actually hindering rather than helping patient response: 'What doing' (e.g. *What's the man doing?*) and 'What happening' (e.g. *What's happening in the picture? Tell me what's happening*). These questions demand verbs if they are to be answered (*He's running, A man's jumping*), and as most of the patients we were analysing had early problems with verbs, these stimuli would only add to their difficulty in replying. An important prior remedial procedure was to teach some verbs, first by imitation, then by using forced alternative questions (*Is he running or jumping?*), before proceeding to the open-ended questions of the 'What doing' type. The interactive section of the chart was designed to draw attention to problems in this area – and in particular to the fact that therapists and patients are engaged in a dialogue, and that any assessment or decision about therapy needed to monitor the evolving discourse relationship between the participants. It is not only the patient's use of language which provides the basis of an assessment; the therapist's use of language has to be taken into account too.

If the chart had been designed a decade later, these sections would probably have looked very different. During the 1980s, pragmatics developed as a branch of linguistics, with its focus on the intentions behind a speaker's choice of utterance and the effects on the listener that these choices convey. Discourse linguistics was also increasingly attracting attention. Both of these perspectives had begun to influence child language studies, and the importance of the type of adult response to a child utterance (e.g. whether the parent expands the child's sentence) had been highlighted as a significant factor in language learning. The second edition of the chart recognizes these trends by adding a Section D, which records the type of reaction of the therapist to what the patient has said. Given the amount of discourse analysis that has taken place in the last 30 years, the classification of utterances in Sections B, C and D is primitive and shows its age. But it is illuminating even in this basic form, and is still an essential part of any investigation.

I always thought of LARSP as a state of mind as much as a procedure. Its aim was to inculcate a way of thinking – a linguistically informed view of language disability which prioritizes three dimensions of grammatical investigation: the comprehensive description of a patient's utterances; the assigning of utterances to a developmental level; and the analysis of the interaction between patient and clinician. The initial aim was to get clinicians, and later remedial teachers, to appreciate the central role of these dimensions in any clinical or educational enquiry and to begin to see patients and pupils within this frame of reference. The chart was simply a way of operationalizing these insights. I used to say, tongue in cheek, that to be a LARSPer you didn't really need the chart – and then stopped saying this when I realized that some people were taking me literally! In fact one does need the chart, as there are too many variables to hold in mind (there are over 150 possible information points on the chart), and a formal record of a patient's achievement at a particular point in time is standard practice in case histories.

The ultimate success of the procedure, I felt, would depend on the extent to which it offered insight into the character of someone's language disability, which would not have been possible using traditional therapeutic paradigms. The insights would be productive if they identified patterns of assessment, suggested paths of remediation, and eventually contributed to diagnosis. But there was a second aim: to introduce an element of conscious control into a clinical or teaching situation. The task facing all involved in language therapy is not solely to obtain progress, but to be sure that the progress is due to their intervention. That is what everyone, from practitioners to parents to purse-holders, needs to be confident about. I believe that linguistic profiling is a powerful way of achieving that level of confidence. When samples are well chosen and charts regularly made and completed, LARSP makes a contribution to efficacy and thus to the skill base that defines professionalism in language intervention.

Notes

(1) *Speech Therapy Services* (London: HMSO, 1972), §6.60.
(2) GALD was first published by Edward Arnold in 1976. A second edition, published by Cole & Whurr, appeared in 1989. In the meantime, a fuller methodological guide with associated papers on the application of LARSP in clinical and remedial settings, had appeared in 1979: *Working With LARSP* (Arnold). All books are now out of print, but GALD is available online at <http://ir.canterbury.ac.nz/handle/10092/5483>; *Working with LARSP* at <http://ir.canterbury.ac.nz/handle/10092/5482>; and *Profiling Linguistic Disability* at <http://ir.canterbury.ac.nz/handle/10092/5510>. Further online exposition can be found in the papers under Clinical Linguistics at <www.davidcrystal.com>: 'Profile analysis of language disability' (with Paul Fletcher), 'Psycholinguistics', 'Putting profiles into practice' and 'Towards a bucket theory of language disability'.
(3) See the site at http://childes.psy.cmu.edu/.
(4) For the other profiles, see Crystal, D. (1992) *Profiling Linguistic Disability* (2nd edn). London: Edward Arnold.
(5) The period is documented in my (2006) *The Fight for English*. Oxford: Oxford University Press. See Chapter 28.
(6) Our grammatical description was based on the approach presented in Quirk *et al.* (1975) *A Comprehensive Grammar of the English Language*. London: Longman. Having worked on the Quirk Survey of English Usage, I was very familiar with this approach, which (most conveniently, from our point of view) was published while we were putting LARSP together.

2 LARSP Thirty Years On
Paul Fletcher, Thomas Klee
and William Gavin

Introduction

It is over three decades since LARSP (Language Assessment, Remediation and Screening Procedure) for English was published (Crystal et al., 1976). This text, along with a revision (Crystal et al., 1989), and other relevant publications (e.g. Crystal, 1979, 1982, 1992) are now out of print.[1] But as a framework for profiling the development of grammar, LARSP has not been superseded. It continues to be taught to student clinicians, and to be used in clinics for assessment and as a basis for intervention. The lapse of time since the profile's emergence has not dramatically altered our view of the broad outline of grammatical development in English, but we have learned a good deal more about the detail of first language learning, in particular about *variability* in the rate of development across typically developing (TD) children, and about children's *gradual* accretion of grammatical competence. We are also much better informed about *faultlines* in the grammars of children with language impairment. In this chapter we explore the implications of this information for assessment and intervention using LARSP, in selected areas of the profile.

Variability

The construction of the initial LARSP profile, in the early 1970s, had a limited range of data on language development in English to draw on. However, even then we knew, from Roger Brown's pioneering work, that some children learned their native tongue more quickly than others. There is a classic graph in his book (Brown, 1973: 57), which plots the mean length of utterance against age in the children he studied. Adam and Sarah reach a mean length of utterance (MLU) of 4.0 at around 42 months, whereas Eve's utterances average four morphemes at the age of 26 months. Given that only these three children were involved in the research, it was impossible to tell at the time whether Eve was unique as a precocious language learner, or a representative example of a much larger group of children. We had to wait until the 1990s, and the advent of studies with larger samples, to get a clearer idea of the variation in rates of development.

The first intimation came from parent report instruments such as the MacArthur-Bates Communicative Development Inventory (MBCDI – Fenson *et al.*, 2007). The MBCDI and similar protocols have been developed for English and for more than 40 other languages (see www.sci.sdsu.edu/cdi/adaptations_ol.htm). They have been widely used over the last two decades to examine lexical development and some aspects of morphosyntactic development between eight and 36 months. The norming study on the MBCDI (carried out in the US) sampled 75 children in each month of the age range – 1800 children in all. It reveals that at 24 months, the mean expressive vocabulary figure for two-year-olds is 312 words. However, children at the 10th centile are reported to have 89 words, while those at the 90th centile use 534 (Bates *et al.*, 1995). A study by Stokes and Klee (2009), which looked at parent-reported vocabulary in over 200 British children between 24 and 30 months of age, confirms this variability in lexical development. Stokes and Klee found that the number of words known expressively by the children in their sample ranges from a low of 15 to a high of 666. Variations in vocabulary size are also revealed by longitudinal studies, such as those by Huttenlocher *et al.* (1991) and by Hart and Risley (1995). Not surprisingly, if the number of words available to two-year-olds can vary so dramatically, their grammatical competence can vary widely also. The MBCDI also contains a grammatical complexity scale including bound morphemes, function words and early-emerging complex sentence forms, for which children receive a composite score. At two years of age the 10th centile score on this scale is zero, while at the 90th centile children score 20 (the maximum score is 40, which children at the 90th centile approximate at 30 months).

Large sample studies based on parent reports thus lead us to expect extensive individual differences in TD children's language abilities. These expectations are confirmed when we examine language samples. Klee and Gavin (2010) constructed a reference database for LARSP categories based on spontaneous language samples obtained from children in play situations. Their sample involved 152 children from 24 to 47 months, half from the US and half from the UK. If we take just one construction, SV (as in *he running, mummy gone*) posited in LARSP to be available to children by the age of 2;0, we find that this is used by two-thirds of the children in the 24–26 month age group. The VO structure (*want drink, hit teddy*) is available to only just over half of the children in the same age group. The immediate lesson for LARSP users, in terms of the individual variation in language learning revealed by large sample studies, is that the age estimates associated with particular stages on the chart may need to be interpreted flexibly. As we shall see, the relative order of the development of constructions outlined in the profile does remain valid, but in assessing a child's grammatical capability, we need to be aware of just how variable 'typical' language development can be, especially in the early stages.

The gradual character of language development

As David Crystal in his introduction (Chapter 1, this volume) makes clear, there are sound reasons for making grammar, rather than vocabulary, the point of entry for the assessment of a child's language competence: vocabulary has to be organized into constructions that are 'legal' in the language in order to make or qualify statements, ask questions, issue requests or commands, and so on. Learning grammar is fundamental to language acquisition, and grammatical deficits define language impairment. It was common parlance in the early modern era of developmental research, under the influence of Chomskyan theory, to emphasize the speed with which children acquired grammar – over a few short years, with no direct instruction, in the context of a language environment that was not ideal. As the data accumulated it became difficult to maintain that the child's language environment was not adapted to support early language development, though there was still no evidence of direct teaching – caregivers seem to modify their utterances to children unconsciously. It has also become clear that a child's mastery of a particular construction is not achieved overnight – gradual and often lexically specific progress towards competence is the norm.

A major proponent of the view that the route to abstract categories is a relatively stately affair is Tomasello (2003: 127). In relation to a construction such as the one LARSP labels SVO, he points out that there is good evidence in the form of overgeneralization errors, such as *she falled me down*, that the SVO structure is productive for the child. The use of the intransitive verb *fall* as used in the transitive SVO frame is not something that the child could have heard and repeated. But it is rare to find these 'errors' prior to three years of age, even though many utterances with SVO form are to be heard prior to the third birthday. And experimental approaches involving novel verbs presented in a sentence frame other than transitive (intransitive, imperative) reveal that it is only by about four years of age that the majority of typically developing children demonstrate the ability to generalize the novel verb to a transitive frame (Tomasello, 2003: 130). Longitudinal studies of speech samples from 12 children between one and three years of age have also indicated a selectivity of construction type for particular verbs, and little evidence that children knew how to reliably mark subjects and objects syntactically via pronoun case (Tomasello, 2000: 3).

The implication of this research is that – while we will want to continue to use LARSP categories as the point of entry to the assessment of children's grammatical capabilities – in relation to transitivity particularly, we will need to be alert to the lexical dimension of their productions, and the diversity of verbs they are able to deploy in the various LARSP-defined constructions. In what follows we will bear this in mind, while examining the impact of research subsequent to the profile's development on our current interpretation of it in some selected areas.

A full version of the LARSP chart appears in Figure 2.1. Here we will concentrate on aspects of the grammatical structures listed under 'Statement', especially in Stages II, III, and V.

Revisiting LARSP

Stages II and III clause structure

Verbs and argument structure

Central to the organization of the simple sentence is the main or lexical verb. Sentences have to have verbs, and verbs have arguments – noun phrases (NP) or sometimes prepositional phrases (PP) – that they mandate. A distinction is made between *internal* arguments and *external* arguments.[2] Internal arguments are those that are required by the verb. So the verbs *break* and *give* differ in their internal arguments, with *break* requiring only a single NP (*break the cup*), while *give* requires either an NP + PP sequence or NP + NP (*give the bone to the dog / give the dog the bone*). The subject NP, obligatory in most English sentences, is an external argument. If a child understands that subjects are obligatory, and is aware of the internal argument requirements for a particular verb, then the basic syntactic structure of the simple sentence falls out automatically. Further, as Pinker (1989: 179ff) points out, children can be guided to internal argument structure by a verb's semantics. The semantics of *put*, for instance, entails something located and a location, which has to be expressed respectively in an NP and a PP (*He put the bread on the table*). The syntax-enabling potential of verb semantics has come to be known as *semantic bootstrapping*. This intimate relationship between lexis and simple sentences implies that if a child developing language normally learns a verb, aspects of syntax will fall out naturally. And conversely, deficiencies in verb learning in children with language impairment will have syntactic consequences.

This close relationship between verbs and syntax suggests that it would be helpful to know more about the verb vocabulary typically found in early childhood as a guide to intervention. A multi-child diary study by Naigles *et al.* (2009) provides some useful information. Eight mothers kept detailed records of their children's first ten uses of verbs from a set of 35. The children ranged in age from 18 to 20 months when they were first recorded, and were followed for periods from 3 to 13 months depending on how quickly they produced the appropriate number of verb-containing utterances. Six of the eight children produced the same 21 verbs from the list. These are displayed in Table 2.1. These verbs fall into three categories: transitive, which require subject and object NPs; intransitive, which require subject NPs only; and alternating,[3] which can be either transitive or intransitive. In LARSP terms, the transitive verbs would be used in VO (*Want juice*) or SVO (*I push that*) structures; the intransitive in SV (*I sit*); and

16 Assessing Grammar

Name   Age   Sample date   Type

A	Unanalysed			Problematic		
	1 Unintelligible	2 Symbolic Noise	3 Deviant	1 Incomplete	2 Ambiguous	3 Stereotypes

B	Responses			Normal Response						Abnormal	
					Major						
	Stimulus Type	Totals	Repetitions	Elliptical			Reduced	Full	Minor	Structural	∅	Problems
				1	2	3+						
	Questions											
	Others											

C	Spontaneous

D	Reactions		General	Structural	∅	Other	Problems

Stage I (0;9–1;6)

Minor	Responses	Vocatives	Other	Problems
Major	Comm.	Quest.	Statement		
	'V'	'Q'	'V'	'N'	Other	Problems

Stage II (1;6–2;0)

Conn.	Clause				Phrase		Word
	VX	QX	SV	AX	DN	VV	-ing
			SO	VO	Adj N	V part	
			SC	VC	NN	Int X	pl
			Neg X	Other	PrN	Other	

Stage III (2;0–2;6)

	X + S:NP	X + V:VP	X + C:NP	X + O:NP	X + A:AP	-ed
	VXY	QXY	SVC	VCA	D Adj N	Cop	-en
	let X Y		SVO	VOA	Adj Adj N	Aux$_O^M$	
	do X Y	VS(X)	SVA	VO$_d$O$_i$	Pr DN		3s
			Neg X Y	Other	Pron$_O^P$	Other	gen

Stage IV (2;6–3;0)

	XY + S:NP	XY + V:VP	XY + C:NP	XY + O:NP	XY + A:AP	n't
	+ S	QVS	SVOA	AAXY	NP Pr NP	Neg V	
		QXY'+	SVCA	Other	Pr D Adj N	Neg X	'cop
	VXY+	VS(X+)	SVO$_d$O$_i$		cX	2 Aux	
		tag	SVOC		XcX	Other	'aux

Stage V (3;0–3;6)

	and	Coord.	Coord.	Coord.	1	1+	Postmod. 1 clause	1+	-est
	c	Other	Other	Subord. A	1	1+			-er
	s			S C O			Postmod. 1+ phrase		-ly
	Other			Comparative					

(+)				(−)			
NP	VP	Clause	Conn.	Clause		Phrase	Word

Stage VI (3;6–4;6)

				Element	NP	VP	N V
Initiator	Complex	Passive	and	∅	D Pr Pron^P	Aux^M Aux^O Cop	irreg
Coord.		Complement.	c	⇆	D∅ Pr∅		
		how what	s	Concord	D ⇆ Pr ⇆	∅	reg
Other						Ambiguous	

Stage VII (4;6+)

Discourse		Syntactic Comprehension
A Connectivity	it	
Comment Clause	there	Style
Emphatic Order	Other	

Total No. Sentences	Mean No. Sentences Per Turn	Mean Sentence Length

© D. Crystal, P. Fletcher, M. Garman, 1981 revision, University of Reading

Figure 2.1 LARSP profile for English

Table 2.1 Verbs used by six of the children in Naigles *et al.* (2009). (Verbs in bold are 'early' verbs – used before 21 months on average.)

Transitive	Intransitive	Alternating
want	come	**bite**
hold	go	cut
like	look	**eat**
need	cry	jump
see	run	kiss
	sit	**open**
	walk	**push**
		roll
		wash

the alternating verbs can appear in all three: *Eating sweet, Me eating sweet* and *Daddy eating*. Of course all three types of verbs can appear on their own, as Stage I 'V' – for example, *want, go, eating*. The figures for co-occurrence of verbs with arguments from the Naigles *et al.* study indicate however that verbs appeared on their own in only about 25% of instances. Subjects occurred with 32% of verb tokens, and direct objects in 46% of instances. And 24% of transitive or alternating verb tokens appeared in SVO frames. But verbs varied in their propensity to occur in particular frames. For instance, the percentage of tokens that occurred in SVO frames varied from 73% for *want*, to 0% for *jump, open*.[4] There was also variation among the children. One child produced transitive or alternating verb tokens in an SVO frame 59% of the time, whereas another child only used the SVO frame with 2% of tokens.

These data underline both the gradual nature of the early unfolding of grammatical ability, and the individual differences to be found among typically developing children in rate of development. They also underline the need to pay close attention to lexis in both assessment and intervention. Klee and Gavin (2010) reveal that SVO is the most frequent clause structure to appear in their samples from 2;6 onwards, at around 12% of the total (up from 7% at 24 months). But the attribution of control of a structure such as SVO to a child requires, as well as relatively frequent use, the appearance in these structures of a range of different verbs, and also diversity in the lexical realization of the arguments of those verbs. Otherwise there is a risk of over-estimation if we attribute SVO structure to what is in fact a stereotype – a repeated, learned sequence (Crystal, 1979: 61ff). A clear implication of this for practitioners is that evaluation of a child's grammatical capabilities via LARSP should be augmented by an assessment of vocabulary, with particular attention to the size and composition of the verb lexicon, for which a valid and reliable approach would be a parent report instrument such as the MBCDI (cf. Hadley, 2006: 181; see also Crystal, 1992: 139 ff. for a description of PRISM, a systematic analysis of vocabulary for clinical purposes, with particular emphasis on semantics).

Verbs and argument structure in children with language impairment

There is ample indication of problems with the learning of verbs, and with argument structure, in children with language impairment.[5] For example Olswang et al. (1997) examined the nature of the lexicon of a group of children with specific expressive language impairment, with particular attention to verbs, over a nine-week period, three of which involved treatment. Results showed a moderate correlation between lexicon size/composition and the emergence of word combinations. The data also suggested that children in the group who had more intransitive verbs, and verbs which can be transitive or intransitive ('alternating' in Table 2.1), made greater progress.

Experimental evidence suggests that children with LI are not as adept as age controls in fast-mapping names for actions, and have problems retaining information about verbs that they have initially acquired after a limited number of exposures (Rice et al., 1994). Chiat (2000: 147) suggests reasons why verbs present a particular challenge for inefficient language learners. She points out that verbs rarely occur in isolation, and that they typically receive less stress than the words around them, which may affect the integrity or specificity of verbs' phonological representations and hence their identification and recognition (see also Leonard & Deevy, 2004: 223). Further problems may result from limited understanding of the perspectives verbs impose on the events they characterize, especially as these events are often of relatively brief duration.

There are also reports of difficulties with both internal and external arguments in children with language impairment. Fletcher (1991), in a report on a group of 15 school-age children with SLI, reports errors of omission of internal arguments (e.g. *he puts webs*, where an obligatory location PP is omitted). In a study of argument structure use in spontaneous language samples, Thordadottir and Ellis Weismer (2002) report that children with specific language impairment (SLI) use fewer argument structure types and verb alternations than age-matched controls. The issue of alternations was also explored in a video elicitation task (King et al., 1995). Their method exploited the alternating argument structures available with certain verbs to compare children with SLI, and younger typically developing children matched on vocabulary test scores. Included in the set of verbs used were those permitting causative-inchoative – verbs like *bounce, move* (Levin, 1993). These verbs have either a transitive or an intransitive form. The video scenes were designed to elicit one of the possible argument frames for a word. So for the causative-inchoative pair *The boy was bouncing the ball / The ball was bouncing*, the scene for the first item in the pair shows the agent, the boy, setting off the bouncing of the object, the ball, across a patio. In the second scene the boy is edited out of the scene, and just the bouncing ball is visible. In contrast to the younger typically developing children, across all alternations the children with SLI tended to prefer one description – the transitive one – for both scenes

Stages II and III clauses: Some descriptive statistics

Clause structures listed at Stages II and III are the major forms the child has to learn in order to construct simple sentences. Klee and Gavin (2010) provide some helpful guidance on the relative importance of structures, but their data suggests that the age estimates originally provided in LARSP are on the optimistic side. If we take the two types of information Klee and Gavin (2010) provide (frequency of structures in a sample of 100 'major' utterances, in LARSP terms, and the proportion of children using a structural type), this is the picture that emerges for Stage II structures[6]:

(1) At 24–26 months, one quarter of all utterances are still Stage I 'N'. By 30 months, this has decreased to 10%.
(2) Just over half of children aged 24–29 months use VO structures. By 30 months 90% of them use the structure, declining to 43% at 47 months. About two thirds of those in the sample use SV at 24–29 months, again rising to 90% at 30 months and then remaining between 90% and 100% through to 47 months. One implication of these values is that for a substantial number of TD children, 2;0–2;6 is a more likely period for the development of Stage II clauses than the 18 months to 2;0 year span estimated in Figure 2.1. The decline of VO structures can be attributed to the child's growing understanding that subject NPs are generally obligatory except in responses to interrogatives: (Q. *What are you doing?* A. *Washing my hands*).
(3) Some structures occur at very low frequencies – all of the following at less than 1% of the total throughout the age range 24–47 months: SO, VC, NegX and II Other.

For Stage III statement clauses we find:

(1) In terms of frequency of occurrence in 100 major utterances, the two most frequent types, SVO and SVC, increase their share of the total from 30–32 months on. And from 30–32 months on, we find very high proportions of the children using them – between 90% and 100%. However, 50% of the sample are using SVC at 24–26 months, and 75% at that age are using SVO. SVA clauses show an increase in frequency at 33–35 months, with a concomitant increase

in the number of children using them (from 33 months on, between 93% and 100% of children use this form).

(2) Some clause types listed at Stage III Statement have either very low frequencies of occurrence (VOA, IIIOther) or have frequencies at or close to zero (NegXY, VCA, VO$_d$O$_i$).

The data available from the Klee and Gavin (KG) database suggest that the age ranges given for Stage II and Stage II structures may err on the optimistic side, at least for a number of TD children. But the data underline a point made in Crystal *et al.* (1989): it is appropriate to think of children not as being at a particular stage at a particular age, but as moving from a preference for Stage II clauses to a preference for Stage III clauses at a particular age, likely to be around 2;6 for the majority. Development, as it is revealed by the KG data, is quite clearly not a matter of leaving behind clauses of one stage to move to clauses of a later stage, except, for example, in the decline of VO structures with increased grammatical sophistication. Crystal *et al.* make the point thus:

> It is therefore possible – and indeed expected – for the signs of development of the linguistic processes falling within a stage to be seen before the chronological onset of that stage; and of course, many of .... the structures which have emerged within a stage will continue to be used after that stage and [into] the adult language. (1989: 61)

Stage II and III expansion

Children not only have to expand their repertoire of clause types in their third year, but also to learn a range of phrase types. The grammatical framework on which LARSP is based (Quirk *et al.*, 1985) recognizes a distinction between clause and phrase levels in the analysis of sentences. This distinction is honoured in the clause and phrase types listed in the LARSP profile. The decision was also made at the time of the profile's construction to link clause types and phrase types by means of two sections, after Stage II and Stage III, which record the integration of phrases into clauses. Although this is a little-researched area of language development, it is one that seems to be an important feature of children's growing competence. There seems to be a difference in the grammatical ability displayed between *Daddy open door* and *Daddy open the front door*, though both are SVO sentences. In the second case the child would be credited with having produced a D Adj N sequence (Stage III phrase). But without the section in the LARSP chart that allows the recording of an elaboration of the O element, the integration of the phrase into the clause would go unsung. The presence of an NP in O position is logged at the end of Stage III, where 'XY + O:NP' reads as 'an NP occurred at O, and there were two other elements of clause structure in the

Table 2.2 Mean percentages of S and O clause elements at Stages II and III showing phrasal expansions

	Stage II % expansions			Stage III % expansions		
	24–26m	30–32m	36–38m	24–26m	30–32m	36–38m
S	14	26	14	14	13	21
O	74	82	76	43	50	70

clause' (in this case S and V). The KG database allows us to examine how the integration of phrase structure into clause structure operates in children between 24 and 47 months. In Table 2.2 we see the proportion of S and O clause elements that have phrasal realizations in both Stage II and Stage III clauses.

It is immediately obvious that, for both Stages II and III, there is a discrepancy between the values for subject and object elements across the board. Subject expansions occur between 13% and 26% across the period and are proportionally much less frequent than the elaborations of O elements. The most obvious explanation for this is the language they hear around them. Leech (2006: 39), following Quirk *et al.* (1985), refers to a tendency in English called 'end-weighting':

> End weight is the principle by which longer and more complex units tend to occur later in the sentence than shorter and less complex units. For example, in sentences consisting of subject, verb and object, the subject is likely to be short and simple in comparison with the object.

The tendency in young children's speech to limit noun phrases in subject position may simply be a reflection of the character of the utterances they hear from their conversational partners.

The other feature of Table 2.2 that merits attention is the difference between O expansions in Stage II and Stage III. The phrase structure values in Stage II clauses are high and stable. In Stage III across the same age range, the expansions start lower and increase over time. This suggests an initial trade-off between clause and phrase structure complexity, with the ability to elaborate object NPs not immediately transferable as the number of clause elements increases.

Stage III: Auxiliary and tense marking

In light of the very close attention paid to finiteness in children with SLI in recent research, the use of verb marking by TD children in the KG database merits inspection. Demonstrations of verb inflection deficits in children with SLI are legion (for a review see Oetting & Hadley, 2009: 342ff.). Of particular significance are studies which show that children with SLI

Table 2.3 Percentages of children between two and four years of age, showing use of auxiliaries in 20-minute language samples

	24–26m	30–32m	36–38m	45–47m
Aux-M	25	36.4	90.9	100
Aux-O	64.3	100	100	100

perform at a lower level on finiteness morphemes than language-matched younger TD children (usually about two years younger). Hadley (2006) summarizes the empirical evidence available on TD children and indicates that we can expect to see present tense marking first, between 24 and 26 months, with past tense a little later. KG database values concur: although both forms, regular past -ed and present tense -s, are present in the 24–26-month samples, -s is much more frequent and is available to a greater proportion of the children. Present tense verb forms outnumber regular past tense by about 13:1 at the 24–26-month level. And three-quarters of the children of this age use present tense, while only about a quarter use past tense. By 33 months, all the children are using present tense as against 60% using past tense. The incidence of past tense does increase over time, so that by 36 months the ratio of present to past usage is around 7:1, and by 47 months, 4:1.

In addition to learning verb inflections, children also have to come to terms with the auxiliary system of English. The TD children in the KG database again show an increasing use over the age range of both modal auxiliaries (Aux-M – *can, could, will, would, might etc.*) and what are labelled 'other auxiliaries' (Aux-O) in the LARSP system – *be, have* and *do*. Verbs in around 6% of major utterances are accompanied by an auxiliary verb at 24–26 months, rising to 22% at 36 months. This percentage remains constant thereafter. At all points, 'other' auxiliaries are more common than modals. Table 2.3 lists the percentages of children using Aux-O and Aux-M at approximately 2, 2;6, 3, and 4 years of age. Both the frequency trajectories for the two types of auxiliary, and the proportion of children using them, suggest that the peak periods of development are later than on the 1981 revised LARSP chart for modal auxiliaries. For Aux-M there is a moderate increase in frequency at 33 months, and a sharp increase at 42 months. Table 2.3 shows that it is 45 months before all children are using modals.

Stage V: Complex sentences

Stage V structures in typically-developing children

In addition to the syntactic structure of simple sentences, somewhat later in their development children also have to master the devices in the language for combining sentences. There are two main types of linkage

(Clark, 2003: 245). One, referred to as coordination, using conjunctions like *and* or *but*, links two or more sentences which are not syntactically dependent on one another. In the LARSP profile, these structures are logged under *Coord* at Stage V Clause. The second type of linkage, subordination, does have one sentence syntactically dependent on the other. The subordinate structure is embedded in the main sentence and dependent on it. Subordinate clauses can have various forms and functions. They can fill one of the grammatical elements in the matrix clause (e.g. *Mummy thinks I've been naughty)*, which is logged as *Clause: O*. A subordinate clause can act as a postmodifier, in this case a relative clause, in a noun phrase, as in *Esme broke the toy that Mama gave me*. Such structures register on the LARSP profile as *Postmod clause*, under Stage V Phrase. And the subordinate structure can operate as an adverbial modifier of a verb phrase: *I had a lot of hair when I was a baby*. This example would be entered as *Subord. A* under Stage V Clause. These linking devices permit the child to:

> convey more complex information in a single utterance and to produce coherent sequences of utterances when ... recounting an adventure, telling a joke, or explaining how a toy came to be broken. (Clark, 2003: 245)

For the TD child, the journey towards mastery of complex syntax begins relatively early. Sentences linked with *and* are typically the earliest to appear. Of the subordinate structures, relative clauses are reported for some children soon after the second birthday. However, many of these early relative clauses lack relative pronouns. This tendency to omit grammatical markers of subordination is also seen in other prototype structures. Certain complement-taking verbs such as *want* require the verb in the complement structure to be preceded by *to*: *I want that man to go now*. The earliest attempts at such structures tend to omit *to*. Other subordinating constructions do not omit the linking forms, but are initially restricted in the range of forms they can deal with. Typically developing pre-school children begin to express temporal and causal relations in their third year, most commonly with *when* as the subordinator for the former and *'cause* for the latter. Conditional constructions can also appear in the second half of the third year, as this example (Clark, 2003: 267) demonstrates: *If I get my graham cracker in the water, it'll get all soapy*.

The KG database indicates relatively low numbers of Stage V structures. Coord, Subord O, and Subord A are the most frequent, but only appear at frequencies of 1–2%. The proportions of children using the forms are more revealing. Few children use a Stage V structure before 33 months, when Subord O, Subord A, and Postmod clause structures appear. Children begin to use Coord structures in this data at 36 months. The data suggest that the age estimates for Stage V on the LARSP chart (36–42 months) are not too wide of the mark. This is borne out by a large-scale study by Diessel (2004), which reveals (Figure 1.1: 10) that complex constructions are infrequent at 36 months but show a strong upward trajectory over the next year. However, language sampling based on play may not be the optimum source of complex sentence structures, and contexts such as narrative may be more conducive to their elicitation.

Stage V structures in children with language impairment

Stage V structures have not been extensively researched in impairment, but for a detailed account of the kinds of problems that can arise see Crystal (1983: 8ff). More recent large sample and small scale reports confirm that Stage V structures can cause problems for children with language impairment. In a cross-sectional study of 65 children aged 6–11 years, Hesketh (2004) used sub-tests from a standardized procedure, *Assessment of Comprehension and Expression 6–11* (Adams et al. 2001), to explore complex sentences. Many of the children tested, but not all, were using the constructions of interest. Approximate percentage values for children using the constructions were as follows: coordination, 75%; Postmod. clause, 75%; subordination (Subord O, temporal or causal Subord A) 65%; Subord A conditional, 45%. Hesketh (2004: 170) gives values for both structured elicitation and narrative, as both methods were used in the study. The percentages quoted are for whichever value is the higher.

There is some indication in examples quoted in the study of the omission of obligatory grammatical markers, which means that a useful complement to the large sample cross-sectional study is a longitudinal case study of MM, a boy with SLI, between the ages of 3;3 and 7;10 (Schuele & Dykes, 2005), in which a dozen samples of conversational speech were analysed. The MLU range from the first to the last sample was 1.91 to 5.46. There is little evidence of the availability of complex constructions until sample 6 (age 4;8, MLU 3.12), when coordinating and subordinating conjunctions appear. Sample 8 (age 5;9, MLU 4.27) sees sentential verb complements (Stage V *Clause: O*), relative clauses (*Postmod. Clause*) and conditionals (*Subord: A*). The percentage of complex sentence use increased from Sample 6 onwards, with 31% of utterances in sample 12 consisting of complex constructions. The data from MM confirm the persistence of grammatical marker omissions within these complex constructions as they develop. For example, the obligatory relative marker in subject Postmod clauses (e.g. *that* in *I was scared of the boy that chased us*) was omitted in every instance, over a long period. A 'subject' relative is one in which the matrix sentence noun which is postmodified functions as the subject noun of the Postmodifying clause, as in the example above. For subject relatives, a grammatical marker *who* or *that* is obligatory. In object relatives – those in which the modified matrix noun functions as the object of the Postmod clause, as in *I was scared of the boy (that) you chased* – the relative marker is optional, and often omitted. This vulnerability of obligatory markers in subject relatives is confirmed by Schuele and Tolbert (2001). They compared a group of children with SLI between five and seven years, and a younger TD group aged from three to five years. The younger TD children never omitted the marker from subject relatives, but the children with SLI left them out of 63% of the time (see also Schuele & Nicholls, 2000).

As with other areas of grammar, the course of complex sentence development in children with language impairment starts later than it does in typically developing age peers. This is particularly apparent in a longitudinal study of a child with SLI (Schuele & Dykes, 2005), where the fifth year, rather than the third year, sees these constructions emerge. A majority of school-age children with language impairment appear to be able to produce a range of complex constructions (Marinellie, 2004). However, a consistent finding is that these children tend to omit obligatory grammatical markers. This is reported by Schuele and Dykes (2005) in their longitudinal study for infinitival *to* in *Clause: O structures* (but see Eisenberg, 2003), *wh*-pronouns in embedded clauses and subject relative markers. Examples of subject relative marker omissions appear in a study of three children with SLI in one family by Schuele and Nicholls (2000):

> She's got all the dishes ____ need to be washed
> And the man ____ owns it, he said
> We got one girl ____ have a birthday in March

Envoi

The LARSP profile for English continues to find extensive application clinically, and, as the chapters in this book attest, it has been widely used as a model for profiles in other languages. The concept has also been robust enough to stand the test of time. A major reason for this is that, in contrast to some other selective approaches to grammar, the profile provides, at a particular level of abstraction, a *comprehensive* taxonomy of clause and phrase constructions. The profile defines all that the child needs, by way of syntactic structures and inflection, to be grammatically competent. But as we have indicated, the attribution of control of a structural type to a child, from sample data, involves an interpretive leap that requires justification in terms of token frequency and lexical variety. In simple clauses especially, lexis has to be taken into account in estimating a child's grammatical ability. This is as true for the other languages represented in this volume as it is for English. Influential current conceptions of grammatical development see the child moving from concrete, lexically-based items to abstract constructional schemas that support productive use (Tomasello, 2003; Diessel, 2004). And if this hypothesis is a reliable guide to the trajectory of grammatical development in the TD child, it is entirely possible that the child with language impairment will be either be lagging well behind, or immobilized somewhere along the route.

Other issues raised here – problems with inflection, the integration of phrase into clause structure, and the late evolution of complex sentences, will not be restricted to English either, and will bear attention in adaptations of the profile to other languages. But there seems no reason why LARSP and its cousins, informed by contemporary language acquisition theory and data, should not continue to function as approaches of first resort to the grammatical analysis of clinical data. It wil be interesting to see what the next 30 years brings.

Notes

(1) They are available electronically via a web archive at the University of Canterbury. See Chapter 1, note 2.
(2) This distinction is not explicit in the grammatical framework used for LARSP, but is formally recognized in grammatical models which identify a VP (Verb Phrase). See Crystal (2003: 32) and Trask (1992: 144).
(3) The term 'alternating' or 'alternation' is applied not only to verbs which can be transitive or intransitive, but for any systematic argument structure variation with a set of verbs. See Levin (1993).
(4) The inclusion of *jump* in the alternating set by Naigles *et al.* (2009) is perhaps debatable. It is true that this verb can be transitive as in *jump the fence*, but it is more likely to be used either intransitively, or followed by a prepositional phrase (Huddleston & Pullum, 2002: 299).
(5) See Crystal (1985) for a discussion of intervention approaches with verbs for children with language impairment.
(6) The data for Klee and Gavin (2010) was collected in a play context. We should bear in mind the possibility that other sampling contexts could produce different results. The criterion Klee and Gavin (2010) apply for 'using a structure' is that the child produces two or more instances per 100 'major' utterances (in LARSP terms).

References

Adams, C., Cooke, R., Crutchley, A., Hesketh, A. and Reeves, D. (2001) *Assessment of Comprehension and Expression 6–11*. Windsor: NFER-Nelson.
Bates, E., Dale, P. and Thal, D. (1995) Individual differences and their implications for theories of language development. In P. Fletcher and B. MacWhinney (eds) *The Handbook of Child Language (pp. 96–151)*. Oxford: Blackwell.
Brown, R. (1973) *A First Language*. London: George Allen and Unwin.
Chiat, S. (2000) *Understanding Children with Language Problems*. Cambridge: Cambridge University Press.
Clark, E. (2003) *First Language Acquisition*. Cambridge: Cambridge University Press.
Crystal, D. (1979) *Working with LARSP*. London: Edward Arnold.
Crystal, D. (1982) *Profiling Linguistic Disability*. London: Edward Arnold.
Crystal, D. (1983) Psycholinguistics. *Folia Phoniatrica* 35, 1–12.
Crystal, D. (1985) Some early problems with verbs. *Child Language, Teaching and Therapy* 1, 46–53.
Crystal, D. (1992) *Profiling Linguistic Disability* (2nd edn). London: Cole and Whurr.
Crystal, D. (2003) *A Dictionary of Linguistics and Phonetics* (5th edn). Oxford: Blackwell.

Crystal, D., Fletcher, P. and Garman, M. (1976) *The Grammatical Analysis of Language Disability*. London: Edward Arnold.
Crystal, D., Fletcher, P. and Garman, M. (1989) *The Grammatical Analysis of Language Disability* (2nd edn). London: Cole and Whurr.
Diessel, H. (2004) *The Acquisition of Complex Sentences*. Cambridge: Cambridge University Press.
Eisenberg, S. (2003) Production of infinitives by 5-year-old children with language impairment on an elicitation task. *First Language* 24, 305–321.
Fenson, L., Marchman, V.A., Thal, D.J., Dale, P.S., Reznick, J.S. and Bates, E. (2007) *MacArthur–Bates Communicative Development Inventories (CDIs): User's Guide and Technical Manual* (2nd edn). Baltimore, MD: Brooks Publishing.
Fletcher, P. (1991) Evidence from syntax for language impairment. In J. Miller (ed.) *Research on Child Language Disorders: A Decade of Progress* (pp. 169–87). Austin, TX: Pro-Ed.
Hadley, P. (2006) Assessing the emergence of grammar in toddlers at risk for specific language impairment. *Seminars in Speech and Language* 27, 173–86
Hart, B. and Risley, R.T. (1995) *Meaningful Differences in the Everyday Experience of Young American Children*. Baltimore: Paul H. Brookes.
Hesketh, A. (2004) Grammatical performance of children with language disorder on structured elicitation and narrative tasks. *Clinical Linguistics & Phonetics* 18, 161–82.
Huddleston, R. and Pullum, G. (2002) *The Cambridge Grammar of the English Language*. Cambridge: Cambridge University Press.
Huttenlocher, J., Haight, W., Bryk, A., Seltzer, M. and Lyons, T. (1991) Early vocabulary growth: Relation to language input and gender. *Developmental Psychology* 27 (2), 236–48.
King, G., Scheletter, C, Sinka, I., Fletcher, P. and Ingham, R. (1995) Are English-speaking SLI children with morpho-syntactic deficits impaired in their use of locative-contact and causative alternations? *Reading Working Papers in Linguistics* 2, 45–65.
Klee, T. and Gavin, W.J. (2010) *LARSP reference data for 2- and 3-year-old children*. Retrieved from University of Canterbury Research Repository: http://hdl.handle.net/10092/4980
Leech, G.N (2006) *A Glossary of English Grammar,* Edinburgh: Edinburgh University Press.
Leonard, L.B. and Deevy, P. (2004) Lexical deficits in specific language impairment. In L.Verhoeven and H. van Balkom (eds) *Classification of Developmental Language Disorders: Theoretical Issues and Clinical Implications* (pp. 209–33). Mahwah, NJ: Lawrence Erlbaum.
Levin, B. (1993) *English Verb Classes and Alternations*. Chicago: University of Chicago Press.
Marinellie, S. (2004) Complex syntax used by school-age children with specific language impairment (SLI) in child-adult conversation. *Journal of Communication Disorders* 37, 517–533
Naigles, L., Hoff, E. and Vear, D. (2009) Flexibility in early verb use: Evidence from a multiple-N diary study. *Monographs of the Society for Research in Child Development* 74, 2.
Oetting, J. and Hadley P. (2009) Morphosyntax. In R.G. Schwartz (ed.) *Handbook of Child Language Disorders* (pp. 341–64). New York and Hove: Psychology Press.
Olswang, L., Long, S. and Fletcher, P. (1997) Verbs in the emergence of word combinations in young children with specific expressive language impairment. *European Journal of Disorders of Communication* 32 (2), 15–33.
Pinker, S. (1989) *Learnability and Cognition: The Acquisition of Argument Structure*. Cambridge, MA: MIT Press.

Quirk, R., Greenbaum, S., Leech, G. and Svartvik, J. (1985) *A Comprehensive Grammar of the English Language*. London: Pearson Longman.

Rice, M.L., Oetting, J., Marquis, J., Bode, J. and Pae, S. (1994) Frequency of input effects on word comprehension of children with specific language impairment. *Journal of Speech and Hearing Research* 37, 106–22.

Schuele, C. and Dykes, J. (2005) Complex syntax acquisition: A longitudinal case study of a child with specific language impairment. *Clinical Linguistics & Phonetics* 19, 295–318.

Schuele, C. and Nicholls, L. (2000) Relative clauses: Evidence of continued linguistic vulnerability in children with specific language impairment. *Clinical Linguistics & Phonetics* 14, 563–585.

Schuele, C. and Tolbert, L. (2001) Omissions of obligatory relative markers in children with specific language impairment. *Clinical Linguistics & Phonetics* 15, 257–74.

Stokes, S.F. and Klee, T. (2009) Factors that influence vocabulary development in two-year-old children. *Journal of Child Psychology and Psychiatry* 50, 498–505.

Thordardottir, E. and Ellis Weismer, S. (2002) Verb argument structure weakness in specific language impairment in relation to age and utterance length. *Clinical Linguistics & Phonetics* 16, 233–50.

Tomasello, M. (2000) Acquiring syntax is not what you think. In D. Bishop and L. Leonard (eds) *Speech and Language Impairments in Children* (pp. 1–15). Hove: Psychology Press.

Tomasello, M. (2003) *Constructing a Language*. Cambridge, MA: Harvard University Press.

Trask, R. (1992) *A Dictionary of Grammatical Terms in Linguistics*. London and New York: Routledge.

3 'Computerized Profiling' of Clinical Language Samples and the Issue of Time[1]

Steven Long

Introduction

Profiling is a procedure for describing language usage based on the data of a clinical sample. The procedure has been developed to handle data at several linguistic levels (grammar, prosody, phonology, semantics) so that individuals exhibiting different types of language disability can be profiled, or so the same individual can be profiled in different ways. The clinical purpose of profiling is 'to enable an accurate assessment of P's disability to be made, sufficient to provide a basis for remedial intervention' (Crystal, 1982: 1).

Clinical Difficulties with Profiling

Profiling is designed as a 'compromise' between the theories and methods of academic linguistics and the needs and abilities of the everyday language clinician. To this end, profiling avoids most of the intricacies of formal linguistic notation and does not aim for nearly the same level of detail. In spite of this effort to make the procedure usable, when compared to most other clinical practices it is difficult and time-consuming to learn. The profiling method for grammar, LARSP, assumes a familiarity with a reference grammar (Quirk *et al.*, 1972) as well as a number of special rules for analysing immature language forms. The profile for prosody, PROP, uses a specific transcriptional system for recording intonation patterns. PRISM-L, the procedure for analysing lexical semantic structure, uses a rather complex classification scheme that involves nearly 300 categories. The PROPH procedure for segmental phonological analysis employs a 'broad phonetic' transcription, but also makes analytical decisions on the basis of syllable stress, position of the phones, certainty of the word gloss and frequency of the phonetic form within the sample. The user must be familiar with all of these notions in order to construct a profile accurately.

Even when the technique has been mastered, profiling can take an extraordinary amount of time to do. Crystal (1981: 9–11) is aware of this problem and suggests that the extra time is justified by (a) the complexity of the problem(s) being treated; and (b) the long-term value (i.e. over the entire course of therapy) of the information derived.

Computerized Profiling

Computerized Profiling is an attempt to alleviate (but not eliminate) the problems of 'learnability' and time. The software is designed so that it guides the user step-by-step through the profiling process, provides analytical support by offering 'tentative' analyses of data, and contains instructional text ('help files') to acquaint or re-acquaint the user with procedural details. It performs nearly all the necessary tallies and calculations, thereby speeding profile construction. When the profile is complete, the program allows the user to rapidly search through data in order to evaluate clinical hypotheses (for example the productivity of pronoun usage or the consistency of phonological substitutions). The software is not a substitute for linguistic knowledge and clinical skill, but is intended as a tool for teaching the profiling method, for constructing profiles within a more clinically practicable span of time, and for improving the interpretation of those profiles.

Hardware

Computerized Profiling operates on PC computers running 32-bit versions of Windows. To run under Windows 7 it requires the installation of Windows XP mode. The program can be configured to read and write data files from the computer's hard drive, or from external media such as flash drives.

Software

The software is available for free download from the website http://www.computerizedprofiling.org. Documentation can be accessed from within the program. The documentation, however, serves only to explain the operation of the program. It is assumed that the user is generally familiar with the procedures for profiling.

The software is organized into different modules corresponding to the different types of linguistic analysis they perform. To carry out a LARSP analysis, two of these modules are used, and they are briefly described below:

(1) *CORPUS* is a module for creating a transcript file that can then be analysed by LARSP and each of the other modules in CP. Sentences are entered into a text-processing program, observing some simple

conventions for capitalization, punctuation, and the identification of speakers (T and P). The text file is imported into CORPUS and converted into a format that CP uses for its analysis. In this process, certain types of editing required for grammatical analysis (for example the division of contracted forms into two morphemes separated by a space: CAN'T → CAN'T) are performed automatically. All files are stored on disk and can be recalled for editing.

(2) *LARSP* is a module for the grammatical analysis of spontaneous speech samples utilizing the 1981 revision of the Language Assessment, Remediation, and Sampling Procedure (Crystal *et al.,* 1981; Crystal, 1982). The program automatically performs a tentative parse of each sentence and displays it in the conventional format. For example:

```
              I     'M    GOING  TO   PLAY   THE   OTHER   GAME   NOW
CL            S     V                       O                     A
SC
PH            PP    AO    V      V          D     AJ      NN     AV
WD                  AX    NG
ER
AI            FL
Spontaneous
```

The symbols below the words in the sentence indicate the elements at different levels of structure: S = SUBJECT, PP = Personal Pronoun, AX = Contracted Auxiliary, FL = Full Sentence, and so on.

The algorithm for parsing each sentence is hierarchical (i.e. it first analyses clause structure, then analyses phrase structure based upon that presumed clause structure, then word structure based on the preceding two levels). Decisions are made on the basis of a 35,000-entry dictionary that identifies the possible grammatical roles of each word. For example, *outline* is listed as both the base form of a verb and a singular noun, while *outfits* is the 3s (3rd person singular present tense) form of a verb as well as a plural noun.

As the decision-making of the program is sequentially dependent, if a misanalysis occurs at Clause level, it will affect the analysis at Phrase and Word level. The results can be seen in the following sentence:

```
              THAT  DOES  N'T    SOUND  LIKE  A    COW    TO    ME
CL            S                         V     D           A
SC
PH            D     AO    NE     V      V     D    NN     PR    PP
WD                  3S    NT
ER
AI            FL
Spontaneous
```

As the program's dictionary contained LIKE as a lexical verb but did not contain SOUND, the Verb element was misassigned at clause level. The user must scan each sentence for mistakes like this and then correct the analysis. The task of correcting is made easier, though, by the fact that the program works hierarchically. In the example above, if the clause line is changed to:

```
     THAT   DOES   N'T    SOUND   LIKE   A   COW   TO   ME
CL   S      V                            A                A
```

the program will automatically revise the phrase line to:

```
     THAT   DOES   N'T    SOUND   LIKE   A   COW   TO   ME
CL   S      V                            A                A
SC
PH   PO     AO     NE     V              PR  D   NN   PR   PP
```

As each sentence in the corpus file is reviewed and, if necessary, corrected, it is also possible to enter codes that indicate the presence of Stage VI Errors. When the review is complete, the program passes the data through a tabulation routine. This routine examines each sentence, identifies the units at each structural level (for example Clause: SVAA; Phrase: Pron-P, Aux, Neg V, PrDN, PrPron-P; Word: 3s, n't), determines the appropriate stage assignments, interprets the Interaction data (for example S: Spontaneous, R: Full) and then tallies the results. When all of the sentences have been examined, the data are formatted to produce a LARSP profile chart identical to that obtained when the procedure is done by hand.

A set of supplementary programs allows the user (1) to search the examples of utterances with particular constituent features (for example all sentences of SVO clause structure or all sentences containing modal verbs); (2) to construct Verb Valency and Verb-form Profiles (Fletcher, 1985); (3) to compare separate analyses of the same corpus file (for example a student's and an instructor's, or that of two researchers wishing to check their reliability); and (4) to change the dictionary of lexical verbs or Minor sentences that the program uses during its automatic parse.

Program Evaluation

As an implementation of existing procedures, Computerized Profiling can best be judged by its success rate, by its speed in comparison to profiling by hand, and by the ease with which it can be learned.

Learning the software

No measurement has been made of how quickly Computerized Profiling can be mastered. Individuals who are familiar with profiling typically have little trouble, once they have adjusted to the program's symbols (for example, IV for Verb$_{imp}$ AJ instead of Adj for Adjectival). As with virtually all software that relies on keyboard data entry, the program favours those who are skilful typists. Students, and others who are first learning to profile, often find that the program promotes systematic work habits and helps to maintain motivation by eliminating the tedium of counting and tallying.

The issue of time

The authors of LARSP have consistently made mention of the time requirements for this and other clinical profiling procedures. However, a good deal of variation can be found in their time estimates, as they focus more or less on different factors likely to slow down the process. In their first text on LARSP, Crystal *et al.* (1976: 24) admit that 'The hard fact of the matter is that if one wants to achieve a complete and accurate understanding of a syntactic disability, there is no alternative but to spend analytic time on it—perhaps three or four hours, in order to obtain a reasonably full analysis of a half-hour sample'. Three years later, Crystal (1979: 21) concluded that 'If T does all the work herself, it will take the best part of a morning to get from transcription to complete profile, and this is impracticable in several clinical settings'. Two years after that, Crystal (1981: 10) made clear the range of possibility by stating, 'While it is possible to do certain types of analyses on certain types of patient in an hour or so, anything at all complex will regularly require a commitment of a half-day or a whole day'.

To investigate in more detail the time required by LARSP, a study was organized to compare manual and computerized implementation of the procedure (Long, 2001). The participants were 256 students and practising speech-language pathologists from the USA and Australia. All participants had received university-level instruction on the analysis procedures they performed for this study. That instruction had occurred as recently as two months and as remotely as 11 years prior to participation. Participants were allowed to select the number and type of analyses they performed, and were cautioned to choose only those analyses with which they felt 'familiar and confident' as a result of previous instruction and practice with the procedures.

All participants reported previous experience in using computers, though no attempt was made to quantify this experience. Given the number of participants, their relatively young age, and their university education, it can be safely assumed that they were generally accustomed to computer technology but that their specific experiences had been diverse, as is characteristic of any cohort of individuals.

Language samples

Grammatical analyses were performed on three language samples. All the samples were typed according to normal orthographic conventions. Decisions regarding utterance boundaries, sentence types (i.e. final utterance punctuation), proper nouns (i.e. capitalized words), mazes and lexical boundaries had been made in the transcripts, and participants were asked to abide by these decisions in their analyses. All the samples were elicited in conversational interactions. Sample G1 was obtained from a girl of 4;3 years being seen for therapy in a university clinic. Her diagnosis was simply 'language disorder'. Sample G2 was a boy of 2;10 years with specific expressive language impairment. He was identified as Child 7 in Long *et al.* (1997). Sample G3 was a typically-developing girl of 8;3 years who was a participant in Channell and Johnson (1999). The variation in sample size, complexity/severity, utterance variability, and suitability for different grammatical analyses is shown in Table 3.1.

Manual analysis procedures

For every sample they were to analyse by hand, participants were given the printed transcript, an instruction packet detailing what was to be included in the completed analysis, a time log, and a form to be used for recording and tabulating the analysis data. Participants were allowed to use hand calculators and to complete the analyses whenever and wherever they chose. They recorded the starting and stopping time of each analysis to the nearest minute. They could take breaks of any duration as long as these were noted in the time log.

The recording form used was developed especially for this study, but was similar in design to that shown in Crystal (1981). Although the use and

Table 3.1 Size and complexity/severity of grammatical samples analysed

	Sample G1	Sample G2	Sample G3
Syntactic utterance types (C&I)	63	25	98
Syntactic utterance tokens (C&I)	67	33	98
All utterance types (C&I)	74	67	99
All utterance tokens (C&I)	99	126	99
Statements (C&I)	86	125	83
Questions (C&I)	4	1	8
Commands (C&I)	9	0	8
MLU	3.64	1.33	7.63

Note. C&I = complete and intelligible.

purpose of the form was explained in the instruction packet, participants could choose to use their own form and procedures if they thought these would be more efficient. Any time devoted to creating or modifying record forms was not added to the time log. The only requirement was that the final form of the analysis had to be as shown in the instructions. When they had completed the analysis, participants turned in their analysis results, their recording and tabulation form, and their time log. If the analysis results were not in the proper form, they were returned for correction and the additional time was added to the log. Final time measurements were calculated from the log.

Computer analysis procedures

All language analyses performed by computer utilized the relevant modules of Computerized Profiling (CP: Long *et al.*, 1996–2000). Participants were introduced to the software either in the context of a university course or a professional workshop. After completing a brief tutorial exercise, all participants had performed at least one full analysis with CP prior to the analysis done for this study.

As this study was primarily focused on the *analysis* phase of language sample analysis, participants were given grammatical samples as electronic text files. Thus, they had to follow the procedures for importing a text file into CP, but did not have to type in the transcript itself.

As they did with their manual analyses, participants recorded their starting and stopping times and all breaks they had taken in a time log. At the conclusion of the analysis they turned in this log and the hard copy or disk file output from CP. An example of the computer-generated LARSP profile is shown in Figure 3.1.

LARSP analysis

A LARSP profile was constructed following the procedures described by Crystal *et al.* (1976) and elaborated by Crystal (1979, 1981). The 1981 revised profile chart was used, but Section D ('Reactions') was not completed. When the LARSP was done by hand, the totals at the bottom of the chart were not calculated and participants were only asked to record occurrences with tally marks on the profile chart. They did not have to record which structures were tallied for each utterance.

Order of analyses

For every language analysis undertaken, participants analysed the same transcript twice, once by hand and once by computer. This allowed for direct comparison of manual and computer times without introducing variation due to individual knowledge and experience. However, it also

36 Assessing Grammar

```
                              LARSP Profile

Filename: G3
Age: 4 years 3 months
Date: 11-16-1995
Type: conversation between clinician and child
Tabulation Method: Standard
Range of Utterances: All
Error Set: Standard LARSP Errors
```

A	UNANALYZED:	Unintelligible 3	Symbolic Noise ·	Deviant ·
	PROBLEMATIC:	Incomplete 3	Ambiguous ·	Stereotypes 1

B RESPONSES   NORMAL RESPONSE   ABNORMAL
                           ——Major——
      TOTALS   Repet-   Elliptical   Red-
               itions   1   2   3+   uced   Full   Minor   Struc-   Prob-
      26 Quest 11   6   5   tural ∅   lems
      45 Other 12   5   3   2   1   18   15
                                                        16
C 28 Spont   2   1   1   24   2

I 0;9-1;6   II 1;6-2;0   III 2;0-2;6   IV 2;6-3;0   V 3;0-3;6   VI 3;6-4;6   VII 4;6+

MINOR   Responses 25   Vocatives 2   Other 6   Problems ·

	COMM	QUEST	STATEMENT		
	'V' 2	'Q' ·	'V' ·	'N' ·	Other · Problems ·

CONN	CLAUSE		PHRASE		WORD
—	VX 3	QX ·	SV 6 AX 5	DN 11 VV 6	-ing 5
—			SO · VO ·	AdjN 1 VPart 1	
—			SC 1 VC ·	NN 2 IntX 5	pl 10
			Neg X · Other ·	PrN · Other 15	
					-ed 2
	X+S:NP 5	X+V:VP 4	X+C:NP 1 X+O:NP ·	X+A:AP 4	reg ·
					irr 2
—	VXY 1	QXY ·	SVC 2 VCA ·	DAdjN · Cop 10	
—		VS(X) 4	SVO 12 VOA ·	AdjAdjN · Aux-M 9	-en 2
—	Let XY ·		SVA 4 VOdOi ·	PrDN 6 Aux-O 10	
	Do XY ·		NegXY · Other 2	Pron-P 43 Other 11	3s 5
				Pron-O 29	reg ·
					irr 5
	XY+S:NP 4	XY+V:VP 11	XY+C:NP 2 XY+O:NP 7	XY+A:AP 3	gen ·
>	+S ·	QVS 1	SVOA 7 AAXY 1	NPPrNP 1 NegV 4	
—		QXY+ ·	SVCA · Other 1	PrDAdjN · NegX 1	n't 3
—	VXY+ 1	VS(X)+ 2	SVOdOi ·	cX · 2 Aux ·	
		tag ·	SVOC ·	XcX · Other	'cop 2
and 16	Coord ·	Coord ·	Coord-1 2 -1+ ·	Postmod Phr-1+ ·	'aux 2
c 2	Other ·	Other ·	Sub A-1 -1+ ·		
> s 4			Sub S ·		-est ·
Other ·			Sub C · Sub O ·		-er ·
			Comparative ·		
			Postmod Cl-1 ·		-ly ·
			Postmod Cl-1+ ·		

	(+) Passive ·	Complement-C ·	Initiator 3	Complex VP 3
	how ·	what ·	Coord NP 1	Complement-P ·
—	(-) and- ·	conn- · sub- ·	Elem∅ 20 Elem-> ·	Conc- · Det- ·
>	D∅ ·	D-> · Prep- ·	Pr∅ · P-> ·	Pron- · Modal- ·
	Aux- ·	Aux∅ · Cop- ·	Irr N- · Reg N- ·	Irr V- · Reg V- ·
	Other ·		Ambiguous ·	

it ·   there 1   A Connectivity 1   Comment Clause ·   Emphatic Order ·

```
             Complete & Intelligible      Total           LARSPed
P Sentences               99                105              98
                                   (3 Incomplete, 3 with Xs)
P MLU in words          3.44               3.50             3.43
P MLU in morphemes      3.64               3.68             3.62
P MSL (Klee, 1992)      4.84              -----            -----
Spontaneous Sentences   -----              -----            23.5%
Adequate Responses      -----              -----           100.0%
Mean P Sentences/Turn                      1.48
Mean T Sentences/Turn                      1.41
P Sentences/T Sentences                    1.05
T Sentences                                100 (25 Question, 46 Other)
T MLU in words                             4.38

              Number   % of Clauses                 Number    % of Phrases
Stage   I Clause   11    16.2%    Stage   I Phrase    78         31.3%
Stage  II Clause   15    22.1%    Stage  II Phrase    41         16.5%
Stage III Clause   25    36.8%    Stage III Phrase   118         47.4%
Stage  IV Clause   13    19.1%    Stage  IV Phrase     5          2.0%
Stage   V Clause    2     2.9%    Stage   V Phrase     0          0.0%
Stage  VI Clause    0     0.0%    Stage  VI Phrase     7          2.8%
Stage VII Clause    2     2.9%
Mean Clausal Complexity 2.91      Mean Sent Complexity - Phrase  8.73

Major sentences that are complex    2/ 66     3.0%
Clauses with 2+ expansions         14/ 68    20.6%
Verb phrases expanded              24/ 55    43.6%
Syntactic complexity score (Blake & Quartaro, 1990):  2.84
```

Figure 3.1 LARSP profile generated by Computerized Profiling software

meant that an order effect was inevitable. As it was anticipated that computer analysis would prove more time efficient, the decision was made to bias the study *against* this effect. Therefore, participants always performed the computer analysis first, thereby ensuring that any advantage gained through previous exposure to the sample would serve to reduce the times for manual analysis.

Accuracy of analyses

A computerized procedure for LARSP analysis, even if it was time-efficient, would be meaningless if the gains in efficiency occurred at the *expense* of accuracy. A comparison was therefore made on six of the separately timed analyses performed for this study. For each of the six analyses, the manual and computerized results were compared to a key prepared by the author. Grammatical analyses were compared by reviewing each of the LARSP profiles and awarding a point to the procedure – manual or computerized – that was found to be more accurate. In the case of ties, half a point was awarded to each procedure.

Although this procedure did not yield point-by-point comparison of all the linguistic judgements rendered in performing manual and computerized analysis, it did provide a clear picture of their relative accuracy. Out of a possible six accuracy points, the computerized procedure received five of them. The only accuracy points going to the manual procedure were the result of ties.

Efficiency of analyses

Table 3.2 shows the time spent by participants completing LARSP analyses on the three different samples. There is no question of the time efficiency of computerized grammatical analysis relative to manual

Table 3.2 LARSP analysis: Manual and computerized times

	Sample G1				Sample G2				Sample G3			
	N	Range	Mean	Max: Min	N	Range	Mean	Max: Min	N	Range	Mean	Max: Min
	33.0				37.0				32.0			
Manual		77.0–305.0	185.0	4.0		34.0–155.0	97.2	4.6		80.0–334.0	199.1	4.2
Computerized		18.0–71.0	44.8	3.9		15.0–50.0	32.0	3.3		37.0–98.0	64.3	2.6
Manual: computerized		2.8–7.6	4.2*	2.7		1.6–6.3	3.1*	3.9		1.7–5.0	3.1*	2.9

Note. All times are in minutes; max:min = ratio of maximum to minimum time.
* $p < 0.0001$.

Table 3.3 Correlations between manual and computerized times

	Sample G1	Sample G2	Sample G3
LARSP	0.82*	0.65*	0.78*

*$p < 0.001$

analysis. In general, the least grammatically complex sample, G2, was the fastest to analyse.

The relationship between manual and computerized analysis times among the individual participants is revealed in Table 3.3, which shows the correlation between the two times for each analysis of each sample. As can be seen, they are strongly and significantly correlated for the manual and computerized LARSP analyses.

Discussion

Foremost among its findings, this study quantifies exactly how much time clinical language sample analysis requires. It should be recalled that, because of the order in which the two analyses were performed, the time taken for manual analysis may have been somewhat underestimated, and the time for computerized analysis somewhat overestimated. Nevertheless, any bias in estimation that may have occurred would merely add support to the conclusions derived here.

Although there was variation in the amount of time needed for different analyses and different samples, it is clear from this study's results that language analysis, if it is done by hand and is intended for use in treatment planning, is a procedure that will not be possible to implement regularly in most clinical schedules. Regrettably, this finding contravenes the need for language analysis.

The clinical need for grammatical analysis can be seen in caseload data. Caseload statistics reveal that developmental language disorders make up a sizeable percentage of cases seen. Developmental language cases are seen by 75.4% of all clinicians and each of those clinicians sees an average of 13.9 such cases in a school year.[2] We do not know how often or how extensively grammatical analysis is being performed. We might assume, pessimistically, that the only analyses performed routinely are MLU and descriptive statistics, such as the number of different sentence types and the number of complete and intelligible utterances, even though these are general measures that cannot serve as the basis of treatment planning (Crystal *et al.*, 1976; Paul, 1995; Miller, 1996). A study conducted with the same group of clinician participants has indicated that these tasks can be completed on a sample of about 100 utterances in 6–16 minutes by an efficient clinician, and in no more than 41 minutes by an inefficient one (Long, 2001). The time range for an efficient clinician seems to fit comfortably into a typical work schedule. Whether the analysis time could be absorbed by an inefficient clinician is less certain. Either way, it bears repeating that these are the times for a minimal grammatical analysis, which will not address many of the treatment needs raised by patients with language disorders.

If those needs are to be met, a more extensive type of grammatical analysis, such as LARSP, is required. LARSP is a procedure best applied to children somewhere between productive word combinations and elaborated complex sentences. It can be used to establish a profile of a child's abilities across grammatical processes such as negation, question formation, noun and verb phrase elaboration, and pronominalization. LARSP is very carefully graded developmentally, which leads the clinician smoothly from analysis to the formulation of treatment goals based on developmental logic (Fey, 1986).

The time needed for manual LARSP analysis of a 100-utterance sample can be estimated from this study, with consideration given to the factors of clinician efficiency and sample complexity/severity. When performed on a linguistically immature child, it could be accomplished in 12 minutes to 2.5 hours, a range that begins within most clinicians' comfort zone for time but finishes well outside it. On more mature samples (G1 and G3), LARSP shows an even greater range, from 19 minutes to over 5.5 hours.

Based on all the manual analyses performed for this study, three conclusions appeared warranted. First, there is a clear effect of sample complexity/severity on analysis time. A clinician evaluating the grammar of a linguistically immature child is in a far better position to fit a manual language analysis into a busy clinical schedule.

Second, the effect of clinician efficiency is considerable for grammatical analysis. This can be seen in the ratios of maximum:minimum times for manual analyses, shown in Table 3.2. These ratios were 2 or greater for all samples and surpassed 5 in the most extreme case. It is as a result of these large ratios that the performance times for grammatical analysis fell so clearly both inside and outside of practical time limits for clinical application. The implication of this finding is that clinicians whose early experiences with manual grammatical analysis are inefficient – and therefore discouraging – might reasonably conclude that the procedure is unfeasible for clinical use.

The third conclusion to be drawn from this study's manual analyses is that the time requirement for language analysis varies with the kind of analysis performed. In particular, those analyses that provide information most useful to treatment planning, because of their structural and developmental organization, are also the analyses that consume the most clinician time. Thus, if these analyses are to be attempted by hand, the justification must be that they will allow clinicians to construct principled programmes of therapy that will prove, in the long-term, to be both more effective and time efficient (Crystal, 1981).

Put together, these three conclusions suggest that the only manual grammatical analysis procedures likely to be time efficient are simple structural counts performed by efficient clinicians on samples obtained from children with very young language ages. But is the picture really this bleak? In many commentaries on clinical language analysis, it is mentioned or even advocated that 'shortcuts' be used to reduce the time of the task (Crystal, 1979; Paul, 1995; Tyack & Venable, 1999). These shortcuts include such steps as scanning for but not tallying structural forms, omitting parts of an analysis procedure that have less relevance to the designated objective of assessment or treatment planning, or putting a ceiling on tallies when either productivity or a linguistic problem area have already been clearly identified. Where the rub comes with these recommended shortcuts is that, in most instances, they rely on the experience of the individual doing the analysis. In other words, a shortcut is most likely to be implemented by someone who recognizes patterns in the linguistic data early on and can draw an appropriate conclusion without completing all the tallies or including all portions of the procedure. Such skills of recognition are usually nurtured by experience, meaning that students and new practitioners will find shortcuts difficult to apply.

Another solution to the problem of time is to perform language analysis with the aid of software. The results of this study are unmistakable: language analysis software saves time for every clinician who uses it. The only question is how much time and, as with manual analysis, we find the factors of individual efficiency and type of analysis to be pertinent. If we use the ratio of manual:computerized time as an index of the time saved by using software, it is apparent that some individuals benefited more than others, as the maximum:minimum ratio for LARSP analyses ranged from 1.6 to 7.6.

What, then, can be said to a clinician who wants to employ clinical language analysis but fears – justifiably, as the findings from this study have shown – that it might consume too much time out of a clinical schedule? The best news is that computerization has brought language analysis within reach of nearly all clinician timetables. The longest average time to perform a computer-assisted LARSP analysis on one of the three samples was 64 minutes. Even the maximum times were under an hour, with the exception of two LARSP analyses that took as long as 71 and 98 minutes, respectively. That said, the decision to use software should probably be based on consideration of factors other than time alone. Clinicians who are proficient at linguistic analysis are able to perform manual procedures such as LARSP more efficiently. This study found that those same clinicians will achieve the lowest times for computerized analysis. These individuals should find themselves able to perform grammatical analysis on the computer in 10–45 minutes, depending on the specific procedure and complexity/severity of the sample. However, clinicians who perform these analyses inefficiently by hand may need as much as 98 minutes even when software is used. Computerization may not bring a more comprehensive grammatical analysis such as LARSP into the time budget of such clinicians.

Ultimately, what may most influence a clinician's decision to use grammatical analysis software is the belief in non-standardized assessment as the basis for treatment planning and as a repeated measure to judge the effectiveness of treatment. One of the main benefits of computerized grammatical analysis, beyond the time it saves, is the capability it provides the clinician to evaluate productivity through a variety of search and sort operations (Long, 1999). This study did not directly measure the time savings that can be achieved by performing productivity analyses on the computer, but the efficiency of this approach seems beyond question. The argument that clinicians will reap the rewards of comprehensive grammatical analysis in the long-term efficiency of therapy is only made more persuasive when the time needed is markedly reduced, the level of accuracy remains the same or better, and the analytical power of the procedure is extended.

The most obvious limitation of the use of computerized language analysis is the availability of the computer itself. At least some clinicians, or their employers, have yet to view the computer as an essential clinical tool. However, if non-standardized procedures are considered to be an important component of language assessment, the results of this study provide a straightforward rationale for computer acquisition. By using the manual to computerized time ratios in Table 3.2, the potential time savings can be calculated for any clinical caseload. This time, it can be argued, should be put to better clinical use.

Notes

(1) This includes only cases classified under Childhood Language Disorders as 'Other (including specific language impairment)'. Additional cases for which grammatical analysis might be appropriate fall under the ASHA (1999) survey categories of Autism/PDD, disorders resulting from attention deficit hyperactivity (ADHD), and learning disabilities.
(2) Earlier versions of this chapter were published in the journal *Clinical Linguistics and Phonetics*. This revised and expanded version is published with the permission of Informa PLC.

References

American Speech-Language-Hearing Association (1999) *1999 Omnibus Survey Caseload Report: SLP*. Rockville, MD: ASHA.
Channell, R.W. and Johnson, B.W. (1999) Automated grammatical tagging of child language samples. *Journal of Speech, Language, and Hearing Research* 42, 727–34.

Crystal, D. (1979) *Working with LARSP*. London: Edward Arnold.
Crystal, D. (1979) *Clinical Linguistics*. New York/Vienna: Springer-Verlag.
Crystal, D. (1982) *Profiling Linguistic Disability*. London: Edward Arnold.
Crystal, D., Fletcher, P. and Garman, M. (1976) *The Grammatical Analysis of Language Disability*. London: Edward Arnold.
Crystal, D., Fletcher, P. and Garman, M. (1981) *The Grammatical Analysis of Language Disability* (revised edn). London: Edward Arnold.
Fey, M.E. (1986) *Language Intervention with Young Children*. Boston: College-Hill Press.
Fletcher, P. (1985) *A Child's Learning of English*. New York: Blackwell.
Long, S.H. (2001) About time: A comparison of computerised and manual procedures for grammatical and phonological analysis. *Clinical Linguistics & Phonetics* 15 (5), 399–426.
Long, S.H. (1999) Technology applications in the assessment of children's language. *Seminars in Speech and Hearing* 20 (2), 117–32.
Long, S.H., Brian, J., Olswang, L.B. and Dale, P.S. (1997) Productivity of emerging word combinations in toddlers with specific expressive language impairment. *American Journal of Speech-Language Pathology* 6, 35–48.
Long, S.H., Fey, M.E. and Channell, R.W. (1996–2000) *Computerized Profiling*, Versions 9.0.3–9.2.7 (MS-DOS) [Computer program]. Cleveland, OH: Department of Communication Sciences, Case Western Reserve University.
Miller, J.F. (1996) Progress in assessing, describing, and defining child language disorder. In K.N. Cole, P.S. Dale and D.J. Thal (eds) *Assessment of Communication and Language* (pp. 309–24). Baltimore: Paul H. Brookes.
Paul, R. (1995) *Language Disorders from Infancy through Adolescence*. St. Louis: Mosby.
Quirk, R., Greenbaum, S., Leech, G. and Svartvik, J. (1972) *A Grammar of Contemporary English*. London: Longman / New York: Harcourt Brace Jovanovich.
Tyack, D. and Venable, G.P. (1999) *Language Sampling, Analysis, and Training: A Handbook* (3rd edn). Austin, TX: Pro-Ed.

4 HARSP: A Developmental Language Profile for Hebrew[1]

Ruth A. Berman and Lyle Lustigman

Introduction

This section outlines the history of the study from which the present chapter is derived and describes its database, and it also provides a brief introduction to relevant features of the structure of Israeli Hebrew. The original study was conducted over a period of several years in the late 1970s and early 1980s by the first author in cooperation with Anita Rom, a senior lecturer and researcher on speech pathology and atypical language development, and Myrna Hirsch, a speech clinician then living on Kibbutz Yizrael where she collected much of the data on which the study is based. This is a revised and updated version of an unpublished booklet produced by Berman et al., entitled *Working with HARSP: Hebrew Adaptation of the LARSP Language Assessment Remediation and Screening Procedure* (February 1982) and presented to the Israel Association of Speech Clinicians during a visit to Israel in 1981 by Michael Garman from the University of Reading. Since that time, the language of Hebrew-acquiring children with both normal and atypical development has been the topic of extensive research, part of which is referenced below. However, while the analyses presented below are considerably modified from the 1982 version of HARSP, our presentation adheres to the format stipulated in Crystal et al. (1989), combined with the 2005 updated manual, in order to be consistent with the overall goals of this volume.

Database

The materials underlying the original HARSP analyses derive from nearly 150 transcripts of adult-child conversations with normally developing Hebrew-speaking children. The interviews conducted by Myrna Hirsch were extended by materials collected under the auspices of Ruth Berman and Anita Rom (by graduate students of Tel Aviv University's departments of Linguistics and of Communications Disorders respectively), and were subsequently checked, revised and edited in standardized format by Ruth Berman. This yielded a set of computerized transcripts available on CHILDES (MacWhinney, 2000), based on adult-child conversational interchanges of

100 Hebrew-speaking pre-schoolers, 20 at each of the following age-groups (in years;months): 1;0–1;11, 2;0–2;11, 3;0–3;11, 4;0–4;11 and 5;0–5;11.[2] These cross-sectional materials were supplemented for present purposes by longitudinal samples of Hebrew child speech recorded and transcribed in the Berman lab at Tel Aviv University for four children between ages 1;3 to 3;6 in interaction with their mothers and other caretakers.

Brief outline of Hebrew grammar

This section focuses on features of Hebrew that are most relevant to the language of children in the age-range dealt with in this chapter (0;9–4;0), relying largely on studies by child language researchers dealing with relevant domains. Brief English-language overviews of the historical development and structure of Modern Hebrew are available in Berman (1985: 257–63; 1997), Berman and Neeman (1994), Ravid (1995a: 3–26) and Schwarzwald (2001).

A major task for Hebrew-acquiring children is mastery of the rich inflectional systems of their language: animate nouns alternate morphologically for gender (compare *iš ~ iša* 'man ~ woman', *xayal ~ xayélet* 'soldier ~ female soldier', *par ~ para* 'bull ~ cow', *tarnegol ~ tarnególet* 'cock ~ hen'), while inanimate nouns are inherently marked for gender as either masculine or feminine (compare masculine *šulxan* 'table' ~ feminine *mita* 'bed', *séfer* 'book' ~ *xovéret* 'notebook').[3] Count nouns can be either singular or masculine in number, with masculine nouns typically taking the suffix *–im* and feminine nouns ending in *–ot* (e.g. *talmidim* 'schoolboys' ~ *talmidot* 'schoolgirls', *parim* 'bulls' ~ *parot* 'cows'). The system is replete with lexical exceptions (including idiosyncratic structural alternations such as *iš ~ anašim* 'man ~ people', *iša ~ našim* 'woman ~ women') and, as the last example shows, cases where a masculine noun takes a feminine plural ending in *–ot* and vice versa (e.g. *šulxan ~ šulxanot* 'table-s', *kir ~ kirot* 'wall-s', and *beyca ~ beycim* 'egg-s', *mila ~ milim* 'word-s' respectively). Different morphological subclasses also entail various stem-changes when a suffix is attached to mark gender or number shifts, and also possessive case (e.g. *yéled ~ yalda ~ yeladim* 'boy ~ girl ~ children', *báyit ~ batim ~ beyti* 'house ~ houses ~ house-my' > 'my house'). Thus, while children acquire the basic systems of number and gender by around the age of three years, it takes them well into school age and sometimes beyond before they master all the different morphophonological alternations and lexical exceptions that these involve in Hebrew.

Moreover, these systems play an important role in the rich array of grammatical agreement in the language – from subject nouns to verbs and predicative adjectives, and from head nouns to their associated adjectives and determiners – as illustrated in (1) and (2).[4]

(1) a. *xaruz gadol nafal* 'bead big fell' > 'A big bead fell'
    b. *ha-xaruz ha-gadol ha-ze nafal* 'the-bead the-big the-that fell' > 'That big bead fell'

c. *(ha)xaruzim (ha)gdolim (ha)eyle naflu* 'beads big + Pl these fell + Pl' > 'These big beads fell'
(2) a. *kubiya gdola nafla* 'block + Fm big + Fm fell + Fm' > 'A big block fell'
b. *ha-kubiya ha-gdola ha-zot nafla* 'the-block + Fm the-big + Fm the-this + Fm fell' > 'That big block fell'
c. *ha-kubiyot ha-gdolot ha-eylu naflu* 'the-block + FmPl the-big + FmPl the-this + FmPl fell + FmPl = those big blocks fell'

These sentences show that agreement cuts across a range of syntactic and lexical categories in Hebrew, and that adjectives are inflected like the nouns they modify in number, gender and definiteness. The latter is marked by the unvarying prefixal clitic *ha-* 'the', while indefinite count nouns, both specific and non-specific, are marked by zero (e.g. *kadur* ~ *ha-kadur* 'a ball ~ the ball'). The 3rd person masculine singular represents the basic, morphologically unmarked form of open class items (nouns, verbs and adjectives), and children typically acquire marking of plural before gender alternations, and of subject-verb agreement before NP-internal agreement.

Verbs also agree with their subject nouns in number and gender and, in past and future tense, in person, cf. singular *nafál-ti* 'fell + 1st' > 'I fell', *nafál-ta* 'fell + 2nd Ms', *nafal-t* 'fell + 2nd Fm', *nafal* 'fell + 3rd Ms', *nafl-a* 'fell + 3rd Fm', plural *nafal-nu* 'fell + 1st' > 'we fell', *nafál-tem* 'fell + 2nd' > 'you (all) fell', *nafl-u* 'fell + 3rd Pl' > 'they fell'. Verbs are inflected for five categories of mood / tense (infinitive, imperative, present, past, future), while aspect is not marked grammatically in Hebrew. All verbs occur in one or more of seven morphological patterns, termed *binyanim*, literally 'buildings', constructed out of consonantal roots plus stem-internal vowels and external affixes. These roots are either full, in which case all three (sometimes four) radical consonants occur in all words constructed out of them, or else defective, containing one or more 'weak' radicals like the glides *y, w,* or low consonants like historical glottals and pharyngeals – in which case, the surface form of verbs (and also nouns and adjectives) that are based on these roots show various and quite complex morphophonological alternations.[5] The sets in (3) show various such possibilities, listing examples from the three patterns with highest (type and token) frequency. It thus excludes the P2 *nif'al* and P4 *hitpa'el* patterns, used mainly for intransitive, change-of-state, or 'unaccusative' verbs, and the two typically passive patterns, which are rare in children's speech. Illustrated in (3) are four different inflectional categories – infinitive, present, past and future (based on four different verb roots), the full, non-defective roots *r-q-d* 'dance', *g-d-l* 'grow', and the defective or weak roots *y-c-'* 'go out, exit', *b-w-'* 'come'. Tense-marked items are listed in the morphologically simplest form of 3rd masculine singular.

(3) Examples of tense / mood forms in three verb *binyan* patterns

Pattern	Root	Gloss	Infinitive	Present	Past	Future
P1 *pa'al*	r-q-d	dance (intr)	*li-rkod*	*roked*	*rakad*	*yi-rkod*
	g-d-l	grow (intr)	*li-gdol*	@*godel*	*gadal*	*yi-gdal*
	y-c-'	go out	*la-cet*	*yoce*	*yaca*	*ye-ce*
	b-w-'	come	*la-vo*	*ba*	*ba*	*ya-vo*
P3 *pi'el*	r-q-d	skip	*le-raked*	*me-raked*	*riked*	*ye-raked*
	g-d-l	raise	*le-gadel*	*me-gadel*	*gidel*	*ye-gadel*
	y-c-'	export	*le-yace*	*me-yace*	*yice*	*ye-yace*
	b-w-'	import	*le-yave*	*me-yave*	@ *yive*	*ye-yave*
P5 *hif'il*	r-q-d	make-dance	*le-harkid*	*ma-rkid*	*hi-rkid*	*ya-rkid*
	g-d-l	enlarge	*le-hagdil*	*ma-gdil*	*hi-gdil*	*ya-gdil*
	y-c-'	take out	*le-hoci*	*mo-ci*	*ho-ci*	*yo-ci*
	b-w-'	bring	*le-havi*	*me-vi*	*he-vi*	*ya-vi*

Note: Items marked with @ indicate forms that are non-normative in prescriptive terms, but are accepted in everyday Hebrew usage, including child input and output.

The syntax of simple clauses is relatively straightforward in Hebrew, with transitive verbs typically occurring in the surface pattern of {NVPrepN}, as illustrated in (4), where *et* indicates the accusative marker (labeled *et* at phrase level) occurring before all and only definite direct objects. For example:

(4 a. *ha-iš ra'a* **et** *ha-iša* 'The man saw *et* the woman'
  b. *ha-iš histakel* **ba**-*iša* 'The man looked at the woman'
  c. *ha-iš azar* **la**-*iša* 'The man helped to-the woman'
  d. *ha-iš paxad* **me-**ha-iša* 'The man feared from > was afraid of the woman'

As the examples in (4b) and (4c) show, definiteness marking is incorporated into the basic prepositions *be-* 'in, at' and *le-* 'to' (and also *k-* 'like'), but is marked separately by *ha-* (typically pronounced without an initial *h*) before other prepositions (e.g. *me-ha-báyit* 'from the-house, *im ha-kélev* 'with the-dog', *al ha-šulxan* 'on the-table'). Hebrew has numerous predicate-initial constructions, of two main types. (i) Existential and possessive constructions with the verb *haya* in past and future and the invariable existential particle *yesh* (or its negative counterpart *eyn*) in the present tense. For example, *yeš óxel ba-mitbax* 'Be food in-the-kitchen' > 'There's food in the kitchen'; *yeš lanu óxel* 'Be to-us food' > 'We have food'; *haya hamon ra'aš* 'Was much noise' > 'It was very noisy'; *hayta le-Ron be'aya* 'Was+Fm to-Ron problem+Fm' > 'Ron had a problem'. These examples also show that Hebrew is a non-*habere* language, having no special verb for 'have'.

(ii) VS order with a lexical verb preceding a lexical subject noun is another, less common type of predicate-initial construction, favoured mainly by change-of-state or unaccusative verbs. For example, *nišpax (li) ha-xalav* 'Spilt (to-me) the-milk' > 'The milk got-spilt (on me)'; *nišbera*+Fm *le-Ron ha-yad*+Fm 'Was-broken to-Ron the-hand' > 'Ron's hand broke / got broken'; *hofia pit'om dmut* 'Appeared suddenly figure' > 'A figure suddenly appeared'.

Hebrew also has a range of subjectless constructions, so that it is basically an (S)VO language. Two such constructions are particularly relevant to early child grammars: person-marked verbs in 1st and 2nd person, past and future tense (e.g. *gamár-ti* 'Finished+1st' > 'I (have) finished'; *ni-gmor* '1st+Pl–finish' > 'We'll finish'); and impersonal constructions with 3rd person plural verbs (e.g. *oxlim et ze im kapit* 'Eat+Pl it with (a) teaspoon' > 'We /you / people eat it / it is eaten with a spoon'; *eyx osim et ze?* 'How do+Pl that?' > 'How do you / does one make that / how is that made?'). This last example also demonstrates that question-formation is quite straightforward, since Hebrew has no structures corresponding to the auxiliary systems of English and other European languages: information questions are formed by placing the question-word initially, and *yes/no*-questions are marked merely by intonation, not syntactically. Relatedly, negation does not involve special syntactic operations, but is nearly always marked by the negative particle *lo* 'no, not' in preverbal position (e.g. *hu lo ohev léxem* 'He not likes bread' > 'He doesn't like bread'; *mi lo ohev shokolad* 'Who not like chocolate' > 'Who doesn't like chocolate?', *hem lo ra'u oto* 'They not saw' > 'They didn't see him'). Since negation by *lo* involves no more than an optional addition to the indicative clause structure, Neg is indicated throughout the chart in parentheses, to show that it may but need not occur.

As indicated by several of these examples, past and future tense verbs are marked not only for number and gender but also for person – by suffixes in the past and by prefixes in the future tense. In contrast, present tense (both immediate or progressive and habitual) is expressed by the so-called *beynoni* 'intermediate' forms that are inflected like nouns and adjectives for number and gender, but not for person.[6] Use of the present tense also differs from past and future in copular constructions, where tense is marked either by zero or by a pronominal copy of the subject rather than, as in past or future, by some form of the verb *haya* 'be' (e.g. *Ron (hu) ba-báyit* 'Ron (he) at-home' > 'Ron is at home' ~ *Ron haya ba-báyit* 'Ron was at-home' ~ *Ron yiheye ba-báyit* 'Ron will-be at-home'; *ha-aruxa*+Fm *(hi) te'ima*+Fm 'The-meal (she) tasty' > 'The meal is tasty' ~ *ha-aruxa hayta te'ima* 'The meal was tasty'). Moreover, as reflected in the preceding examples, a special existential particle is used in existential and possessive constructions in the present, as against past and future tense.

As these examples indicate, word order is quite straightforward, since it is mainly subject-initial, except for the predicate-initial constructions noted earlier. Word order is also relatively flexible, since non-subject nouns are typically marked by prepositions, and the rich system of agreement also provides cues to grammatical relations, with the subject noun, as noted, controlling predicate agreement for number, gender, and person. Internal noun-phrase ordering is consistently post-nominal or right-headed: except for quantifiers, all modifying elements occur after the head noun (e.g. *šney ha-yeladim ha-ktanim ha-éyle im se'ar šaxor še-ra'ínu šam* 'Two the-children the-little the-those with hair black that-saw+1stPl there' > 'Those two little boys with black hair that we saw there'). This example also shows that complex syntax is relatively straightforward as well: relative clauses are marked invariably by the same general subordinating conjunction *še-*'that'. This same basic element is also used to mark complement clauses (e.g. *hu ra'a še-ha-yéled boxe* 'He saw that-the-boy cries' > 'He saw that the boy was crying') as well as – following a prepositional – in most adverbial clauses (e.g. *biglal še-ha-yéled baxa* 'Because (that) the boy was-crying'; *lamrot še-ha-yeled baxa* 'Even that > although the-boy was-crying').

Finally, personal pronouns manifest a complex interplay between inflectional morphology and syntactic function. Pronouns in the nominative case (i.e. surface subjects) occur in the free form, while all other pronouns are suffixed to case-marking or adverbial-marking prepositions (e.g. *hu diber ito alav bil'aday* 'He spoke with-him about-him without-me' vs. *ani dibárti ita aléha bil'adav* 'I spoke with-her about-her without-him').

Terminological notes

The term *sentence*, as an abstract theoretical construct, is often inapplicable to units of speech in general and to early child language in particular. Consequently, throughout this chapter, the term *utterance* is used to refer to segments of children's speech output in preference to sentence. Here, an utterance refers to a piece of verbal output that can be defined behaviourally by its intonational contours irrespective of whether it is grammatically well formed or syntactically complete. The term *construction* refers to grammatical units such as phrase, clause, or sentence. Following the definition of a clause as 'any unit that contains a unified predicate ... expressing a single situation – activity, event, state' (Berman & Slobin, 1994: 660–62), we adopt this term for any utterance that contains a predication, whether or not it can be grammatically defined as a 'sentence' in normative or model-theoretic terms. The proportion of utterances other than those that can be defined as clauses (that is, as containing predications) increases significantly as a function of age in children's interactive speech output (Dromi & Berman, 1986), as does the proportion of clauses with lexical verbs rather than with copular or existential-possessive verbs (Berman & Slobin, 1994: 137n).

Design of the profile chart (see Appendix A)

The chart is divided into two main parts: *Types of Utterances* – relating to Sections A to D in the profile chart (see below) – and *Grammatical Analyses* (described at Clause-, Phrase-, and Word-Level, divided developmentally between Stages I through VI). The blocs headed A to D (Part One) in general correspond closely to the LARSP conventions specified in Crystal *et al.* (1989) and the Users' Manual of Boehm *et al.* (2005), while other levels of analysis are adapted to suit Hebrew morpho-syntax.

At the top of the second part of the chart, preceding detailing of the developmental stages, is a bar headed *Minor* that specifies the following types of non-expandable utterances: *Responses* – typically single-element responses to input (e.g. *ken* 'yes', *káxa* 'just so' in response to the query *láma?* 'why?'); *Vocatives* – addressing or calling a person or animal by name; *Other* – routine elements, as in counting or saying the letters of the alphabet; and *Problems* – cases where it is unclear whether the utterance is minor or grammatically analysable. Utterances defined as *Major* form the bulk of the chart, divided into stages from I to VI.

Types of Utterances: Child and/or Adult[7]

This heading refers to types of children's responses in relation to surrounding discourse. As detailed in Sections A to D of the original LARSP chart in *Working with LARSP* (Crystal, 1979) and further elaborated by Crystal in the present volume, these types of speech output are not language-specific, but apply to the pragmatics of adult-child conversational interchanges in general (at least in Western-type industrialized societies), and so are only briefly illustrated below for Hebrew.

Bloc A includes utterances that are not fully grammatically analysable, of two kinds – unanalysed strings and ones characterized as problematic. As examples of unanalysed strings, *ababu* could stand for a meaningful string like *ába bakbuk* 'Daddy bottle' or *ába šabur* 'Daddy broken', but is uninterpretable as it stands; and *a da še a ze* 'xxx that this one' – where the string *ada* could, but need not, stand for the girl's name *Ada*. The string *ni yaxol lex im ze yuxal* 'I can go with this will-be-able' is not analysed since it is *Unintelligible*, being uninterpretable because it contains recognizable words but with no identifiable syntactic structure.

Child output characterized as *Problematic* includes utterances that are only partially compositional (cf. the analysis in Berman & Slobin of children's narratives, dividing data in five different languages into 'uncoded versus coded clauses' (1994: 26, 658–9)). Child utterances that are unanalysed because they are *Incomplete* are illustrated in (5):

(5) a. Ad: *le'an haláxtem* 'Where-to you went' > 'Where did you-all go to?'
      Ch: *ani lo* 'I not' > 'I don't, didn't ...'

b. Ad: *hine macat ugiya kazot* 'Look, you-found (a) cookie like that'
   Ch: *po etmol* 'Here yesterday'

Note: The HARSP Section A differs from the original LARSP profile in that it does not include the category *Deviant*. We have also done away with the Error Box that appears as part of Stage VI in LARSP. Instead, we introduce an *Error Line* that applies to each stage from Stage III on.

Blocs B and C refer to the relationship, if any, between adult input and child output, divided between elicited and spontaneous child responses, while *Stimulus Type* records the total number of adult input utterances in the form of questions and other types of stimuli (e.g. utterance-initiation, shaping utterances) that the adult provides as prompts for the child.

– *Elicited Responses* include direct or partial repetitions of an utterance just produced by the adult, as in (6):

(6) a. Ad: *ze lo tov* 'It not good' > 'That's no good'
       Ch: *ze lo tov* [parroting, with same intonation]
    b. Ad: *éyfo Xanan?* 'Where (is) Chanan?'
       Ch: *Xanan?* 'Chanan?' [again, no change in intonation]

– *Elliptical responses* are grammatically analysable utterances that omit information available from the input (e.g. the adult asks *éyfo ha-xatul?* 'Where('s) the-cat?' and the child responds with *ba-sal* 'In-the-basket').
– *Reduced responses* omit clausal elements that are not retrievable from the preceding input (e.g. Adult: *ma kore?* 'What's happening?', Child: *yalda ba-xanut* '(A) child (is) in-the-store').
– *Minor Responses* are single-unit utterances, occurring usually but not only in Stage I (e.g. *lo* 'No', *uwa* 'Wow!').
– *Abnormal Responses* are unexpected or inappropriate given the input stimulus (e.g. to the question *ma ose ha-xatul?* 'What does the-cat' > 'What is the cat doing / What noise does a cat make?' the child responds with *ken* 'Yes'. *ni yaxol lex im ze yuxal* 'I can go with this will-be-able').
– *Zero Responses* are indicated when the child fails to provide a response to a question or some other elicitation on the part of the adult.

Bloc D Reactions relate to the impact of the adult's reactions on the child's speech output.

Note: Importantly, many early child utterances that would be defined as elliptical, incomplete, or telegraphic in English in fact constitute complete or well-formed clauses in Hebrew. For example, the two strings *hine mazleg* 'Here (is a) fork' and *ze adom ve ze adom* 'This (is) red and this (is) red' would be analysed as non-elliptical, hence analysable at clause level since Hebrew copular sentences in the present tense do not have an overt verb, nor does Hebrew have a morpheme corresponding to the indefinite article of English or Romance languages. Items given in parentheses (...) in the English glosses stand for elements that have no surface form in Hebrew; in representing children's speech output, they stand here for elements that occur in adult usage but were omitted or not pronounced by the child.

Grammatical Analyses

This heading refers to constructions that are treated as analysable at three main levels of lexico-grammatical structure – Clause, Phrase and Word (as summarized below) – corresponding to what were termed *major categories* in the original HARSP chart. From Stage IV, complex syntax is dealt with at the additional level of Connectivity.

Categories and levels of analysis

Analysis is confined to grammar in the narrow sense of morpho-syntax (i.e. the focus is on morphology and syntax as grammatical domains that in Hebrew are closely interconnected). In general, morphology refers to two main types of word-internal structure – grammatical inflections and derivational word-formation processes. In the present context, the concern is mainly with inflectional morphology as relevant to different aspects of early grammar, rather than with derivational processes that apply mainly to the developing lexicon. Syntax relates to structural processes of combining words into phrases and clauses, focusing mainly on the simple-clause level. Complex syntax is dealt with under the heading of Connectivity in combining clauses by processes of coordination, complementation and subordination at clause level (Diessel, 2004) from Stage IV, and in combining phrases – mainly by coordination – at phrase level from Stage V. Grammatical analysis is conducted at three main levels for Stages I through III – Clause, Phrase and Word – as defined below for Hebrew – with clause-combining Connectivity added from Stage IV.

As noted earlier, there is no equivalent to the LARSP Error Box in the HARSP chart. The Error Line that appears from Stage III serves for deviations from grammatical usages that are expected to be acquired by the relevant stage – and so corresponds to the LARSP category of Deviant. The variety of Hebrew serving as our target language is the colloquial spoken usage of adult speakers of standard Hebrew (Ben-David & Berman, 2007), so that we do not count as errors usages that are typical of the adult input to normally developing Hebrew-acquiring children, even if they violate normative prescriptions of the Hebrew language establishment. These include: (i) non-observation of subject-verb agreement in verb-initial contexts (e.g. *koev li ha-bēten* 'Hurts+Ms to-me the-stomach+Fm' > 'My tummy hurts, I have a tummy-ache'; *haya šam hamon anašim* 'Was there many people' > 'There were lots of people there'); (ii) levelling of the distinction between prepositions marking comitative and instrumental case in the form of *im* 'with' and *be-* 'in, at' respectively (e.g. *oxlim et ze im kapit* '(You / people) eat it with (a) teaspoon' vs. normative *be-kapit* 'in (a) spoon'); and (iii) levelling of the 1st person and 3rd person masculine prefix in future tense (e.g. *ani ya'ase et ze* 'I-3rd-Ms will-do it' > 'I will do it').

For Hebrew, usages counted as grammatical errors are marked for each level (Connectivity, Clause, Phrase, Word). These involve mainly: (i) non-congruent agreement (e.g. plural subject with singular verb, feminine noun with masculine adjective, with special treatment of errors that overextend feminine gender on numbers), and (ii) omission of grammatical items (e.g. definite marker, preposition). Imprecise or incomplete use of morphophonological processes like stem-changes (e.g. *simlot* for *smalot* 'dresses', *kélevim* for *klavim* 'dogs') are counted as errors only from Stage VI, and so are other 'creative errors' like mixing of *binyan* verb patterns (e.g. *nifrak* for *hitparek* 'fell apart' or *mizaher* for *nizhar* 'take care' are not treated as errors if they occur before Stage VI). The criterion here for not indicating an error is that children show productive use of grammatical rules (for, say, adding agreement- marking inflections) or derivational morphology (such as an alternation between transitive and intransitive verbs). Errors of this kind are only indicated if they occur at a stage beyond when the target adult forms are described as already acquired (as discussed subsequently).

Clause-level categories

Clause level refers to how major constituents are organized inside (not between) clauses in terms of different types of grammatical relations: predicates and the syntactic constituents associated with them – typically in the form of noun phrases and prepositional phrases. Predicates take the form of verb phrases headed by: (i) a lexical verb [V] that can be identified as made up of a combination of consonantal root and one out of the seven morphological *binyan* verb patterns; (ii) by the copular verb *haya* alternating in the present tense with the existential particle *yeš* in existential and possessive constructions; or (iii) in copular constructions by the same verb *haya* alternating in the present tense with zero or a pronoun [Cop]. Other syntactic constituents include grammatical subjects and different types of objects associated with particular types of predicates. Subjects [S] alternate between: (i) lexical noun phrases (e.g. *yeladim* 'children', *ha-kadur* 'the-ball'; *kol ha-yeladim ha-ktanim ha-éyle* 'all those little children'), (ii) pronouns in the nominative case (e.g. *ata* 'you MsSg', *hu* 'he', *hem* 'they'), or (iii) zero – in impersonal or verb-inflected subjectless constructions.

Objects take the form of: (i) direct objects [O] marked by the accusative preposition *et* when the object NP is definite; (ii) oblique objects [Obl], when the verb governs a preposition (e.g. *histakel be-* 'look at'; *hirbic le* 'hit to

= hit'; *ka'as al* 'angered on' > 'was angry with'); or (iii) indirect [dative] objects [IO] in the case of three-place predicates (e.g. *Ron natan et ha-séfer le-Rina* 'Ron gave *et* the-book to-Rina'). Other clause-level constituents cover a range of adverbial constructions, typically in the form of prepositional phrases. These are associated with the predicate in expressing relations such as manner (e.g. *bi-mhirut* 'with quickness' > 'quickly'), time (e.g. *lifney ša'a* 'before hour' > 'an hour ago'), place – location or direction, source (e.g. *me-ha-báyit* 'from the house'), and goal, and they may be more or less obligatory, depending on the particular verb that serves as the predicate.

Phrase-level categories
Phrase level refers to the internal structure of clause-level constituents consisting minimally of a head, often with associated modifying elements. Thus, a noun phrase (NP) consists minimally of a pronoun or a lexical noun (e.g. *yéled* '(a) boy') expandable by different types of modifiers which in Hebrew typically follow the head noun (e.g. *ha-yéled ha-katan ha-ze* 'that little boy'). NPs can function either as subject (e.g. *ha-yéled ha-katan ha-ze hirbic li* 'that little boy hit me'), as direct object (e.g. *ra'íti et ha-yéled ha-katan ha-ze* 'I-saw that little boy'), as indirect object (e.g. *natáti et ha-séfer la-yēled-katan ha-ze* 'I gave the-book to that little boy'), or as oblique object (e.g. *ha-iš histakel al ha-yéled ha-katan ha-ze* 'the-man looked at that little boy').

A Verb Phrase (VP) functioning as predicate can be realized: (i) as a lexical verb in intransitive clauses (e.g. *ha-yéled boxe* 'the-boy cries' > 'is crying'; *ha-yéled nafal* 'the boy fell (down)') and with an object in transitive clauses (e.g. *ha-yéled maca séfer* 'the-boy found (a) book'; *ha-yéled histakel ba-séfer* 'the-boy looked in-the-book'; *ha-yéled natan et ha-séfer la-axot šelo* 'the boy gave *et* the book to sister-his' > 'his sister'); (ii) as an 'extended predicate' with modal and aspectual verbs (e.g. *ha-yéled yaxol la-vo* 'the-boy can to-come'; *yodéa lisxot* 'knows (how) to-swim'; *hitxil le-daber* 'began to-talk'); and (iii) in copular sentences, as zero or a pronoun in the present tense and as a form of the verb *haya* 'be' in the past and future, followed by a complement in the form of an NP (e.g. *ha-yéled 0 ~ hu / haya talmid tov* 'the-boy is / was (a) good student'), an adjective or adjective phrase (e.g. *ha-sipur haya acuv me'od* 'the-story was very sad'), or a locative expression, often in the form of a prepositional phrase (e.g. *kulam ba-báyit* 'everyone (is) at home').

Prepositional phrases (PPs) consist of a preposition + NP (e.g. *al ha-šulxan* 'on the-table'; *le-xeyfa* 'to Haifa'; *im ha-xaver šeli* 'with my friend'; *bli ezra mi-afexad* 'without help from anybody'). These typically function as oblique or dative objects and as various kinds of adverbials.

Word-level categories
Word level analyses refer to how words are grammatically modified by a range of inflectional categories, as outlined earlier. These include: number and gender marked by suffixes on nouns and their associated verbs and

adjectives; person marked on verbs in the 1st and 2nd person by suffixes in the past tense and prefixes in the future tense (e.g. *haláx-ti* 'went-1stSg' > 'I went' ~ *ne-lex* '1stPl+will-go' > 'We'll go'); and mood/tense marking on verbs as differentiating between the five categories of infinitive, imperative, present, past and future number – by internal vowel alternations (e.g. *halax* 'went' vs. *holex* 'goes') and suffixes and/or prefixes (e.g. *medaber* 'talks, is-talking', *diber* 'talked', *yedaber* 'will-talk'). Pronouns are inflected as suffixes on their associated (case- and adverbial-marking) prepositions except when they are nominative, that is, functioning as grammatical subjects (e.g. *ha-yéled diber im axiv al ha-séfer* 'The boy talked with his-brother about the-book' ~ *hu diber <u>ito alav</u>* 'he talked <u>to-him on-him</u> = about-it'; *ha-séfer nafal me-ha-madaf al ha-roš šel ha-yéled* 'The-book fell from-the-shelf on(to) the-head of the-boy' ~ *hu nafal <u>miménu alav</u>* ~ *al ha-roš <u>šelo</u>* '<u>it </u>fell <u>from-it onto-him</u>' ~ 'onto head his' > 'onto his head').

The varied word-formation devices represented by the rich derivational morphology of Hebrew are considered here only in relation to the *binyan* verb-pattern conjugations, since these go beyond the means for extending vocabulary, and are criterial for evaluating clause-grammatical development (e.g. compare *ha-yéled **šavar** et ha-xalon* 'The-boy broke the-window' ~ *ha-xalon **nišbar*** 'The-window broke' from the shared root *š-b-r*, *ha-yéled **raxac** et ha-dúbi* 'The-boy washed the-teddy' ~ *ha-yéled **hitraxec*** 'The-boy washed (himself)' from the root *r-x-c*).

Speech act categories

Each utterance that is analysed can be assigned to one of three main classes of grammatical constructions: imperative, interrogative, indicative. In pragmatic terms, these serve to express different types of speech acts: requests or commands, queries and questions, or statements and propositions respectively.

Imperatives express three main kinds of acts: requests, commands and, in the negative, prohibitions. In colloquial Hebrew, these take the same inflected form as verbs in the future tense, 2nd person (singular or plural, masculine or feminine) either: (i) consisting of the verb stem alone (e.g. *zuz* 'Move!', feminine *zúzi*, plural *zúzu*; *lex* 'Go (away)!', feminine *léxi*, plural *léxu*); or (ii) with a person-marking prefix (e.g. *te-sapri li* 'Tell+Fm me!'; *ta-vi lánu* 'Bring to-us!'). (For details of these alternations, see Berman, 1985: 288–90). In the usage of younger children and their caretakers, commands and prohibitions may also take the form of the infinitive (e.g. *axšav kulam la-šévet* 'Now everyone to-sit' > 'Now everyone sit down!'), or in the negative (e.g. *lo le-daber axšav* 'Not to talk now' > 'No talking now!'). Negative commands expressing prohibitions and using future rather than infinitive forms of the verb take a special imperative negator in the form of *al* (e.g. *al ta-zúzu* 'Not-2nd move+2ndPl' > 'Don't move'; *al te-daber* 'Not-2nd will-talk+2nd' > 'Don't talk, you mustn't talk'; *Al ta-azru la* 'Not-2nd help+2ndPl her' > 'Don't help her').

Interrogatives in Hebrew as in other languages express two types of question: *yea/no* and information.

– *Yes/no questions* do not have a special grammatical construction or lexical marker in colloquial Hebrew, but are realized in speech by a rising intonation on statements (e.g. *ata roce glída¿* '(Do) you want ice-cream¿' ~ *ken, ani roce (glida)* 'Yes, I want (ice-cream)'). As these examples show, Hebrew has nothing corresponding to the dummy auxiliary *do* of English short answers. Nor does Hebrew have auxiliaries marking aspectual categories corresponding to progressive or perfect in English or Spanish, so there is no room for inversion either. Thus *yes/no*-questions have the same surface form as statements in Hebrew (e.g. *ha-tinok boxe¿* 'The-baby cries' > 'is crying' ~ 'Is the baby crying'; *ába kvar halax¿* 'Daddy already went' > 'Has Daddy gone already¿', 'Did Daddy go already¿' – except, as noted, for being marked by intonation).

– *Information questions* are formed by fronting a question word (e.g. [Q S] *éyfo ha-séfer* 'Where (is) the-book¿'; [Q V Obl] *ma kara le-Ron¿* 'What happened to-Ron¿'; *le-an hu halax¿* 'To-where he went' > 'Where did he go to¿'; [Q S V] *láma ha-tinok boxe* 'Why the-baby cries' > 'Why is the baby crying¿'). As these examples show, question-formation in Hebrew does not require any inversion operations, although information questions may but need not trigger VS order (e.g. [Q V S] *le-an halax ha-yéled¿* 'To-where went the-boy' > 'Where did the boy go¿'; *eyx nigmar ha-sipur* 'How ended the-story¿' > 'How did the story end¿'). Note, too, that Hebrew does not have a set of grammaticized WH-operators like English, such as *who, what, why, where,* and so on, but a group of morphologically unrelated question words (e.g. *éyfo* 'where', *le-an* 'to-where', *lama* 'why', *eyx* 'how').

Statements are propositions constructed in the basic or unmarked indicative mood, serving to describe situations or to express ideas. They are either affirmative or negative, in the latter case marked simply by the general negating morpheme *lo* 'no, not' (e.g. *Dani halax ha-báyta* 'Danny went home' ~ *Dani lo halax ha-báyta* 'Danny not went home' > 'didn't go home'; *haya hamon rá'aš ba-xéder* '(There) was lots-of noise in-the-room' ~ *lo haya šam rá'aš bixlal* 'Not was there noise at-all' > 'There wasn't any noise there at all'). In existential and possessive constructions in the present tense, the general existential particle *yeš* alternates with the negator *eyn*. For example, *yeš šam rá'aš* '(There) be noise there' ~ *eyn šam rá'aš* '(There) not-be noise there'; *yeš li na'aláyim xadašot* 'Be to-me new shoes' > 'I have new shoes' ~ *eyn li na'aláyim xadašot* 'Not to-me new shoes' > 'I don't have new shoes').

Note: Since Hebrew does not have syntactic operations such as auxiliary inversion differentiating these three types of constructions, we eliminate these categories except for Stage I. Instead, Questions are marked [Q] if and only if they contain an overt question-word, and imperatives are marked morphologically at Word level.

Developmental Analyses

Six developmental stages are specified below, defined in age-related terms so as to accord with the overall approach of LARSP-based analyses. Each type of structure is entered at the levels of Clause, Phrase and/or Word (from Stage IV, also at the level of inter-clausal Connectivity), by the developmental stage at which it typically emerges in the language of normally developing Hebrew-acquiring children. The stages specified below derive from three main sources: preliminary analyses undertaken for the original 1982 HARSP study of Berman *et al.*; analysis of materials collected subsequently by the authors and their associates in the Berman lab; and findings of other research on Hebrew child language. These yielded the following broad stages of morpho-syntactic development characterizing early Hebrew child grammar defined, as noted, by chronological age, from one to four years of age.

(8) Stage I – Single-unit utterances [c. 0;9–1;6]
 Stage II – Early combinations [c. 1;6–2;0]
 Stage III – Early clause structure [c. 2;0–2;6]
 Stage IV – Extended modification [c. 2;6–3;0]
 Stage V – Complex syntax [c. 3;0–3;6]
 Stage VI – Early grammar consolidation [c.3;6–4;0]

It must be borne in mind that age ranges are essentially approximate in relation to language as to other developmental domains.[8] While the same overall progression tends to be shared by most normally developing children, there is bound to be great individual variation from one child to the next, and from one linguistic domain to another. Thus, different children will demonstrate different developmental patterns: some may start late and then catch up rapidly with their peers; some children may move gradually from one 'stage' to the next, while others may appear to skip a stage; and transitions from one stage to the next may be clearly demarcated by some children, while being blurred in the case of others.

Stage I [c. 0;9–1;6]

Under this heading, we refer to what appears to be a universal stage in children's initial pairing of strings of sounds with semantic content.

Following Peters (1983), the term 'single-unit' is preferred to the more familiar 'one-word stage', since at this developmental phase children may combine into single, unanalysed strings elements that constitute two or more words in the target language. Examples in Hebrew are: (i) the string pronounced something like *eze* standing for target *et ze* – the accusative or direct object [Acc] marking preposition *et* plus the deictic pronoun *ze* 'it, that' – when pointing to an object; or (ii), *máze* 'wazzit' from the question word *ma* 'what' plus the deictic *pronoun ze* 'it, that' representing the question *ma zeʔ* 'What's that' common in adult input as well as children's output for the purpose of labelling objects; (iii) the string *ápam* from target *od* 'another' + *pa'ám* 'time' > 'again', when a child wants to repeat an activity; (iv) common 'multi-word' requests like *níli* or *víli* from *tni* 'give+Fm!' + *li* ' to-me' for 'give (it) to me' or *tavíli* 'bring (it) to-me' analogously to English *gimme*; and (v) lexicalized compounds that children typically treat as single words (e.g. *yəmulédet* for *yom hulédet* 'day birth' > 'birthday' or *becéfer* for *bet séfer* 'house (of) book' > 'school').

Following research on developmental phases in Hebrew, the type of knowledge represented by such usages is analysed as 'pre-grammatical' in the following sense. Although in using them, children are attributing appropriate (quite restricted) senses to given strings of sound, they fail to reflect any structure-dependent analysis. Relatedly, words that may consist of more than a single morpheme in the target language are not yet analysed for inflectional categories such as number, gender, or (pronominal) case-marking. Common examples are words that (for pragmatic reasons) typically occur in early child Hebrew only in the more marked forms of plural number (e.g. *na'al-áyim* 'shoe-s'; *ca'acu-im* 'toy-s'; *kubiy-ot* 'block-s') or feminine gender (e.g. *par-a* 'cow'; *tarnegól-et* 'hen'). Further, at this stage the child cannot be said to have grammatical, structure-based knowledge of part-of-speech categories. This is reflected by the use of single quotes for categories listed for Stage I (e.g. 'V' stands for verb-like element in the child's initial use, 'N' stands for something like a noun, and so on).

Working across the Profile Chart in Appendix I, the following three types of utterances are identified: Command-Type, Question-Type and Statement-Type. Categories identified specifically for this initial stage by single quotes include: 'V' for an utterance with a verb-like or predicating function; 'N' for one with a labelling function or to refer to a person or object; 'D' for deictic, pointing elements; 'F' for elements resembling closed-class function items like pronouns or prepositions; and 'Other' for situational or evaluative elements that are hard to classify.

– *Command-Type*. 'V': any verb-like utterance the child uses in making a request or giving an order. These may take one of three forms, often only distinguished by the extralinguistic situation: (i) 'V-Imp': an imperative or truncated 'bare-stem' form. For example, *zuz* 'move!', *kax* 'take', *šev!* 'sit (down)', *ten(li)* 'give (me)' – or their feminine alternants of such forms, often favoured by girl-children (*zúzi, kxi, švi, tni* respectively) – *stalek* 'go away', *bo-héna* 'come here' (unless the child also produces *bo* 'come' alone, in which case it counts as a two-element structure); (ii) 'V-Fut': future-tense forms with 2nd person *t-* prefixes. For example, *tir'e* 'look!', *tavi* 'bring' (me)!', *tafsik* 'stop!', again sometimes used with a feminine suffix, especially by girls (*tir'i, tni, tafsíki* respectively); (iii) 'V-Inf': a truncated form of the infinitive, grammatically marked by an initial *l* + vowel meaning 'to' that is typically omitted at this initial stage. For example, *éde* '(I want to) get down' (cf. infinitive *larédet*), *xol* 'eat!' (cf. infinitive *le'exol*), *šon* '(go to) sleep!', 'lie down!' (cf. *lišon*).

- *Question-Type.* 'Q': any single-element utterance with the force of a question, typically one-word information questions (e.g. *éyfo* 'where', *ma* 'what', *máze* 'what's that' and occasional *yes/no*-questions).
- *Statement-Type.* 'V': a single-element utterance that is verb-like in form and content, making a statement about an activity or situation (e.g. *halax* 'went, has-gone, has left', *roce/roca* 'want Ms/Fm'; *(ya)šen* 'sleep, is-sleeping', *boxe* 'cry, is-crying', *(na)fal* '(it) fell', *(niš)bar* 'broke, got broken', *(hit)pocec* 'burst'); 'N': a single-element utterance that is noun-like, referring to people or objects (e.g. *ába* 'daddy (for any man)', *ima* 'mommy', *(ti)nok* 'baby', *may(im)* 'water', *buba* 'doll', *(ci)por* 'bird', *(mixna)-sáyim* 'pants', *(ka)dur* 'ball'); 'D': a deictic element, typically some form of *ze* 'it, this, that', (e.g. *eze, edze, etze* or *híne* 'here('s), lookit'); 'F': an element resembling function words or closed-class items (e.g. *eyn* 'not, none, allgone' to express absence or disappearance, *day* 'enough' to protest or reject, *od* 'more, another' for addition or recurrence); 'O': all other single-element utterances that cannot be classified as one of the above, including 'situational' and nursery terms (e.g. *am* for 'food, eating, meal', *áyta* 'go out, take a walk, buggy', *pípi* 'wet, diaper, urine', *yófi* 'great!, nice', *tov* 'good, okay, alright').

Stage II [c. 1;6 – 2;0]

This stage takes the form of initial combining of two or three elements, without as yet involving fully grammaticized syntactic relations or lexical categories. These elements are combined at clause level to serve generalized syntactic functions (in subject- or predicate-like roles) and are not as yet specified for part-of-speech categories. Hebrew Stage II does not as yet involve phrase-level expansions, although it can include some initial word-level combinations of stem plus inflection or an adjective in a non-syntactically specifiable position. Note, again, that many Stage II utterances are grammatically well-formed in Hebrew, which does not have an indefinite article or a present tense form of the copular *is, are*.

Clause-level combinations

- *Stage I expansions*: use of elements labeled 'D', 'F', or 'O' at Stage I, in combination with another element (labelled X, as non-specified for lexical class) plays a critical role in the transition to Stage II (e.g. [D X] *híne kadur* 'Here ('s a) ball'; *ze dúbi* 'It ~ that's (a) teddy'; [F X] *eyn xalav* 'Not ~ none ~ allgone milk'; *od kúku* 'More, another peekaboo').
- *Transitional copular constructions*: the general deictic or demonstrative pronoun *ze* 'it, this, that' with a noun used in a labelling function, specified as [ze 'N'] to indicate that *ze* serves as precursor of a grammatical subject (e.g. *ze sus* 'It (is a) horse'; *ze ába* 'That (is) Daddy'; *ze cipor* 'It ('s a) bird'; *ze kos* 'It('s) a cup'). Note that these are grammatically well-formed strings in Hebrew.
- *Q-word + X*: interrogatives functioning as information questions, often also using elements from Stage I (e.g. [Q V] *ma kara?* 'What happened?'; *mi ba* 'Who('s) coming/came?'; [Q X] *éyfo ába Tali* 'Where ('s) Daddy Talli' > 'Where's Tally's Daddy?').
- *'N' + C*: 'N' here is a lexical noun in subject position in present-tense copular constructions (so-called 'nominal sentences') with different types of complements – labelled C (with the label Comp used for complement clauses under Connectivity). These include mainly labelling constructions in the form [*ze* 'N'] as above, and also [N C] lexical N + locative (e.g. *ába avoda* 'Daddy's (at) work ~ went to work'; *tinok agala* '(The) baby (is in the) buggy').
- *'V' Constructions*: combinations of a verb or verb-like element either before or after some other element (e.g. [X 'V'] *lo roca ~ roce* 'Not want+Fm ~ Ms' > 'I don't want to'); or ['V' X] (e.g. *ába ba* 'Daddy is-coming ~ came'; *halax (ha)báyta* 'Went ~ gone home'). These also include commands, requests and prohibitions (e.g. [X 'V'] *lo (laš)évet* 'Not (to) sit' > 'Don't sit down'; ['V' X] *sími po* 'Put (it) here'; *Od (li)rkod* 'More to-dance' > 'I want to dance some more').

Word-level combinations

These refer to the first instances of stem + inflection, or inflection + stem combinations, showing a clear expansion from Stage I usages.

- *In verbs*. A child who formerly used only a bare-stem form of a verb now adds the infinitive-marking *l-* [Inf], as in *lašévet* 'to-sit', *lirkod* 'to dance'; the imperative-marking prefixal *t-* [Imp] in *tatxil* 'you-will-start' > 'begin!'; *torídi (li)* 'you-will-take-down+Fm' > 'take (something) down ~ off (for me)!' when asking to have clothing removed; or a person- or gender-marking suffix as in past tense [1stPa] *nafál+ti* 'fell+1stSg' > 'I fell' or present tense *oxél-et* 'eat+FmSg' > 'eats / is eating' when talking about something done by a girl or woman.

- *In nouns.* Here we see marking of the (masculine) plural suffix [Pl] on a noun the child also uses in the singular (e.g. *kadur-im* 'ball-s', *xatul-im* 'cat-s'); initial alternations of pronominal suffixes on the possessive marker [Poss+1stSg ~ 2ndSg], (e.g. *šeli* ~ *šelxa* 'of-me' > 'my' ~ 'of-you' > 'your'); or on prepositions [Prep + 1st ~ 3rd] (e.g. *tni li* ~ *tni lo* 'give to-me' ~ 'give to-him / it').
- *In adjectives.* This stage reflects the emergence of the two distinct syntactic positions (predicative and attributive), with predicative adjectives occurring mainly in subjectless clauses, and attribute adjectives in headless constructions such as *ani roce et ha-gadol* (I want Acc the-big (one)).

Stage III [c. 2;0 – 2;6]

At this stage, children can be credited with at least partially grammaticized syntactic relations (subject, predicate, adverbial, etc.) and lexical categories (noun, verb, etc.). Accordingly, from Stage III on, errors are entered in a special line at the end of each stage, as specified earlier.

Clause-level structure

Importantly, by Stage III, Hebrew clause-level structures cannot be evaluated by counting, because the number of surface elements is often not indicative of increased grammatical complexity – particularly since grammatically well-formed clauses may lack a surface subject or verb. Instead, the grammatical structures that occur at this stage are indicated as such, ranging from one to three and occasionally even four surface elements. Note further that, at this stage, the negating element *lo* [Neg] 'no, not' may be added to any or all of the clause-level structures listed below.

- *Subjectless clauses*: grammatically well-formed clauses may lack a surface subject in cases of: (i) verbs inflected for person (e.g. [V] *hitraxácti* 'Washed+1stSg' > 'I washed (myself)'; [V O] *ra'ínu oto* 'Saw+1stPl 'We saw him'; [V A] *haláxti habáyta* 'Went+Past 2ndMsSg to-home' > 'You went home'); (ii) impersonal constructions with a verb in 3rd person masculine plural (e.g. [V O] *šavru et ze* 'Broke+Pl it' > 'It got-broken, someone broke it'; [Q V A] *ma ro'im po?* 'What see+Pl here' > 'What do we / people see here?'); (iii) commands, requests and prohibitions (e.g. [NegV O] *lo leharbic la-kélev* 'Not to-hit the-dog' > 'Don't hit the dog'); (iv) weather expressions (e.g. [Adj A] *Xam po* '(It's) hot here'); and sensations with a dative experiencer (e.g. [V Dat] *ko'ev li* 'Hurts to-me' > 'I hurt'; [Adj Dat] *kaše lánu* 'Hard to-us' > 'It's hard for us'). (Subjectless constructions with a modal or evaluative operator plus complement occur later, in Stage IV).

  Note: Further grammatical complexity of the V element from Stage III on is marked at Word level (e.g. past tense + 1st person *baxíti* 'I

cried'; *rác-nu* past tense + 1st person plural 'we ran'; *yašan-tem* past tense + 2nd person plural 'you slept'; *yavo* 3rd person singular + future 'I'll come'; *nistader* 1st person plural + future 'we'll manage').
- *Copular constructions* [S (Cop) C (X)]: these are clauses with the copular verb *haya* in the past and future tense or with a zero surface form of the verb in the present tense ('nominal sentences'), sometimes realized by a pronoun linking subject and complement (e.g. [S Cop C] *hu haya ba-báyit* 'He was at-home'; *ha-mic ze šeli* 'The-juice it (is) mine' – most typically at this stage [S C] as in *ha-tinok ra'ev* 'The-baby (is) hungry'; *aba ba-avoda* 'Daddy's at-work'). These may also include an adverbial, as in [S C A] *Ze adom po* 'It (is) red here'; *ha-kadur šavur axšav* 'The-ball (is) broken now' or [S A C] *éyle kvar beséder* 'These (are) already okay'.
- *Existential and possessive constructions* [Ex (Dat) $S_{ex \sim poss}$]: clauses with the existential operator *yeš* '(there) be' or its negative counterpart *eyn* 'not (be)' in the present tense, or a form of the copular verb *haya* 'be' in the past and future are used to express: (i) existence [Ex S_{ex} A] as in *yeš xol bifnim* 'Be > There is sand inside', or non-existence [(Neg)Ex S_{ex} A] as in *eyn oxel hayom* 'None food today' > 'There's no food today'; and (ii) possession – with the dative marker *le-* indicating the possessor [(Neg)Ex Dat S_{poss}] as in *Yeš lo kadur* 'Be to-him ball' > 'He has a ball'; *Lo haya li sefer* 'Not was to-me (a) book' > 'I didn't have a book'. In order to differentiate these two constructions from languages with: (a) a surface marker of existence like English *there*, or (b) a special verb of possession like English *have*, pronouns and NPs that follow the existential markers are specified as special kinds of subjects: S_{ex} for existential and S_{poss} for possession. When S_{poss} is definite, the accusative object-marker *et* may be added (e.g. [Ex Dat S_{poss}] *haya lo et ha-séfer* 'Be to-him *et* the-book' > 'He had the book'). This is not counted as an error, since it is common in colloquial adult usage.

Verb-initial utterances, with a lexical (not existential or possessive copula) are also possible in Hebrew, mainly with verbs that are semantically change-of-state, syntactically unaccusative, as in [V S] *nafal kise* 'Fell (a) chair'; *nišpax xalav* 'Got-spilt (the)-milk'. Children sometimes overuse this construction inappropriately (often with a definite subject NP). For example, [V S] *halax ába* 'Went daddy', *boxe ha-tinok* '(Is)-crying the baby', and these may be marked as errors. Another common deviation from normative forms is the use of the basic masculine singular form of the verb when the subject N that follows is feminine or plural (e.g. [V Dat S] *ko'ev li ha-béten* 'Hurts+Ms to-me the tummy+Fm' > 'I've got a tummy ache'; *nafal lo pit'om kol ha-kubiyot* 'fell+Sg to-him suddenly all the-blocks+Pl' > 'All his blocks fell down suddenly'). These neutralizations in verb-initial constructions occur in adult Hebrew as well, so should not be marked as errors.

- *Intransitive clauses* [S (Neg)V (X)]: most typically at this stage these are bare subject + verb [S V], as in *ába ba* 'Daddy comes ~ is-coming ~ has come'; *(ha-)tinok yašen* '(The-)baby sleeps' > 'is-sleeping'; *ani (lo) baxíti* 'I cried ~ was-crying ~ didn't cry, wasn't crying'; *aba šeli yix'as* 'My daddy will-be-angry', also sometimes expanded to [S V A] as in *ha-yeladim barxu mi-šam* 'The-children ran-away from-there'. As noted above, some intransitive verbs also occur in [(Neg)V S] verb-initial constructions.
- *Transitive clauses* [(S) (Neg)V O (X)]: verbs in transitive clauses take three main types of objects: (i) a non-definite direct object, [S V O] *ani roce kadur* 'I want (a) ball'; *hu (lo) šata xalav* 'He drank ~ didn't drink milk'; *tecayri praxim* '(You) will draw+2ndFm flowers'; (ii) a definite direct object taking the accusative case-marking preposition *et* [S V AccO], as in *ani roce et ha-kadur* 'I want *et* the-ball'; *ha-yeladim yecayru et ha- praxim* 'The children will-draw *et* the-flowers'; and (iii) an oblique object that governs another preposition [S V Obl], as in *hi mistakélet alav ~ al ha-tmuna* 'She is-looking at him ~ at the-picture'; *hu hirbic li ~ la-xaver šelo* 'He hit to-me ~ to-his friend'.
- *Bi-transitive clauses* [(S) V O IO]: these require two objects, a direct object and a dative-marked indirect object [IO], not necessarily in that order, in the construction [S V IO O], as in *ába natan ~ kana li matana* 'Daddy gave to-me ~ bought for-me (a) book'; *heví'u lánu et ha- séfer* '(They ~ someone) brought to-us *et* the-book'. The indirect object is always marked by *le-* standing for both English 'to' or 'for', in constructions with verbs of transferring to or producing for someone, and it is typically a pronoun, certainly at this developmental stage. Ordering of the direct and indirect objects is flexible, but the *le-* prepositional marker is always retained on the indirect object in Hebrew.
- *Question clauses* [Q (S) X Y]: all of the above five constructions can occur with an initial question-word (e.g. [Q S (Neg) V] as in *láma ába lo ba¿* 'Why Daddy not came¿' > 'Why didn't Daddy come¿'; [Q S V O] as in *éyfo hu sam et ze¿* 'Where (did) he put *et* it¿').

Clause-level agreement

Initial Stage-III marking of grammatical agreement between subject and predicate is marked both at the clause (constituent) level and at the word (inflection) level: masculine 3rd person singular present tense is taken as neutral and unmarked; any other marking of agreement (plural number, feminine gender, 1st or 2nd person) is marked at the clause level by a subscript on the predicate (e.g. *yeladim boxim* 'Children are-crying' [S V_{agr}]; *ha-iša yafa* 'The-woman (is) pretty' [S C_{agr}]; *hu axal* 'He ate' [S V_{agr}]; *ani lakáxti* 'I took+1st' [S V_{agr}]). Each instance of correct agreement marking (for plural number, feminine gender, 1st or 2nd person) is entered as a separate clause-level value for SV or SC from Stage III on. Incorrect marking of agreement is indicated in the Error Line. The specific inflections that mark clause-level agreement are listed in the word-level column.

Phrase-level constructions

Stage III Phrase-level expansions in Hebrew include the following.

- In *lexical noun phrases* (subject or object), we find the addition of quantifiers (before the head noun) and/or of the definite marker *ha-* 'the' and/or possessive and/or demonstrative modifying elements (after the head noun). Relative constructions include [Quant N] as in *harbe yeladim* 'many children'; [Det-N] as in *ha-yeladim* 'the-boys', *ha-yéled ha-ze* [Det-N Dem], *ha-kadur šeli* [Det-N Poss] 'the-ball of-me ' > 'my ball', and *ha-kadur šel Dani* 'the-ball of Danny' > 'Danny's ball'. Omission of definite marking in grammatical or extralinguistic contexts where it is required should be marked in the Error Line from Stage III.
- *Prepositional marking* includes different kinds of objects and adverbial relations: (i) with lexical nouns (e.g. [Pr Det N] (*ka'as*) *al ha-yeled* '(was-angry) at the-boy'; (*šaxav*) *ba-mita* [Pr N] 'lay in-the-bed'; *nasa li-rushayalim* 'went to-Jerusalem'); and (ii) suffixed to pronouns (e.g. (*sixáknu*) *ito* [Pr P]'(we-played) with-him'; (*yašávti*) *alav* 'I sat on-it').

Word level

From Stage III on, some inflections are assumed to be productively used. This is shown, for example, when the same noun is used in both singular and plural or with both masculine and feminine gender, or the same verb is used in more than one tense-mood form (e.g. both infinitive and present, both present and past) or more than one person (e.g. both 1st and 3rd). Some of these may appear only in Stage IV, and can be transferred to the Stage IV section on the chart. Stage III inflections are as listed:

- *Nouns*: (i) Masculine plural – *im appears* on regular nouns, including those with no stem change (e.g. *kadur-im* 'ball-s', *kélev-im* 'dog-s') and also on masculine nouns that take the feminine plural *-ot* (e.g. *kir-im, xalon-im*). These are evidence of initial productive use of inflections and should not be marked in the Error Line before Stage V. (ii) Gender alternations appear on a few high-frequency animate nouns (e.g. *iš ~ iša* 'man ~ woman', *yéled ~ yalda* 'boy ~ girl', *tarnególet ~ tarnegol* 'hen ~ cock').
- *Verbs*: (iii) We find the use of infinitival and imperative forms (e.g. *šev ~ švi ~ laševet* 'sit!+Ms' ~ 'sit +Fm' ~ 'to-sit'); (iv) plural number or feminine gender in the present tense (e.g. *holex ~ holxim ~ holéxet* 'go+3rd Sg ~ go+Ms Pl ~ go+Sg Fm'); (v) alternations of present and past tense (e.g. *holex ~ halax* 'goes ~ went', *oxlim ~ axlu* 'eat+Pl ~ ate + Pl'); (vi) partial marking of person in the past tense (e.g. *halax ~ halxa ~ haláxti ~* 'went+3rd Ms ~ went+3rd Fm ~ went+1st Sg')

- *Adjectives*: (vii) Plural and feminine agreement markers on adjectives are used predicatively in copular constructions, e.g. *Ha-praxim yafim* 'The-flowers (are) pretty+Pl'; *Ha-yalda hayta acuva* 'The-girl was sad+Fm'.
- *Pronouns*: (viii) There is transitional non-inflected marking of non-subject pronouns (e.g. *al hu* 'on he' in place of grammatical *alav* 'on-him'; *im at* 'with you+Fem' in place of inflected *itax* 'with you'); and also (ix) inflected marking of a few non-subject pronouns (e.g. alternation of a rote-learned form like *li* 'to-me' ~ *lexa* 'to-you'; *šeli* ~ *šelxa* ~ *šelo* 'of-me ~ of-you ~ of-him' > 'my ~ your ~ his') – including ungrammatical combinations (e.g. *alo* for *alav* 'on-him, on-it').

Stage IV [c. 2;6 – 3;0]

This stage represents consolidation of early grammar en route to the acquisition of complex syntax in Stage V. The main advances at this stage for Hebrew are at clause-level – initial marking of clause-combining connectivity; at clause-and phrase-level – addition of modifying elements; and at word-level – a fuller set of inflectional affixes.

Connectivity

Two main types of constructions indicate that children at this stage are en route to the acquisition of complex syntax, combining two clauses in a single utterance.

- *Truncated coordinate or subordinate clauses*: these are utterances beginning with a conjunction – *ve-* 'and', *še-* 'that', or *ki* 'because' – without being combined with another clause in the same utterance, typically in response to relevant input in an adjacency pair (e.g. [*ve* PP V A S$_{ex}$] *ve le-Uri yeš gam caláxat gdola* 'And to-Uri also is (a) big plate' > 'Uri also has a big plate', in response to an adult's query if the child wants some cake; [*še-* V A A] as in *še-haláxnu im banot la-hagan ša'ašuim* 'That [= where/when] we-went with the girls to-the playground' in response to her mother's query 'What else do you want to tell me?'; and [*ki* V] *ki nafal* 'Cos (he) fell' in response to the question asking why the teddy was crying).
- *Restricted indirect questions*: indirect questions with set, attention-getting opening clauses (e.g. [V [Q V]] *tir'i ma asíti* 'See+Fm [what I-did]'; [V [Q S V]] *stakel eyx hu holex* 'Look how he walks').

Clause level
- *Adverbial constituents*: (i) We find more varied types of adverbial modifiers [A], in addition to time (e.g. *axšav* 'now', *etmol* 'yesterday') and place (*po* 'here', *šam* 'there'): expressions of manner (e.g. *maher* 'quickly',

be-kalut 'with ease = easily'), goal (e.g. le-Ruti 'to Ruthy'), and amount (e.g. harbe 'a lot', kcat 'a little'). (ii) More than one adverbial modifier is used in the same utterance, [SVAA] as in hu rac maher ha-báyta 'He ran quickly home'; ani bone po axšav 'I'm building here now'. (iii) Adverbials are used in transitive clauses, [SVAO] as in ani oxel kol yom marak 'I eat every day soup'. Note: Adverbial position is flexible in Hebrew.
- *Bi-transitive clauses* are used with lexical indirect objects, not only pronouns, [(S)V O IO] as in natáti le-Ruti et ha-séfer 'I-gave to Ruthy et the-book'

Clause-level agreement marking
These are as for Stage III.

Phrase level
- *Extended predicates* [VV]: modal and aspectual verbs modify the main verb in the infinitive form (e.g. [VV] yaxol le'exol 'able to-eat' > 'can eat'; cerixa la-azor 'has-to help' > 'must help'; hitxil livkot 'began to-cry' > 'began crying'). These may also occur as modal operators in subjectless constructions (e.g. [VV] carix le-maher 'must to-hurry' > 'we / they need to hurry'; efšar lakáxat¿'possible to-take¿' > 'can I ~ may we take it¿'; asur leharbic 'forbidden to-hit' > 'don't hit, you mustn't hit').
- *Noun phrase expansions*: this is where all modifiers follow the head noun, except for quantifiers. We find: (i) Noun + adjective [NAdj] in attributive function (in addition to the predicative function as a complement in Stage II), with adjectives – like all noun modifiers except for quantifiers – following the head noun (e.g. kadur agol 'ball round' > 'a round ball'; séfer gadol 'book big' > 'a big book'); (ii) Noun + Possessive [NPoss(N)] (e.g. kadur šeli 'ball of-me' > 'my ball'; séfer šelo 'book of-him' > 'his book'; bakbuk šel tinok 'bottle of baby' > 'baby's bottle', na'aláyim šel íma 'shoes of mommy' > 'mommy's shoes' (typically with an animate possessor)); (iii) Quantifier + Noun [QuantN] (e.g. harbe šókolad 'much > lots of chocolate'; štey yeladot 'two girls'); (iv) Incipient compounding (so-called *smixut* 'construct-state' constructions) by combining two nouns without overt grammatical marking (e.g. [NN] madafim sfarim 'shelves books') (cf. grammatical madafey sfarim 'shelves-Gen books' > 'bookshelves'; mišpaxa pilpilon 'family baby-elephants') (cf. mišpáxat pilpilon 'family-Gen baby-elephants', marked in the Error Line); (v) Definiteness agreement (e.g. [DetN DetAdj] as in ha-yeled ha-katan 'the-boy the-small' > 'the little boy') and use of the definite marker with object noun phrases marked with the accusative preposition et [et Det N], (e.g. (ra'a) et ha-yeled 'saw et the-boy').
- *Prepositional phrases* [Prep NP]: increased use of modifying adverbials (clause-level A constituents) in Stage IV is typically in the form of prepositional phrases (e.g. oxlim et ze **be/im kapit** 'eat+Pl it with (a)

spoon'; *Íma sáma oto **ba-agala** '*Mommy put it in-the-buggy'; *ani roca lašévet **alex*** [adult form = *aláyix*] 'I want to-sit on-you').

Examples of longer and more complexly expanded sentences at this stage include [S NegV O A] *ani lo yilbaš et ha-mixnasáyim ha-éle yoter* 'I not wear+Fu *et* the-pants the-those more' > 'I won't wear those pants any more'; [S A V O] *ába bétax natan la óxel* 'Daddy sure gave to-her food' > 'Daddy gave her food for sure'; [V IO O A] *natnu li et ze la-yomuledet* 'Gave+Pl me *et* it for (my) birthday' > 'They gave it to me ~ I got it for my birthday'; [A A NegV O] *axšav kvar lo crixim oto* 'Now already not need it' > 'We don't need it any more by now').

Phrase-level agreement marking

Initial Stage-III marking of grammatical agreement between subject and predicate is extended here to phrase level, inside noun phrases, to agreement between the head noun and its associated modifiers (e.g. [NA$_{agr}$] as in *yalda yafa* 'girl pretty+Fm' > 'a pretty girl'; [ND$_{agr}$] as in *ha-anašim ha-éle* 'the-people the-those' > 'those people', *šaloš tmunot* 'three+Fm pictures+Fm' [Quant$_{agr}$ N]). Categories of agreement-marking appear at word level, as for Stage III. Normative use of gender marking on numbers in current Hebrew is often violated, including by adult speakers (Ravid, 1995b). Errors in the number system (e.g. *shalosh shkalim* 'three+Fm shekels+Ms') should be marked separately as [Agr-nr] in the Error Line from Stage IV, since they are not only juvenile developmental 'errors'.

Word level

- *Nouns*: (i) The feminine plural suffix *-ot* (e.g. *kubiy-ot* 'block-s', *xatul-ot* 'cat-s+Fm') is used at this stage, often without required changes in the stem (e.g. *simla ~ simlot* 'dress(es)' instead of required *smalot*). This also includes some high-frequency masculine nouns that take the irregular forms of feminine plural *-ot* (e.g. *kir-ot* 'wall-s', *xalon-ot* 'window-s').
- *Verbs*: (ii) Plural past tense suffixes are used (e.g. *patax-tem* '(you) opened+2ndPl'; *sixák-nu* '(we) played+1stPl').[9] (iii) Future tense inflections (e.g. *te-lx-i* 'will-go+2ndFmSg'; *ti-lbesh-u* 'will-wear+2ndPl') are used to express future tense and not imperative mood.
- *Pronouns*: (iv) Additional non-subject pronouns are suffixed to additional prepositions, not necessarily with the correct inflected form: *la-xem* 'to-you+Pl'; *šel-ánu* 'of-us = our(s)'; *al-o* 'on-it/him [correct adult form: *alav*]'.
- *Adjectives*: (v) Agreement markers of agreement are used on predicative adjectives and their subject nouns in copular constructions (e.g. feminine plural *-ot* in *ha-yeladot hayu acuvot* 'the-girls were sad+Pl') and on attributive adjectives and their head nouns in noun phrases (e.g. *yalda ktana nafla* '(a) girl small+Fm (fell+Fm)' > 'a little girl fell').

Stage V [c 3;0 – 3;6]

This is a stage of increased grammatical complexity both within and between clauses. Between clauses, complex syntax takes the form of advances in clause-combining connectivity; within clauses, word-level verb morphology is used to alternate transitivity and valence relations to expression causativity, reflexivity and so on (specified below at word level for this stage).

Clause-combining connectivity

Autonomous clause-combining is self-initiated and involves at least two consecutive clauses, either coordinate or subordinate. Coordinate clauses at this stage are combined with *ve-* 'and' in the form [Cl ve- Cl] (e.g. *maxar ani avo ve- ani yagid la* 'Tomorrow I will-come and I will-tell her') – most typically with an overt subject in the second clause – with same-subject ellipsis in the second, coordinated clause appearing from Stage VI. Three main types of clauses are traditionally identified as subordinate: complements, adverbials and relative clauses, all usually marked at this stage by the invariant subordinating conjunction *še-* 'that'.

- *Complement clauses*: [Cl še Comp] (e.g. *ra'íti še- hu nafal* 'I-saw that it fell'; *ani roce še- yihye músika,* 'I want that there will-be music > to have music').
- *Adverbial clauses*: marked by *še-*'that' in a lexically unspecified way, including for time and purpose, instead of required *kše-* 'when', *kdey še-* 'so that', in the form [Cl še- Adv] (e.g. *tikra la **še- sába yavo*** 'Call her that > when Grampa comes'; *axárkax **še- kulam yoc'im*** *az ha-galgal ha-anak ole od pá'am* 'Afterwards that > when everyone goes out, so the big wheel goes up again'; *asáfnu **še- yihye mesudar*** 'we put together (the blocks) that > so that, in order that it would-be tidy').
- *Reason adverbials:* marked by *ki* 'because': [Cl ki Adv] (e.g. *ha-yéled nafal **ki ha-yanšuf hipil oto*** 'The-boy fell because the owl pushed him down').
- *Relative clauses*: also marked by the invariant subordinator *še-*, [Cl še- Rel] (e.g. *tadlik or menora **še- lemá'la*** 'Put on the lamp that's on-top'; *ani roca léxem **še- ába marax lax***, 'I want bread that Daddy spread for-you'). An example of more than two clauses combined together is this [Cl ve- Cl še- Rel] construction produced by a 3–year-old boy: *laxácti kol ha-zman **ve- hayíti ba- rakévet ha- zot še- raíti šam anašim gdolim*** 'I pressed all the time and I was on that train that I saw there [> where] big people'.

Note: (*a*) At clause-level, each clause in clause-combining constructions is separately analysed for its internal structure (e.g. in a complex sentence like [Cl *še-* Comp] *hu yada še-hi tavo* 'He knew that-she would-come', the main clause is analysed as [S V Comp] and the complement clause is analysed as [*še-* S V]); (*b*) These different types of coordinate and subordinate clauses tend to appear more or less at the same developmental stage, and development concerns the type of coordinate or subordinate clauses that are used (e.g. with or without same-subject ellipsis in coordination, complement clauses with more complex introducing clauses, relative clauses with resumptive pronouns standing for oblique objects as well as with subjects and direct objects). However, some children may reveal more clearly staggered acquisition of clause-combining, so that some coordinate and only complement clauses occur in Stage V or even Stage IV, while other children use a range of such constructions.

Clause level

- *Questions on prepositional phrases* (typically adverbial): [PrepQ (S) V X] (e.g. in addition to lexical *me-éyfo* 'from where' as in *me-éyfo ze ba?* 'From where it came' > 'Where did it come from?', we have **im mi** *hu yašav* 'With who(m) he sat?' > 'Who did he sit with?'; **al ma** *sámta et ha-sir?* 'On what put+2nd *et* the-pot' > 'What did you put the pot on?') (Note that Hebrew does not allow 'dangling prepositions' at the end of question or relative clauses).
- *Comparatives within and between clauses* [Compar]: Note: Comparatives are constructed syntactically in Hebrew, where English may use morphology, by the quantifier / intensifier *yoter* 'more' plus the ablative preposition *mi ~ min* 'from' (e.g. [S V Compar PP] *Dan oxel yoter mi-méni* 'Dan eats more from-me' > 'Dan eats more than I (do)'; [S Compar-Adj PP] *ani yoter gadol mi-ménu* 'I (am) more big from-him' > 'I am bigger than he (is)'; [S V Compar-A PP] *hu rac yoter maher mi-Dan* 'He runs more fast from Dan' > 'He runs faster than Dan (does)'). Some initial, less syntactically complete forms of comparatives without the PP may occur in Stage IV (e.g. [S Compar Adj] *ze yoter yafe* 'That (is) more pretty' > 'That's prettier').

Phrase level

This includes initial, quite limited combining of members of the same grammatical category in a single phrase-level constituent, mainly by means of the coordinating conjunction *ve* 'and' – beyond the formulaic types of such constructions that may appear earlier (e.g. *ába ve- íma* 'Daddy and Mommy'; *Ami ve Tami* 'Hansel and Gretel'). These occur inside subject or object NPs, [N ve N V PP] as in *Roni ve Dana sixaku ba-argaz xol* 'Ronny and Dana played in-the-sandbox', or [S V N ve N] as in *ani roca sukarya ve- mastik* 'I want candy and chewing-gum' respectively.

Word level

A fuller range of inflections, including productive marking of noun compound relations, in the form of nonlexicalized *smixut* 'construct-state constructions' of head + modifier, where Ngen stands for a noun in genitive case in the context [Ngen N] (e.g. *tmunat parpar* 'picture-of butterfly', *bubat jiráfa* 'doll-gen giraffe' > 'a giraffe doll', *gurey klavim* 'puppies-gen dogs' > 'puppy dogs', including where no overt marking is required, e.g. *kadur cémer* 'ball wool' > 'a ball of wool'). If required, genitive marking is omitted and this should be indicated in the Error Line (e.g. [N N] *madafim sfarim* 'shelves books' in place of [Ngen N] *madafey sfarim* 'shelves+Gen books' > 'bookshelves'). In the verb system, alternations between the same verb root in different *binyan* conjugation patterns indicate changes in transitivity (e.g. not only basic *šaxav* 'lie (down)' but also causative *maškiv* 'lay down' > 'put to bed'), and, in the opposite direction, not only causative *hilbiš* 'dress (someone)' but also *lavaš* 'wear, put on (clothes)', intransitive reflexive *mitraxec* 'wash (oneself)' but also transitive *roxec* 'wash (someone or something)'. These are shown as follows: P1 ~ P2 = alternations between the basic *qal* conjugation and the intransitive *nif'al,* P1 ~ P5 = between basic *qal* and *hif'il* causative, P3 ~ P4 = between active transitive *pi'el* and intransitive reflexive *hitpa'el* and so on. Productive command of the system is manifested by unconventional alternations (e.g. *nifrak* 'fell apart' for normative *hitparek* in alternation with transitive *pirek* 'pull apart', reflexive *hitpagšu* 'met (each other)' for normative *nifgešu* alternating with basic *pagaš* 'met'). These are not counted as errors until Stage VI or even later. Use of the two passive *binyan* constructions *pu'al* and *hof'al* are later, Stage VII acquisitions.

These two examples (*smixut* noun compounds and *binyan* verb alternations) are marked at word level since they are realized by inflectional and derivational morphology respectively, but in fact they express phrase- or clause-level syntactic relations.

Stage VI [c. 3;6 – 4;0]

This stage sees considerable expansion in semantic and lexical specification of syntactic relations that emerged in preceding stages, including: (i) more specific and more complex subordinating markers like *ad še-* 'till that' > 'until' and *lamrot še-* 'although'; (ii) a wider variety of cognitive and other verbs introducing complement clauses in addition to basic verbs of saying; and (iii) a wider range of prepositions with pronominal suffixes, including *bli* 'without' and *al ydey* 'by (means of)'. Beyond this, the major advance at this stage is in clause-combining connectivity, as specified below.

Clause-combining connectivity

We find more complex inter-clausal relations, including:

- Coordinate clauses with same-subject ellipsis, [Cl *ve-* ØCoord] (e.g. *az axarkax hu yaca ve hithapex* 'So afterwards he went-out and overturned';

ha-yéled tipes al ha-ec ve-xipes et ha-cfardea 'The-boy climbed the tree and looked for the-frog').
- Other coordinate conjunctions in addition to *ve-* 'and' (e.g. [Cl *aval* Cl] as in *ani raciti xalil aval ima sheli lo, hi nigna be- štey xalilim aval hem lo hayu mangina* 'I wanted (a) recorder but my mother (did) not, she played two recorders, but they were not (a) tune > they didn't make a tune').
- Correlative markers of coordination, [corr CL corr CL] (e.g. *im ata roce še-ani etraxec az ten li et ha-balon* 'If you want that I will wash [> me to wash], then give me the balloon').
- A wider range of complement clauses in the form of embedded or indirect questions, e.g. [Cl Q Comp] (e.g. *hem lo hevínu láma hi ka'asa* 'They didn't understand why he was-angry'; *hi sha'ala oto éyfo sámu et ha-sfarim* 'She asked him where they put the books').
- Clauses embedded inside one another, marked by curly brackets, [NP { še- Rel} VP] (e.g. *ha-yéled {še-ra'ínu sham} raca lavo itánu* 'The boy that we saw there wanted to come with us'), [Cl {ApposI} še- Comp] (e.g. *hu amar lánu, {káxa nidme li}, še- yavo maxar)*.
- Inter-dependencies of two or more clauses to a single main clause, including complements on coordinate clauses, [Cl še- Comp ve Coord še- Comp im Adv] (e.g. *hu amar še- yavo ve- še- gam ani yaxol lavo im erce* 'He said that (he) would-come and that I could also come if I wanted'). This example shows that adverbial clauses also include conditional relations at this stage, while relative clauses are used with oblique objects as well as with subjects and direct objects, that is, constructions that require resumptive pronouns in Hebrew (e.g. *lo ra'íti et ha-yeladim še- hu sixek itam ~ še- dibárta aleyhem* 'I did not see the children that he played with them ~ that you-talked about-them').

Clause and phrase level

At this stage, syntactic development is reflected mainly by additional modification at both clause and phrase level simultaneously. At clause level, this typically takes the form of stringing together several expanded phrases in a single clause (e.g. [S VV O A] as in *íma šeli halxa liknot sfarim la-bet-séfer šelánu* 'My mother went to-buy books for my school'). Adverbial modifiers, including manner adverbs, are mainly in the form of a prepositional phrase (PP) (e.g. [S V IO AA A] as in *hu nixnas lo be-šéket be-šéket la-máyim* 'He went-in by-himself with-quiet with-quiet to-the-water' > 'He went into the water very quietly'). As an example of how increased Stage VI syntactic complexity is reflected at one and the same time in clause-combining, internal clause level *and* phrase level, consider the following utterance of a girl aged 3;7 talking to her younger brother, in a construction [V A še- Cl = S V IO DO = N PP *ve-* NP *ve-* PP *ve-* PP] realized as: *nesaper gam še-íma sipra lánu sipur al tipot ve-ha-rúax ve-al ha-gešem ve-al ha-stav* 'We'll tell also that Mommy told us (a) story about drops and-the-wind and-about the-rain and-about-the-autumn'. An additional phrase-level feature at Stage VI is use of negative indefinite pronouns, as in strings like [NegIndef Neg V] *af exad lo ba* 'No one not came' > 'Nobody came'; [Neg V NegIndef], *lo ra'íti šum davar* 'Not saw=1st no thing' > I didn't see anything'.

Word level

Here we mainly find the lexically conventional use of morphological affixation, including the introduction of the appropriate stem changes before inflectional affixes (e.g. *péca* ~ *pca'im* 'sore-s'; *simla* ~ *smal-ot* 'dress-es'), the non-regularization of affixes on verbs with defective roots (e.g. *baníti* 'built+1st' in place of juvenile *baná-ti*; *nizhar* 'be careful' in place of *mizaher*), and the appropriate use of *binyan* verb patterns (e.g. *hitparek* 'fell apart' and not juvenile *nifrak*; *mexuse* 'covered' and not childish *kasuy*).

Later Acquisition (Beyond Age 4)

These involve mainly morpho-syntactic constructions that have been studied under the heading of 'later language development', mastered only at late pre-school and even at school age. They include: (i) syntactic passive constructions by means of the two passive *binyan* patterns *pu'al* and *hof'al* as well as the earlier acquired *nif'al* used in a clearly passive construction – typically in past or future tense; (ii) the extension of conditional clauses to unreal conditionals, typically by the use of a special conjunction *lu* in place of the general *im* 'if' combined with a complex verb construction of *haya* + *benoni* 'was ~ were + Participle' for marking hypothetical clauses (e.g. the use of the *benoni* participles in non-finite adverbial clauses); (iii) *smixut* construct-state compounds (e.g. *yaldey ha-kita* 'children+Gen the-class' > 'the class children'; *kitat ha-mexunanim* 'class+Gen the-gifted" > 'the class of the gifted (students)'); (iv) nominalizations (e.g. *lemida* 'studying, learning' and *meni'a* 'prevention'), used typically in forming complex NPs, often as heads of *smixut* constructions; and (v) denominal adjectives (e.g. *ta'asiyat-i* 'industrial' and *yecirat-i* 'creative'), used in attributive NA constructions to create the heavy noun phrases typical of more complex Hebrew syntax. These examples demonstrate that increased grammatical complexity in Hebrew is typically reflected by the interplay between morphology and syntax.

Notes

(1) The authors are grateful to Dr Anita Rom, Seminar HaKibbutzim Teacher Training College, Tel Aviv, for her cooperation, to Prof Dorit Ravid for her invaluable feedback on an earlier draft, and to Rona Ramon-Blumberg, Tel Aviv University Linguistics Department, for assistance in producing this chapter.
(2) This was done while the first author was on sabbatical at the University of California, Berkeley, in the mid-1980s. We are indebted to Brian MacWhinney of Carnegie Mellon University for his assistance with scanning and computerization.

(3) Hebrew items are transcribed as follows. Hebrew forms are given in broad phonemic transcription intended to represent how target items are pronounced in the ambient language. Word-stress is on the final syllable unless otherwise indicated by an *accent aigu* on the (pen)ultimate syllable. Hyphens between parts of words are used for morphemes that in English and other European languages are represented by separate words, but in Hebrew are written as part of the next orthographic word: the definite article *ha-* 'the', basic prepositions meaning 'to', 'at', 'in', 'from', 'like' (which may incorporate definiteness marking), the coordinating conjunction *ve-* 'and' and the subordinator *še-* 'that'. Elements that are required in English but are not realized in Hebrew are given in parentheses in the gloss, e.g. *ima ba-báyit* "mommy (is) in-the-house', *iša ba'a le-vaker* '(a) woman came to-visit'. Square brackets are used to explain un-English sounding usages, e.g. in response to the question *Eyfo haya ha-xatul?* 'Where was the-cat?', the response *hu haya ba-báyit* 'He [=it] was at-home' indicates that animals and humans are referred to by the same pronouns, in this case 'he'.

(4) The following is a list of notational abbreviations to specify Hebrew inflectional categories, marked by a plus sign + and separated by a comma if they co-occur: 1st, 2nd, 3rd = Person categories, Fu = Future, Imp = Imperative, Inf = Infinitive, Ms = Masculine, Fm = Feminine, Pa = Past, Pr = Present, Pl = Plural. Labels of other grammatical categories follow the conventions of LARSP (e.g. A = adverb, Adj = adjective, N = noun, Q = question (word).

(5) Many of these alternations are due to historical processes that are no longer realized in current Hebrew pronunciation, including: consonant gemination and the alternation between long and short vowels, the distinction between pharyngeal and velar consonants, where the former but not the latter entail vowel lowering, and the fact that glottal consonants are currently not pronounced in many environments. Despite the lack of phonetic realization, these historical distinctions still have a major impact on morphophonological processes in the language (e.g. vowel lowering), and hence on children's pattern-detection abilities and their acquisition of morphological alternations.

(6) The same forms also serve as non-finite participles. They are used to express habitual past tense or unreal conditionals following past tense forms of the verb *haya* 'be' (e.g. *hayínu **holxim** le-sham ba'avar* 'Were+1stPl go+Pl there in-the-past' > 'We used to go there' or *hayíti ose zot im / lu yaxolti* 'Was+1stSg do that if could+1stSg' > 'I would do / would have done that if I could'). And they also serve as non-finite verbs in complement clauses (e.g. *šamáti otam šarim* 'heard+1stSg them sing+Pl' > 'I heard them singing'). These are both late acquisitions in children's language.

(7) The terms 'child' and 'adult' are used here in preference to 'patient' and 'adult' in order to suit the materials to non-clinical situations and the normal language development charted here.

(8) In the work of the first author, following Karmiloff-Smith's (1986, 1992) developmental models, the term *phases* is used to characterize recurrent cycles consisting of initial data-based rote learning followed by structure-dependent acquisition and eventually discursively appropriate mastery of different systems and subsystems of Hebrew grammar from early childhood (Berman, 1986) across school-age later language development (Berman, 2004) in a range of domains. These include morphological marking of transitivity and voice (Berman, 1993a, 1993b); syntactic constructions such as complex noun phrases, word classes, null subjects, and nominalizations (Berman, 1987, 1988, 1990, 1993b); and narrative text construction (Berman, 1988, 1993).

(9) Plural inflections in past and future 2nd and 3rd person typically neutralize gender distinctions, and are confined to masculine forms (e.g. *halax**tem*** 'went+2ndPl'; *kol ha-yeldadot **yel**xu* 'all the-girls will+3rd Masc-go' prefixes), so should not be marked as errors.

References

Ben-David, A. and Berman, R.A. (2007) Chapter 44: Hebrew. In S. McLeod (ed.) *The International Perspective on Speech Acquisition* (pp. 437–456). Clifton Park, NY: Thomas Delmar Learning.

Berman, R.A. (1985) Acquisition of Hebrew. In D.I. Slobin (ed.) *Crosslinguistic Study of Language Acquisition* (Vol.1) (pp. 255–371). Hillsdale, NJ: Lawrence Erlbaum.

Berman, R.A. (1993) The development of language use: Expressing perspectives on a scene. In E. Dromi (ed.) *Language and Cognition: A Developmental Perspective* (pp. 172–201). Norwood, NJ: Ablex.

Berman, R.A. (1997) Israeli Hebrew. In R. Hetzron (ed.) *The Semitic Languages* (pp. 312–33). London: Routledge.

Berman, R.A. (2004) Between emergence and mastery: The long developmental route of language acquisition. In R.A. Berman (ed.) *Language Development Across Childhood and Adolescence* (pp. 9–34). Amsterdam: John Benjamins.

Berman, R.A. and Neeman, Y. (1994) Acquisition of forms: Hebrew. In R.A Berman and D.I Slobin (eds) *Relating Events in Narrative: A Crosslinguistic Developmental Study* (pp. 285–328). Hillsdale, NJ: Lawrence Erlbaum.

Berman, R.A., Rom, A. and Hirsch, M. (1982) *Working with HARSP: Hebrew Adaptation of the LARSP Language Assessment Remediation and Screening Procedure*. Tel Aviv University.

Berman, R.A. and Slobin, D.I. (1994) *Relating Events in Narrative: A Crosslinguistic Developmental Study*. Hillsdale, NJ: Lawrence Erlbaum.

Boehm, J., Daley, G., Harvey, S., Hawkins, A. and Tsap, B. (2005) *LARSP: Language Assessment, Remediation, and Screeing Procedure: Users' Manual*. http://www.latrobe.edu.au/communication-clinic/attachments/pdf/larsp-manual.pdf

Crystal, D. (1979) *Working with LARSP*. London: Edward Arnold.

Crystal, D., Fletcher, P. and Garman, M. (1989) *The Grammatical Analysis of Language Disability* (2nd edn). London: Cole & Whurr.

Diessel, H. (2004) *The Acquisition of Complex Sentences*. Cambridge: Cambridge University Press.

Dromi, E. and Berman, R.A. (1986) Language-general and language-specific in developing syntax. *Journal of Child Language* 14, 371–87.

Karmiloff-Smith, A. (1986) Stage/structure versus phase/process in modeling linguistic and cognitive development. In I. Levin (ed.) *Stage and Structure: Reopening the Debate* (pp. 164–90). New York: Ablex.

Karmiloff-Smith, A. (1992) *Beyond Modularity: A Developmental Perspective on Cognitive Science*. Bradford, UK: Bradford Books, MIT Press.

MacWhinney, B. (2000) *The CHILDES Project: Tools for Analyzing Talk*. Mahwah, NJ: Lawrence Erlbaum.

Peters, A.M. (1983) *The Units of Language Acquisition*. Cambridge: Cambridge University Press.

Ravid, D. (1995a) *Language Change in Child and Adult Hebrew: A Psycholinguistic Perspective*. New York: Oxford University Press.

Ravid, D. (1995b) Neutralization of gender distinctions in Modern Hebrew numerals. *Language Variation and Change* 7, 79–100.

Schwarzwald, O.R. (2001) *Modern Hebrew*. München: Lincom Europa.

74 Assessing Grammar

HARSP PROFILE CHART

Name   Age   Sample Date   Type

A Unanalyzed

| Unt | Sym |

B Responses

		Partially Compositional					
Repetitions	Incomplete	Ambiguous		Stereotype		Social	Problems
		Normal Responses		Minor		Abnormal	
		Major	Reduced		Full	Structural	Ø
		Elliptical					

Stimulus type   Totals

Question
Others

C Spontaneous

D Reaction

	General	Structural	Ø	Other	Problems

Minor	Responses	Vocatives	Other	Problems

Stage I

Command-type 'V'			Question-type 'Q'		Statement-type			
'V-Imp'	'V-Fut'	'V-Inf'			'V'	'N'	'D'	'F'	'O'

Stage II

Connectivity	Clause	Phrase	Word
	D X		V: Inf *l-*
	F X		Imp *t-*
	Q X		Pa 1ˢᵗ Sg -*ti*
			Pr Fm Sg -*et*, -*a*
	N C		
	'V' X		N: Ms Pl -*im*
	ze X		
			Pron: Poss + 1ˢᵗ Sg, 2ⁿᵈ Sg
			Prep + 1ˢᵗ, 3ʳᵈ

Stage III		(Neg)V
		(Neg)V O
		(Neg)V A
		Q (Neg)V A
		Adj A
		V Dat
		V Dat S
		Adj Dat
		(Neg)Ex S$_{ex}$ A
		(Neg)Ex Dat S$_{poss}$
		S (Neg)V
		S (Neg)V A
		V S
		S (Neg)V O
		S (Neg)V etO
		S (Neg)V Obl
		S (Neg)V O IO
		(S)(Neg) O X
		S C
		S Cop C
		S C A
		Q S (Neg)V O
		, O
			(Neg)V$_{agr}$
			(Neg)V$_{agr}$O
			(Neg)V$_{agr}$A
			Q (Neg)V$_{agr}$A
			(Neg)V$_{agr}$ Dat
			(Neg)V$_{agr}$ Dat S
			S V$_{agr}$
			S V$_{agrA}$
			V$_{agr}$S
			S (Neg)V$_{agr}$ O
			S (Neg)V$_{agr}$ etO
			S (Neg)V$_{agr}$ Obl
			S V$_{agr}$O IO
			S C$_{agr}$
			S Cop C$_{agr}$
			S C$_{agr}$ A
			Q S (Neg)V
				Det-N
				Quant N
				Det-N Dem
				Det-N Poss
				AccDetN
				PrDetN
				PrN
				PrP
					N: Pl Ms -im
					    Fm Sg -et, -a
					V: Inf
					    Imp
					    Suffixes:
					      Pr Ms Pl -im, Fm Pl -ot
					      Pa 1st Pl -nu,
					        2nd Pl -tem,
					        3rd Fm Sg -a,
					        1st Sg -ti
					    Prefixes:
					      Fu 3rd Sg y-, 1st Pl n-
					A: Fm Sg -a
					    Ms Pl -im
					Pron: Prep + 1st ~ 2nd ~ 3rd
					       Non-inflected non-subject [al hu]
					       Poss + 2nd ~ 3rd

Errors		Agreement error	Omission of grammatical item (definite marker or preposition)	

Stage IV	ve PP (Neg)V A S$_{ex}$
	še- (Neg)V A A
	ki V
	V [Q V]
	V [Q S V]
		A
		NegA (Neg)V (O)
		S (Neg)V A A
		S (Neg)V$_{agr}$ A O
		(S) (Neg)V O IO
			NegA (Neg)V$_{agr}$ (O)
			S (Neg)V$_{agr}$ A A
			S (Neg)V$_{agr}$ A O
			(S) (Neg)V$_{agr}$ O IO
				V V
				N Adj
				NPoss(N)
				QuantN
				N N
				DetN DetAdj
				et Det N
				PrepNP
					NAdj$_{agr}$
					Quant$_{agr}$N
					Det-NDem$_{agr}$
						N: Pl Fm -ot
						V: Suffixes
						     Fu 2nd Fm. Sg -i
						     Fu 2nd Pl -u
						     Fu 3rd Pl -u
						    Prefixes
						     Fu 2nd Sg t-
						     Fu 2nd Pl t-
						     Fu 3rd Pl y-
						A: Pl Fm -ot
						Pron: Additional non-subject pronouns suffixed to additional prepositions

Errors		Agreement error (Person, Number, Gender) Agr-nr (in number system)	Omission of grammatical item (definite marker or preposition)	

Stage V	Cl *ve*- Cl Cl *še* Comp Cl *še*- Comp Cl *še*- Adv Cl *ki* Adv Cl *še*- Rel Cl *ve*- Cl *še*- Rel	PrepQ(S)VX S V-Compar PP S Compar-Adj PP S (Neg)V Compar-A PP S Compar Adj	N *ve* N Adj *ve* Adj	N: Ngen N V: **P1 ~ P2** (alternations between the basic *qal* conjugation and the intransitive *nif'al*) **P1 ~ P5** (alternations between basic *qal* and *hif'il* causative) **P1 ~ P5** (alternations between basic *qal* and *hif'il* causative) Unconventional alternations (e.g., *nifrak* 'fell apart' in alternation with *pirek* 'pull apart', reflexive *hitpagšu* 'met (each other)' for normative *nifgešu* alternating with basic *pagaš* 'met').
Errors		Agreement error (Person, Number, Gender) Agr-nr (in number system) Omission of definite marking	Omission of grammatical item (definite marker or preposition)	Error in stem change Plural suffix error Incorrect or omission of required Genitive marker
Stage VI	Cl *ve*- ØCoord Cl *aval* Cl corr CL corr CL NP { *še*- Rel} VP Cl {Apposl} *še*-Comp Cl *še*- Comp *ve*- Coord *še*- Comp *im* Adv Cl Q Comp Cl Q Comp	Clause and Phrase level: stringing together several expanded phrases in a single clause	NegIndef	N: appropriate stem changes before inflectional affixes V: non-regularization of affixes on verbs with defective roots appropriate use of *binyan* verb patterns
Errors		Agreement error (Person, Number, Gender) Agr-nr (in number system)	Omission of grammatical item (definite marker or preposition)	Error in stem change Plural suffix error Incorrect or omission of required Genitive marker

Note: At Word-Level, a comma between forms means that they co-occur; a tilde ~ between forms means that they alternate.

© Ruth Berman and Lyle Lustigman

5 Profiling Linguistic Disability in German-Speaking Children

Harald Clahsen and Detlef Hansen

Introduction

This chapter presents a brief description of a linguistic procedure for assessing language impairments in German-speaking children. The procedure was developed by an interdisciplinary research group at the University of Düsseldorf and published as a book (Clahsen, 1986). Later, a computer-assisted version of the procedure ('COPROF', Computer-unterstützte Profilanalyse 'computer-assisted profile analysis') was developed and published (Clahsen & Hansen, 1991). Since then the procedure has been used in clinical and research contexts for assessing children with language impairments, particularly with regard to grammatical disabilities (Clahsen, 1991; Hansen, 1996).

COPROF was designed on the model of LARSP, the Language Assessment Remediation and Screening Procedure originally developed by Crystal *et al.* (1976) for English (see also Crystal 1979, 1982). In the same way as LARSP, the German version provides descriptive tools for analysing a wide range of syntactic and morphological properties of language. Following LARSP, COPROF distinguishes between different levels of grammatical analysis (word, phrase, clause) and allows the clinician or researcher to analyse child utterances as combinations of constituents or inflectional endings. Furthermore, COPROF offers an analysis of word-order patterns, an important area of developmental changes in early German child language. Overall, COPROF provides for a detailed and comprehensive grammatical analysis of a sample of speech or text.

Another characteristic that COPROF has adopted from LARSP is that the descriptive linguistic categories are graded developmentally according to their emergence in typically developing children. The developmental chart of COPROF is divided into five stages, each of which provides the most commonly used patterns typically developing German children produce. Thus, like LARSP, COPROF is not just a descriptive framework for analysing disordered language, but more importantly, a procedure to identify the developmental level of language acquisition an individual child has reached. Finally, apart from the grammatical categories, COPROF contains labels for separating out utterance types that occur in a sample of spontaneous speech but are not further grammatically analysed – for example, simple yes / no responses to questions, incomprehensible or stereotypical utterances and imitations.

COPROF differs from more standard language assessment tests in a number of ways. One property of COPROF is that it uses oral speech production as a basis for language assessment, rather than for testing comprehension, reading and writing or metalinguistic abilities. The rationale for this is that oral language skills are central to a child's communicative needs. The second guideline for COPROF is that the assessment should be based on a representative sample of spontaneous speech gathered in a natural communicative setting. Highly structured test situations in which specific linguistic responses are targeted are not ideal for examining children with language impairments. Instead, a sample of spontaneous speech is thought to more adequately represent a child's linguistic proficiency. In addition, if deemed necessary – for example to probe for particular linguistic phenomena – data from elicited productions may be used to supplement the spontaneous speech sample.

The third guideline is that COPROF should provide for a comprehensive descriptive analysis of a child's grammar. Instead of selecting particular markers for assessment, the procedure aims at covering a wide range of different word and sentence-level phenomena. COPROF does, however, focus on the evaluation of syntactic and morphological properties of language. The justification for this is threefold. First, syntax and morphology may be regarded as the structural core of a language. Consequently, a meaningful assessment of a child's linguistic proficiency should include syntax and morphology. Furthermore, difficulties in the domain of syntax and morphology are common in different kinds of developmental impairments, not only for children with specific language impairment, but also for those with developmental dyslexia, autism, and Down's syndrome. Hence, an assessment procedure that focuses on syntax and morphology is likely to be widely applicable in clinical practice. Syntax and morphology have also been studied in considerably more detail in German child language than other domains of language, such as phonology or semantics, and this knowledge can be used to provide a sufficiently detailed assessment of impaired language.

Finally, the most important guideline for COPROF is that it grades grammatical structures in terms of the order of acquisition in German child language development. Clearly, to be relevant for clinical practice and to indicate potential goals for therapy, an assessment procedure should not only provide a linguistic description of a child's language, but should also determine its developmental level. Studies of typically developing children have led to the identification of a set of developmental stages for the acquisition of German syntax and morphology. COPROF relies on these stages to assess the developmental level of an individual child's grammar. Before summarising the developmental sequence (see below), we briefly describe the linguistic phenomena of German that are assessed with COPROF.

Linguistic Phenomena Assessed with COPROF

COPROF allows users to analyse all of a child's utterances from a spontaneous speech sample. The core of the profile chart consists of a set of basic elements of German grammar ordered into five phases, which correspond to the sequence in which these syntactic and morphological properties develop in typically developing German-speaking children. The grammatical analysis focuses on five syntactic and morphological properties of German.

The *word and constituent structure* analysis reports on the main word classes, nouns, different kinds of verbs and verb-like elements, articles, prepositions, coordinating and subordinating conjunctions, adjectives, and the internal structure of noun phrases (NPs), prepositional phrases (PPs) and verb phrases (VPs).

The analysis of *inflectional morphology* includes two paradigms that have been studied for German child language, case marking and subject-verb agreement. The analysis of case morphology includes possessive genitives (e.g. *Marias Haus* 'Mary's house'), and accusative and dative case markings required on direct and indirect objects and objects of prepositions, which are spelled out on articles and other kinds of determiners (e.g. *Ich sah [den Mann]* 'I saw [the$_{acc}$ man]'), or on pronouns. The second inflectional phenomenon incorporated in COPROF is the encoding of person and number features of the grammatical subject on the finite verb. In German, person and number marking is found in preterite and present tense forms in the indicative as well as in the subjunctive mood. There are four overt person and number affixes, *-e*, *-st*, *-t*, and *-n*. The paradigm of the weak verb *lachen* 'to laugh' is shown in (1) for illustration.

(1) Inflectional paradigm for *lachen* 'to laugh'

	Present	Preterite	Present Subjunctive	Past Subjunctive
1st sg.	lach(e)	lachte	lache	lachte
2nd sg.	lachst	lachtest	lachest	lachtest
3rd sg.	lacht	lachte	lache	lachte
1st pl.	lachen	lachten	lachen	lachten
2nd pl.	lacht	lachtet	lachet	lachtet
3rd pl.	lachen	lachten	lachen	lachten

The main section of the grammatical profile refers to the analysis of *sentence structure*, which covers the types and position of major constituents (subjects, complements, verbal elements) within sentences. Negation, specifically the position of negation words relative to verbs and other elements in the clause, as well as the internal structure and word order of *wh* and *yes/no* questions, are analysed separately in the profile chart. The core phenomenon that is examined within the sentence-structure analysis is the verb-second (V2) phenomenon of German syntax. V2 includes the following properties. In declarative main clauses and *wh*-questions, the finite verb occupies the second position in the sentence (2a). Crucially, this is not always the post-subject position, as is usually the case in unmarked English clauses of the same type (2b). Moreover, it is always a finite verb or auxiliary that appears in second position (2a, 2b), and it only appears there in main clauses. In embedded clauses, the finite verb appears clause-finally (2c), and in some constructions (e.g. in *yes-no* questions and in imperatives) the finite verb is the initial element of the clause (2d).

(2a) *Pauline hat mittlerweile die Aufgabe gelöst.*
 'Pauline has in the meantime the task solved'
 (= In the meantime, Pauline has solved the task.)
(2b) *Die Aufgabe hat Pauline mittlerweile gelöst.*
 'The task has Pauline in the meantime solved'
 (= As to the task, Pauline has solved it in the meantime.)
(2c) *Der Lehrer bemerkte, daß Pauline mittlerweile die Aufgabe gelöst hat.*
 'The teacher realized that Pauline in the meantime the task solved has'
 (=The teacher realized that in the meantime, Pauline has solved the task.)
(2d) *Hat Pauline die Aufgabe mittlerweile gelöst?*
 'Has Pauline the task in the meantime solved'
 (= Has Pauline meanwhile solved the task?)

The profile chart provides a set of categories that allows the user to assess whether a given child has acquired the V2 phenomenon.

Five Phases of Grammatical Development in German

COPROF comprises a developmental chart that consists of five phases of grammatical development, ranging from the period when children predominantly use one-constituent utterances up to the stage when embedded clauses are produced. For each phase, the developmental chart provides characteristic grammatical patterns reported in empirical studies of typically developing German-speaking children. The developmental profile was derived from a descriptive synthesis of studies of German child language that were available before 1986; see Clahsen (1986) for a detailed description.

Since then, a range of other child language phenomena has been examined for German. Although these new findings may in future be used to supplement the set of phenomena included in COPROF, for the purpose of the present overview we will stick to the original developmental chart, assuming that it represents particular states of the acquisition of grammar in typically developing German-speaking children.

Phase I refers to single-word utterances consisting of nouns (N), verbal particles, and isolated negation words (e.g. *nein* 'no'). In phase II, children produce basic word classes, such as nouns, main lexical verbs, adverbs, adjectives, articles, and syntactic constituents, such as noun phrases (NP), and verb phrases (VP). Another property of phase II is two-constituent sentences consisting, for example, of subject plus verb or verb plus object. Word order is variable in phase II. Subjects preferably appear before verbs, rarely after verbs, and direct objects precede and sometimes follow verbs; see Clahsen (1982) for a detailed description. A further characteristic of phase II is that children's sentences mainly consist of content words, whilst function words (auxiliaries, determiners, etc.) hardly occur. Moreover, subjects and verbs are often left out. Overall, phase II corresponds to the characteristics of Stage I in Brown's (1973) developmental sequence for English child language. Phase III is characterised by several developments which exceed the early two-word combinations of phase II. Children now produce multi-constituent sentences with adverbs and auxiliary+participle and modal verb+infinitive constructions. Children also extend their inventory of inflectional affixes.

Phase IV represents a clear shift towards the adult grammar in the acquisition of German. Word order is now mostly correct, also in complex cases, for example for separable prefix verbs and combinations of different verbal elements. The V2-property of German, with finite verbs appearing in second or first and non-finite verbs in clause-final position, has now been fully acquired. For inflectional morphology, phase IV also sees considerable changes towards the adult system in that the subject-verb agreement paradigm has now been fully acquired. Furthermore, omissions of grammatical function words are now rare. The final phase of the developmental chart, phase V, is characterised by the production of subordinate clauses and double-object constructions, and the use of dative and accusative case markings for (direct and indirect) objects and complements of prepositions (see Clahsen, 1984). Children in phase V have acquired the core elements of German grammar. The time it takes children to go through these phases varies considerably, but it is safe to say that typically developing children reach phase V no later than 3;5 years of age. In terms of the 'mean length of utterance' (MLU), the developmental profile covers the period beginning with an MLU (calculated for words) of approximately 1.0 in phase I to about 4.0 in phase V; see Clahsen (1986: 74) for details.

Description of the Profile Chart

The COPROF chart (see Figure 5.1) allows the user to analyse the utterances a child produces in a sample of speech, with the aim of reconstructing the child's grammar and to assess its developmental level. All utterances produced by the child have to be included in the chart, since each of them may contribute information to the final assessment (a version of the chart in German is available in Clahsen, 1986).

The upper parts A and B provide a preliminary classification of a child's utterances. *Section A* comprises labels for utterances that cannot be further analysed with respect to their grammatical structure because they are 'unintelligible' (e.g. due to outside noise), 'incomplete' (e.g. due to interruptions by others), 'ambiguous' or otherwise incomprehensible. Furthermore, direct 'imitations', 'simple' (yes/no) responses to questions, 'stereotypical utterances' (e.g. *good morning*) and 'formulaic' routinely used phrases or sentences are also registered here. *Section B* provides an overview of all utterances that were entered into the grammatical analysis. A distinction is made between one, two, and multiple-constituent utterances. Non-clausal ('elliptical') utterances (e.g. responses to questions) are further analysed within the word/phrase-structure analysis of the developmental chart. Full clause-level utterances ('Other') are subjected to a complete analysis of both word/phrase and sentence structure. Finally, utterances in which the child repeats her immediately preceding utterance, or part of it, are classified as 'repetitions'. Together with the other quantitative measures provided at the bottom of the profile chart (MLU, and the numbers of one, two and multi-word utterances), Section B provides an overview of the sample size for the grammatical analysis and an overall indication of a child's level of language development.

The *developmental chart* comprises two major components, a word/phrase structure and a sentence structure analysis. Whilst utterances classified as 'Elliptical' in Section B are entered into the word/phrase-level analysis only, all utterances classified as 'Other' in Section B are analysed with respect to both their word/phrase and sentence structure. The former captures the main word classes, such as different kinds of nominals (with and without determiners), verbs, auxiliaries and other verb-like elements, prepositions, adverbials and conjunctions, as well as subject-verb-agreement affixes and case markings. The sentence structure section provides analyses of the combinations and the order of major constituents in a child's spoken sentences. Included are subjects (S), objects (O), adverbials (A), and different kinds of verbal elements, such as main verbs (V), predicative adjectives (Adj), verbs with separable prefixes (PrV), participle constructions with and without auxiliaries, and modal verb plus infinitive constructions. Due to their specific syntax, questions and negation are analysed separately. Additional analyses within the sentence structure section of the developmental chart

Profiling Linguistic Disability in German-Speaking Children 83

Name: Age: Date:

A. Unanalysed utterances

Unintelligible:	Incomplete:
Ambiguous:	Imitations:
Simple replies:	Stereotypes:
Formulaic:	Other:

B. Analysed utterances

	One constituent	Two constituents	Multiple constituents
Elliptical:			
Other:			
Repetitions:			

C. Developmental profile

Word, phrase structure   Sentence structure

I   N: Pr: Question: 'Q':   Negation:'nein':

II   Pro^P : Pro^O :   SV: VS: SO: OS: SA: AS:
      DN   : AdjN   :   VO: OV: VA: AV: OA: AO:
      DAdjN   : NPNP   :   AA: Other:
      Adv   : PNP   :
      V   : Adj   :   Question: QXY: Negation: Neg V:
      PrV   : Other   :   V Neg:

      O: n: t:
      ------------------------ Missing elements Cop: Aux: V: --
III   P :   Art: S:

      Aux   :   SXV   :   XS(Y)V   :   XYV   :   SXY   :
      Mod   :   SXAdj   :   XS(Y)Adj   :   XYAdj :   X(Y)S(Z) :
      Cop   :   SXPr(V) :   XS(Y)Pr(V) :   XYPr(V): XYZ   :
                   SXPt   :   XS(Y)Pt   :   XYPt :   Other   :
                   SVX   :   XSVY   :   (X)VY(Z):
      Gen.suff.:
                                Question: QXYZ: Negation:(X)Neg(Y)V(Z):
      e   :   Other   :
      ------------------------ Argument structure   --
IV   (V)XA: (V)XAA: Other:

      Nominative   (X) Aux Y Pt :   (X) V$_f$ A O :   X V$_f$ S (Y) :
      Acc.con.:   (X) Mod Y Inf:
      Dat.con.:   (X) Cop Y Adj:
                    (X) V$_f$ Y Pr:

      st: Question: (w) V$_f$ S (X):   Negation:(X) V$_f$ Neg (Y):
      Other: Q   V$_f$ S (X):

V   Accusative   (sC)SXV$_f$:   (sC)SV :   (sC)X   :
      Acc.con.:   (sC)XV$_f$:   (sC)SX :   Other:
      Dat.con.:
      Dative: Question:(ob) X: Negation:(sC) X Neg V$_f$:
      Other :   (w) X: (X) V$_f$ Y Neg (Z):
                    Argument structure
      sConj: cConj: 2Obj: 2Obj+A: Other:

      MLU: 1Word-utterances: 2Word-utterances: Multi-Word-utterances:

Figure 5.1 Profile chart

are provided for: (i) 'missing elements' (i.e. omissions of obligatory constituents or grammatical function words, such as copulas, auxiliaries, prepositions, articles, subjects, and verbs), and (ii) argument structure, displaying single and double-object constructions and the number of adjuncts. In addition to the main clause patterns in phases I to IV, phase V of the developmental chart includes an analysis for subordinate clauses and indirect questions for which clause-final placement of the finite verb is required in German.

Word/phrase-structure analysis

Nominal elements

A noun phrase (NP) may consist of single noun (N), a personal pronoun (Pro^P) or other pronoun (Pro^O), such as demonstratives and possessives. Noun phrases may contain a determiner (D) (e.g. an article), or an attributive adjective (AdjN).

Adverbial elements

An adverbial constituent may consist of a single adverb (Adv) or a prepositional phrase (PNP). The NP included in the PNP has to be analysed separately with respect to the subtypes of nominal elements.

Verbal elements

Main lexical verbs (V), verbal particles (Pr, e.g. *auf* 'up'), main verbs containing verbal participles (PrV, e.g. *aufstellen* 'put up'), and predicative adjectives (Adj) are distinguished from closed-class verbal elements (i.e. copulas (Cop), auxiliaries, and modal verbs).

In addition to these major word classes, the numbers of subordinating (sConj) and coordinating conjunctions (cConj) produced by a child are given in the word and phrase analysis section of phase V. Finally, two sets of inflectional forms are included in this part of the profile chart: (i) regular subject-verb-agreement inflections (*-n, -t, -e, -st*, and the bare (0) stem), and (ii) nominative, accusative, and dative case markings, and the possessive genitive marker *–s*. For subject-verb-agreement, the profile chart simply shows the number of occurrences of the five agreement forms. For case markings, the chart additionally displays whether the child produced the correct case-marked forms in contexts that required accusatives/datives or whether (incorrect) nominatives or accusatives forms were produced.

Sentence-structure analysis

The main part of this section of the profile chart consists of categories representing the order and combination of major constituents in the sentences produced by a child. The entries in phases I to IV are for main and those in phase V for embedded clauses.

Sentences consisting of two major constituents are analysed with the labels shown in phase II. These sentences may contain a subject and a verbal element in either order (SV, VS). They may be subjectless, with a verbal element and an object in either order (VO, OV) or a verbal element and an adverbial in either order (VA, AV). Two-constituent sentences may also be verbless, with the subject and an object in either order (SO, OS) or the subject and an adverbial in either order (SA, AS). Finally, they may be both subjectless and verbless, with the object and an adverbial appearing in either order (OA, AO).

Multi-constituent main clauses are analysed using the structures for phases III and IV, and subordinate clauses in phase V. A multi-constituent main clause is assigned to one of the patterns of phase III if it comprises one or more verbal elements placed next to each other with no subject or with the subject placed before the verbal elements. The following distinctions are made:

Sentences with overt subjects and verbal elements

The leftmost subgroup of sentence structures within phase III is for subject-initial sentences with a verbal element in clause-final position (i.e. a main verb (SXV), a predicative adjective (SXAdj), a verbal prefix or prefix verb (SXPr(V)), or (past) participle (SXPt)). Alternatively, a simple main verb may appear after the subject and before any complements or adverbials yielding the kinds of SVX sentences that are common in adult German. The next subgroup of phase III structures to the right (XS(Y)V to XSVY) is for cases with the same structure as subject-initial sentences but with an adverbial or an object preceding the subject.

Sentences with a verbal element but without a subject

These are assigned to the third subgroup of phase III structures (XYV to (X)VY(Z)), again distinguishing between different kinds of verbal element in final position from a simple main verb in first or second position.

Sentences with a subject but without verbal elements

As before, subject-initial sentences (SXY) are analysed separately from complement-initial ones (X(Y)S(Z)).

Sentences without a subject or a verbal element (XYZ)

The sentence structures in phase IV capture cases of verb-second patterns characteristic of main clauses in adult German. The leftmost four patterns are for cases of discontinuous verb placement with a finite verbal element in second and a non-finite one in clause-final position (X Aux Y Pt to X V_f Y Pr). Sentences with an adverbial appearing between a fronted finite verb and an object ((X) V_f A O) and sentences involving subject-verb inversion (X V_f S (Y)) are analysed separately.

Finally, subordinate clauses (which require clause-final placement of finite verbs in German) are covered in phase V, distinguishing five cases: (sC)SXV$_f$ for complete sentences with a subject and a finite verb in clause-final position; (sC)SV$_f$ for simple sentences with a finite verb and a preverbal subject; (sC)XV$_f$ for subjectless sentences and a finite verb in clause-final position; (sC)SX for verbless sentences with a subject; and (sC)X for sentences without a finite verb or subject.

Questions are analysed separately in the profile chart. Intonationally marked questions with or without *wh*-pronouns are assigned to phases I to III, one-constituent questions to 'Q' in phase I, two-constituent ones to 'QXY' in phase II, and multi-constituent questions to 'QXYZ' in phase III. Main-clause questions with correct subject-verb inversion are entered into phase IV: (w) V$_f$ S (X) for *wh*-questions and Q V$_f$ S (X) for yes-no questions. Finally, indirect questions that take the form of subordinate clauses are assigned to phase V: (ob) X for *ob* 'if/whether' sentences and (w) X for indirect *wh*-questions. The internal structure of these sentences is analysed separately using the subtypes of subordinate clause structures in phase V.

For *negation*, the developmental chart also provides dedicated entries. One-constituent utterances with *nein* 'no' are assigned to phase I, two-constituent utterances with a verbal element and clause-initial (Neg V) or clause-final negation (V Neg) to phase II, and multi-constituent utterances with preverbal negation ((X)Neg(Y)V(Z)) to phase III. Main clauses with the negator placed immediately after the finite verb ((X) V$_f$ Neg (Y)) are recorded in phase IV. Finally, the entries in phase V are for advanced structures: main clauses in which (as required in German) the finite verb is separated from the (postverbal) negator by one or more other consituents ((X) V$_f$ Y Neg (Z)) and subordinate clauses with negation in which the negator precedes the finite verb ((sC) X Neg V$_f$).

An Illustration

This section presents an analysis of one sample of spontaneous speech from a language-impaired child using COPROF. This analysis is intended to illustrate the use of the profile chart as an assessment procedure. We chose a transcript from the child 'Wolfgang' (W), for whom a detailed grammatical description based on larger samples is available from Hansen (1983). To be meaningful, COPROF requires a sample of at least 100 grammatically analysable utterances, which, depending on a child's developmental level and the situational context, can be gathered from a 30 to 60 minutes recording of spontaneous or semi-elicited speech. For the example chosen here, 34 minutes of speech from the first sample of W (of the four Hansen (1983) collected) were analysed, during which the child produced 113 consecutive utterances. The profile chart is shown in Figure 5.2

Profiling Linguistic Disability in German-Speaking Children 87

```
Name: Wolfgang        Age: 04;05;10                Date: 10/82
```

A. Unanalysed utterances

Unintelligible:		Incomplete:	
Ambiguous:		Imitations:	
Simple replies:	5	Stereotypes:	
Formulaic:	1	Other:	5

B. Analysed utterances

	One constituent	Two constituents	Multiple constituents
Elliptical:	5		
Other:	17	25	55
Repetitions:	2		

C. Developmental profile

```
Word, phrase structure      Sentence structure

I    N: 27   Pr: 1          Question: 'Q': 2      Negation:'nein': 2

II   Pro^p  :28  Pro^o :30   SV:7      VS:        SO:6      OS:     SA:       AS:2
     DN     :35  AdjN  :     VO:       OV: 1      VA:1      AV:3    OA:4      AO:
     DAdjN  :    NPNP  :     AA:4      Other:
     Adv    :70  PNP   : 2
     V      :46  Adj   : 4   Question: QXY:1      Negation: Neg V:
     PrV    : 6  Other : 1                                  V Neg:

     O:31      n:       t:   -----------------------------------------------
     ---------------------   Missing elements  Cop:6    Aux: 3    V:19       --
III                                            P  :2    Art:19    S:20
                             -----------------------------------------------
     Aux      :              SXV      :13   XS(Y)V     :8   XYV     :5   SXY       :4
     Mod      :              SXAdj    :     XS(Y)Adj   :1   XYAdj   :    X(Y)S(Z)  :3
     Cop      :3             SXPr(V)  :     XS(Y)Pr(V) :2   XYPr(V) :    XYZ       :
                             SXPt     : 1   XS(Y)Pt    :1   XYPt    :    Other     :2
                             SVX      : 4   XSVY       :1   (X)VY(Z):2
     Gen.suff.:
                             Question: QXYZ:          Negation:(X)Neg(Y)V(Z):1
     e        : 1                                              Other         :3
     ---------------------   Argument structure                                --
IV                           (V)XA: 31      (V)XAA:           Other:
                             -----------------------------------------------
     Nominative              (X) Aux Y Pt :    (X) V_f A O : 3    X V_f S (Y) :
     Acc.con.:7              (X) Mod Y Inf:
     Dat.con.:               (X) Cop Y Adj:
                             (X) V_f Y Pr  : 2

     st:20                   Question: (w) V_f S (X):   Negation:(X) V_f Neg (Y): 3
     Other:                            Q  V_f S (X):
     -----------------------------------------------------------------------
V    Accusative              (sC)SXV_f:         (sC)SV:        (sC) X   :
     Acc.con.:               (sC)XV_f :         (sC)SX:        Other:
     Dat.con.: 1
                             Question:(ob) X:          Negation:(sC)  X Neg  V_f :
     Dative:                          (w)  X:                  (X) V_f Y Neg (Z):1
     Other : 14
                             Argument structure
     sConj:      cConj:          2Obj: 1    2Obj+A:      Other:
     -----------------------------------------------------------------------
     MLU:2.92    1Word-utterances:13  2Word-utterances:27  Multi-Word-utterances:63
```

Figure 5.2   Profile chart for Wolfgang

Sections A and B of the profile chart show that almost all of the child's utterances can be grammatically analysed, namely 102 of the total 113 utterances. The proportion of elliptical utterances and simple yes/no responses is small, which means that most of W's utterances can be analysed with respect to both word/phrase and sentence structure. The MLU for the sample under study is close to 3.0, and multi-word utterances are more common than one and two-word utterances, which means that – in terms of these quantitative criteria – W's language has almost developed to the level of phase IV.

The *word/phrase structure* analysis of the profile chart shows that the child produces almost all types of phase I and II level elements, including nouns, pronouns, and combinations of determiners and nouns (DN). Complex noun phrases with determiners and attributive adjectives are not yet present (DAdjN). Furthermore, obligatory articles are often omitted ($N=19$). Furthermore, W produces simple main verbs, but, except for three cases of copulas, none of the functional verbal elements characteristic of phase III and later stages of development. Instead, auxiliaries and copulas are most often missing in obligatory contexts. Subjects are also often omitted ($N=25$) yielding many (incorrect) subjectless sentences. W has not yet acquired the German case-marking system. He over applies nominative forms in contexts that require accusative case marking ($N=7$) and in one case an accusative form in a dative context. These kinds of error are familiar from typically developing German children before phases IV/V. In addition, W has not acquired the subject-verb-agreement paradigm of German. Instead, bare (-0) verb forms are produced almost exclusively ($N=31$), except for one instance with *–e*, and no cases of *–t* or *–st*. This represents an extremely limited set of verb forms, even for a phase II system. Overall, according to the word/phrase structure analysis, W's grammar has not developed further than phase II/III.

The *sentence structure* analysis reveals that W produces the two-constituent patterns characteristic of phase II, as well as 31 cases ((V)XA) with more than one complement. Verbal elements preferably appear clause-finally, as can be seen by comparing the totals for SXV, XS(Y)V, and XYV in phase III to the corresponding ones with V appearing before an object or adjunct (SVX, XSVY, (X)VY(Z)). By contrast, the characteristic verb-second pattern of German (see phase IV) is rarely used by W: two cases of discontinuous verb placement ((X) V_f Y Pr), and three cases of subject-verb inversion (X V_f S (Y)). The profile chart shows that there are several instances in which subject-verb inversion is required in W's utterances. In these cases, however, the verb appears clause-finally after the subject. Overall, W's clause structures correspond to phases II/III.

Negation is represented in a number of W's utterances. In addition to simple instances of *nein* 'no', in multi-word utterances with verbs, W places the negator immediately next to the verb, most often in a postverbal position ((X) V_f Neg (Y)). Overall, W's grammar of negation corresponds to phase III of typical development. *Questions* are rare in the present sample. There were two single-constituent and one two-constituent questions, all of which were marked by intonation only. This represents a phase I/II system.

Taken together, we note that, in all the examined domains, W's development of language is severely delayed relative to his chronological age in that, at an age of 4;5, he performs at the level of phases II/III, which corresponds to an age of 2;0 to 2;5 in typically developing children:

– word and phrase structure: phase II/III
– sentence structure: phase II/III
– argument structure: phase III
– negation   phase III
– question formation   phase II
– MLU   phase III/IV

The analysis also shows that W's language development is not just globally delayed, as his performance across the various domains cannot be assigned to one single phase of typical language development. Instead, particular domains of W's grammar are more affected than others. With respect to quantitative criteria (e.g. MLU), W's developmental level is relatively more advanced than for word and constituent or sentence structures. W's grammar is specifically affected in the domain of verb inflection, for which his grammar is even more limited than in phase II of typical development.

The results of the COPROF analysis do not only provide a detailed description of a child's grammatical performance, but also a set of specific objectives and potential pathways for therapy and remediation. In the case of W, one may focus on the domains of his grammar that were identified as specifically weak or affected, such as verb inflection. In addition, one may use the profile chart to establish a progressive order of grammatical phenomena for therapy and remediation, in which advanced grammatical structures are only targeted once the child has acquired the more basic structures of the earlier phases. In the case of W, a child at an early developmental level (phase II/III) in most areas of grammar, this would mean that therapy should focus on phase IV phenomena before moving on to phase V. Reports of attempts at implementing and testing such a developmental approach for language therapy in German are available from Dannenbauer (1992) and Hansen (1996).

Further Developments

Although the profile chart for German has been positively reviewed by clinicians as providing a detailed assessment of a child's grammar and level of grammatical development (see e.g. Dannenbauer, 1992; Heidtmann, 1988; Rothweiler *et al.*, 1995), the relatively large amount of time and effort required to complete a profile chart for an individual child has turned out to be a major obstacle for its routine use in clinical contexts. In response to that, several attempts have been made at simplifying the original profile chart, by leaving out or streamlining parts of the analysis (see Behrenbeck *et al.*, 1990; Bertz, 1994; Schrey-Dern, 1990). It is true that these reduced versions require considerably less time to administer. However, although the simplified profile charts may serve for initial screening, Behrenbeck *et al.* (1990: 35), for example, noted that the restricted versions lack the detailed diagnostic information that may be required to design specific measures for therapy.

Another related development that may be used to supplement the profile chart for German is ESGRAF (*Evozierte Sprachdiagnose grammatischer Fähigkeiten* 'Evoked diagnosis of grammatical abilities', Motsch, 1999), which provides materials to elicit semi-spontaneous speech from children. In addition, ESGRAF also includes tools for analysing children's speech, but this component is essentially a simplified profile chart with considerably fewer categories than the original one (Motsch & Hansen, 1999).

Finally, the presentation of a computer-assisted version of the original profile chart for German (COPROF, Clahsen & Hansen, 1991) has considerably contributed to making the procedure more suitable for clinical practice. COPROF is a user-friendly, easy to administer, interactive software program which provides a step-by-step guide throughout the analysis. For each child utterance, the user responds to a series of program-generated data queries, in most cases simple yes/no decisions made by keyboard entries. COPROF also provides elaborated HELP functions containing descriptions of grammatical categories and examples of how to analyse problem cases. This prevents errors of analysis and is also useful for training purposes, including self-training (Hansen, 2000). Furthermore, COPROF checks the analysis of each utterance for completeness and internal consistency, which improves the reliability of the procedure. Finally, COPROF contains routines for calculating totals and means, displaying the results, and providing selected reports and lists of examples for any aspect of the analysis. COPROF is a simple MS-DOS based software program, which, except for a PC, does not require any specific hardware components. It is available for free upon contacting the second author.

References

Behrenbeck, B., Junker, D., Langhorst, P., Schneider, P., Türke, K. and Weinmüller, B. (1990) Überprüfung eines Screening-Verfahrens zur Diagnostik des kindlichen Grammatikerwerbs und seine Anwendung in der Praxis. *Sprache – Stimme – Gehör* 14, 34–37.

Bertz, F. (1994) Das Morpho-Syntaktische Entwicklungsgitter. Entstehungsbedingungen und Anwendungsbereiche. Unpublished manuscript: Bad Salzdetfurth.
Brown, R. (1973) *A First Language: The Early Stages*. Cambridge, MA: Harvard University Press.
Clahsen, H. (1982) *Spracherwerb in der Kindheit. Eine Untersuchung zur Entwicklung der Syntax bei Kleinkindern*. Tübingen: Narr.
Clahsen, H. (1984) Der Erwerb von Kasusmarkierungen in der deutschen Kindersprache. *Linguistische Berichte* 89, 1–31.
Clahsen, H. (1986) *Die Profilanalyse*. Berlin: Spiess.
Clahsen, H. (1991) *Child Language and Developmental Dysphasia*. Amsterdam/Philadelphia: John Benjamins.
Clahsen, H. and Hansen, D. (1991) *COPROF – Ein linguistisches Untersuchungsverfahren für die logopädische Praxis*. Cologne: Focus.
Crystal, D. (1979) *Working with LARSP*. London: Arnold.
Crystal, D. (1982) *Profiling Linguistic Disability*. London: Arnold.
Crystal, D., Fletcher, P. and Garman, M. (1976) *The Grammatical Analysis of Language Disability*. London: Arnold.
Dannenbauer, F.M. (1992) Grammatik. In S. Baumgartner and I. Füssenich (eds) *Sprachtherapie mit Kindern* (pp. 123–203). Munich: UTB.
Hansen, D. (1983) *Linguistische Analyse von Spontansprachproben*. Unpublished manuscript: University of Cologne.
Hansen, D. (1996) *Spracherwerb und Dysgrammatismus*. Munich: Reinhardt
Hansen, D. (2000) Die Computerunterstützte Profilanalyse COPROF – Diagnoseinstrument und linguistisches Lernprogramm. *Forum Logopädie* 2, 19–22.
Heidtmann, H. (1988) *Neue Wege der Sprachdiagnostik*. Berlin: Spiess.
Motsch, H-J. (1999) *ESGRAF. Testmanual und Video*. Munich: Reinhardt.
Motsch, H-J. and Hansen, D. (1999) COPROF und ESGRAF – Diagnoseverfahren grammatischer Störungen im Vergleich. *Die Sprachheilarbeit* 44, 151–162.
Rothweiler, M., Pitsch, S. and Siegmüller, J. (1995) Spontansprachdiagnose bei Dysgrammatismus. *Die Sprachheilarbeit* 40, 331–350.
Schrey-Dern, D. (1990) Screening-Verfahren zur Diagnostik des kindlichen Grammatikerwerbs auf der Grundlage der Profilanalyse nach Clahsen. *Sprache – Stimme – Gehör* 14, 31–33.

6 GRAMAT: A Dutch Adaptation of LARSP

Gerard W. Bol

History of Development

In the academic year 1977/8, Folkert Kuiken and the present author, at the time both students of General Linguistics at the University of Amsterdam, participated in a seminar in Developmental Language Disorders (DLD), given by Prof Dr B.Th. Tervoort. The seminar was attended both by students of the university and speech therapy students of the Polytechnic of Amsterdam, which was not common at the time. The initial idea was to create a Dutch version of LARSP. During the seminar, it appeared that this would take far more work than could be done by the students within a few weeks. So, Kuiken and Bol conceived the idea of making a pilot adaptation of a Dutch version of LARSP and writing their MA thesis on the topic. They later decided to write a PhD grant proposal concerning not only normal language development in Dutch children aged one to four, but also analysing the linguistic abilities of three groups of children with DLD by using the LARSP method, adapted for Dutch. These were children with specific language impairment, children with hearing problems and children with Down's syndrome. The grant was awarded, and in 1988 their dissertation was published, entitled *Grammaticale Analyse van Taalontwikkelingsstoornissen* ('Grammatical Analysis of Developmental Language Disorders' – GRAMAT). One of the publications that came from the dissertation is Bol and Kuiken (1990).

A Dutch Adaptation

Like LARSP, the Dutch adaptation GRAMAT contains a profile chart in which the scores of the structures produced by the children can be listed. For Dutch, however, when the profile chart had to be constructed, there was little (if any) information on the language development of children aged one to four, especially concerning the morphosyntactic characteristics of their spontaneous speech. Thus, the first thing to do was to obtain an overview of the most frequently used morphosyntactic structures of typically developing children in this age range. The period was divided into six stages of six months. At each stage, spontaneous language samples were obtained from 12 children equally divided by sex and social class.

To obtain an overview of the morphosyntactic structures produced by the children, a longitudinal design was needed. The data was therefore collected twice with an interval of six months (recording 1 and recording 2). This design made it possible to look at development over a four-year period, without having to collect longitudinal data during this time (see Table 6.1). For instance, children who were 1;3 years old in the first recording and who belonged to Stage I were recorded again half a year later, when they were 1;9 years old and belonged to Stage II. This scheme was then applied to all the typically developing children. The number of subjects in each stage was 12. After transcription, the results of the analyses were used to characterize the development of the morphosyntactic structures produced by typically developing children aged one to four.

The children were selected from playgroups and day-care centres in Amsterdam. They were audio-recorded for one hour in everyday situations in their homes in the presence of at least one of the parents and two observers. After the transcription of the recordings, a hundred successive utterances from the eleventh minute of the recording onwards were used for the morphosyntactic analysis. The notion of utterance was based on the T-unit as defined by Hunt (1970). All utterances were analysed at clause, phrase, and word level. The morphosyntactic framework we used was based on descriptive Dutch grammars (Geerts *et al.*, 1984; Klooster *et al.*, 1974; Pollmann & Sturm, 1980; and Van den Toorn, 1979). In order to determine

Table 6.1 Recording scheme (n = 42 different typically developing children)

Stage (Age)		Sex	Socio-economic status					
			lower	middle	upper	lower	middle	upper
I	1;0–1;6	M	1	1	1	1	1	1
		F	1	1	1	1	1	1
II	1;6–2;0	M	1	1	1	1	1	1
		F	1	1	1	1	1	1
III	2;0–2;6	M	1	1	1	1	1	1
		F	1	1	1	1	1	1
IV	2;6–3;0	M	1	1	1	1	1	1
		F	1	1	1	1	1	1
V	3;0–3;6	M	1	1	1	1	1	1
		F	1	1	1	1	1	1
VI	3;6–4;0	M	1	1	1	1	1	1
		F	1	1	1	1	1	1
			RECORDING 1			RECORDING 2		

what morphosyntactic structures should be included in the profile chart at each specific stage, two criteria were applied. The first was that the structure should be used by at least 50% of the children at a particular stage. This criterion, adopted from Wells (1985), takes into account the requirement that the structure should be used by the majority of the population. The second was a criterion of frequency: the median of the frequency with which a structure is used should have a value of at least 1.0. The application of these productivity criteria has yielded a profile chart in which structures are entered that are the most frequently used by typically developing children between one and four years of age. The chart will be discussed below. No distinction is made on the basis of sex or socio-economic status.

The Profile Chart

The upper part of the profile chart (Figure 6.1) is reserved for general information on the child. The utterances which cannot be analysed morphosyntactically are noted in Section A. Some quantitative measures of the child's language production, like MLU and MLUL (the MLU of the five longest utterances) are marked down in Section B.

Stage I, which covers the period from 1;0 to 1;6 years, is the stage of one-element utterances. We distinguish three kinds of utterances here: (1) those with a nominal character (Noun), indicating objects, (2) utterances with a verbal character (Verb), indicating actions and events, and (3) a category Other, used to indicate all other words that are not nouns or verbs.

In the second stage, from 1;6 to 2;0 years, Dutch children have learned how to combine words, both at clause and phrase level. Children of this age combine subjects, verbs, and adverbial adjuncts to the clause structures: SA, SV, and AV. It is noteworthy that children at this stage already use utterances containing three or even four elements, although these utterances did not meet the productivity criteria mentioned above to be included in the profile chart. At phrase level, demonstrative and personal pronouns are used, besides combinations of a determiner with a noun. At word level, the diminutive appears, as well as the second and third person singular forms of the verb in the present tense.

At Stage III, from 2;0 to 2;6 years, four clause structures consisting of two constituents appear: (1) structures with an object (OV) (e.g. *steen gooien* 'throw stone'); (2) structures with a complement (SC), which is in most cases the nominal part of the predicate (e.g. *hond lief* 'dog sweet'); (3) structures consisting of two adverbial adjuncts (AA), like *daar ook* ('there too') and; (4) imperatives (Imper) of the type VX, in which V denotes the verb and X any other clause element, like *kom hier* ('come here'). At this stage, some three-element utterances (SVA, SAA, OAV, SVC, and SVO) and two four-element utterances (SVAA and SVAO) become productive as well. These clause structures are mostly rather elementary at this point; that is to

Name: Therapist:
Date of birth: Remarks:
Date of recording:
Age:

A. Unanalysed Unintelligible Deviant Minor				Incomplete Ambiguous Repetitions	
B. Analysed utterances MLU				Total number of utterances MLUL	
Stage I 1;0 - 1;6	Noun		Verb	Other	
Stage II 1;6 - 2;0	*Clause*			*Phrase*	*Morphology*
	Imper.	Inter.	Statement		
			SA SV AV	demonstr. pronoun determiner + Noun personal pronoun	diminutive 2/3 singular
Stage III 2;0 - 2;6	VX	VSX	OV SC SVA AA SAA OAV SVC SVO SVAA SVAO	copula auxiliary adjective + Noun prep. + det. + Noun prep. + Noun	plural of Nouns 1 singular adjective -e past participle
Stage IV 2;6 - 3;0		QXY	VC And OA AAV SVAC 4+	poss. pron. + Noun postmodification det. + adj. + Noun interrog. pronoun prep. + pers. pronoun adverb + adverb	past tense
Stage V 3;0 - 3;6		QXYZ	Subordination Co-ordination	adverb + adjective indefinite pronoun	
Stage VI 3;6 - 4;0		VSXY		prep. + poss.pron + Noun repl./part. "er"	
	Other			other	other

Figure 6.1 The profile chart

say, they consist of single words. In the category of interrogatives (Inter), questions of the type VSX appear. At phrase level, the use of prepositions can be noted. Constructions consisting of a preposition, determiner, and noun (e.g. *naar de tuin* 'to the garden') become productive at the same time as those without a determiner, like *naar bed* ('to bed'). The use of copulas is linked with the use of a complement at the clause level at this stage, as in *hond is lief* ('dog is sweet'), resulting in an SVC structure at clause level. Auxiliaries can be found as well. Sometimes these are used in combination with past participles, which are registered at the word level at this stage. Adjectives are used in combination with a noun. At word level, the inflection of the adjective in Dutch (adjective-e) is scored. Other morphemes becoming productive are the plural form of nouns and the first person singular of the verb in the present tense.

At stage IV, from 2;6 to 3;0 years, we see that the children produce the coordinating conjunction *en* ('and'). The two-element utterances VC and OA and the three-element utterance AAV meet the criteria set above. Given the use of SVAA at Stage III, one wonders why AAV meets the criteria only now. When we take a closer look at these structures, we discover that SVAA structures are of a more elementary character than AAV structures, which are more developed at phrase level. The following examples may illustrate this:

SVAA: *ik kan niet bij* ('I cannot reach')

clause: <u>S</u>   V   A   A
phrase: personal pronoun

           AAV: *gaat nu <u>naar de stad</u>* ('goes now to the town')
clause: V   A   A
phrase: preposition + determiner + noun

At this stage we can also see utterances with four elements of the type SVAC (e.g. *ik ben ook ziek* 'I am ill too'), and utterances which contain more than four elements, indicated by 4+. Finally, at clause level, children are using *wh*-questions in utterances with two other clause elements, indicated by QXY. The interrogative pronouns which are used in these questions appear at phrase level in this stage. Possessive pronouns are used in combination with a noun. At this level, we also see that the children produce postmodifications (e.g. *de poes met witte pootjes* 'the cat with white feet'), in which *met witte pootjes* is analysed as postmodification. Children start using phrase structures containing a preposition and a personal pronoun as well. The form of the pronoun in these constructions is the object form, which becomes productive later than the subject form at Stage II. Finally, noun phrases consisting of a determiner, an adjective and a noun are used, as well as constructions consisting of two adverbs, like *heel snel* ('very quickly'). At word level, we see that children between 2;6 and 3;0 years of age produce past tense forms.

At Stage V, at clause level, children between 3;0 and 3;6 years no longer coordinate utterances only with 'and' (Stage IV), but also use other coordinating conjunctions, such as *maar* ('but'), *of* ('or') and *want* ('for'). Subordinating conjunctions appear as well (e.g. *omdat* 'because'). We also see the use of question words, now with three other clause elements, indicated by QXYZ. At phrase level, indefinite pronouns become productive, as well as structures in which the adjective is modified by an adverb (e.g. *heel groot* 'very big').

At Stage VI, between 3;6 and 4;0 years, children produce questions with inversion of verb and subject that contain four clause elements in total, indicated by VSXY. At phrase level we see that the category possessive pronoun plus noun from Stage IV is now preceded by a preposition. Finally, at phrase level, structures with *er* become productive. In Dutch there are two kinds of *er* to be noted here: (1) one with a partitive meaning, as in *ik heb er twee* ('I have got two of them') and (2) the repletive *er*, which introduces an indefinite subject, as in *er zit een poes in de tuin* ('there is a cat in the garden'). Structures that did not meet the criteria to be included in one of the stages are noted in the categories Other/other at the bottom of the profile chart.

Production Frequencies of the Structures in the Profile Chart

In order to determine to what extent children with DLD differ from their typically developing peers in using the morphosyntactic structures from the profile chart, the frequencies are calculated for all structures of the chart. These frequencies indicate the number of times a group of typically developing children in a certain stage has produced a certain structure in 100 analysable utterances. Interquartile ranges of the frequencies of all structures are calculated, indicating the values of each structure between the 25th and the 75th percentile (i.e. the first and the third quartile). The value of the 50th percentile, the median score or the second quartile of each structure is calculated as well. If a child with a language disorder has a score below the 25th percentile, this indicates that three-quarters of the typically developing children in a certain stage have produced the given structure more often. If a child with a language disorder produces a certain structure above the value of the 75th percentile, this indicates that three-quarters of the typically developing children produce this structure less often than the child with the language problem.

It is important to note that a production frequency that is higher compared to typically developing children is not always sufficient for the conclusion that no problems exist. One has to consider whether the frequency of a structure increases or decreases during normal language development. For instance, the number of one-word utterances (e.g. a single

N or V) within 100 utterances has to decrease when a child gets older. So if a child with a language disorder produces a number of one-word utterances that is higher than the 75th percentile, one must not conclude that the frequency of this category is without problems. Likewise, if a child with language problems produces one-word utterances below the frequency of the 25th percentile, this has to be seen as a positive aspect of language development. The interquartile ranges of the structures (in Dutch; see also the Dutch version of the profile chart in Appendix 6.1) produced by the typically developing children are given in Table 6.2. The numbers are given exactly as provided by the output of the SPSS program by which they were calculated. The fact that not all numbers are whole numbers is a consequence of interpolation. Therefore, all numbers except those for MLU(L) should be rounded up or down.

The following provides a step-by-step guide to working with the interquartile ranges. After audio or video recording a child with a language disorder, the researcher has to make a transcript containing 100 analysable utterances. The MLU and the MLUL are calculated, counted in morphemes. The values of MLU(L) are looked up in one of the columns. The column with the value of the MLU(L) that is most close to the MLU(L) of the child with the language disorder is the column with the interquartile ranges of the frequency of the structures of the typically developing children. In this way an MLU(L) match is made between the child with a language problem and a group of typically developing children of the same language age. It is possible to match a child with a language problem on chronological age with a group of typically developing children, by choosing the column according to one of the six stages that are classified by years and months. Working with children with language disorders, one will often see that only the last stages of the profile chart will be suitable for matching on chronological age.

Frequencies of structures that fall outside the range of the 25th to the 75th percentile should be considered as possible goals for intervention. In the next section, a case study of a Dutch boy with specific language impairment is presented and goals for intervention are discussed.

Case Study

Mark is a boy with specific language impairment (SLI). At the time of this recording of his spontaneous speech he was six years of age. His problems concerned both speech and language, the latter involving both production and comprehension difficulties. Mark went to a special school for children with speech, language, and hearing problems in Amsterdam, The Netherlands, for a year and a half. His speech therapist suspected dyspraxia, because of his articulation problems. Mark had a weak auditory memory: he had problems reproducing longer sentences and tasks. His

Table 6.2 Interquartile ranges of the typically developing children (in Dutch)

		I	II	III	IV	V	VI
A	Onb/onv	24,50-46,00-54,50	16,50-42,50-52,75	12,00-19,50-31,75	6,25-13,00-21,25	7,00-11,50-15,75	4,00-8,00-14,50
	Afwijkend	0,00-0,00-0,00	0,00-0,00-0,00	0,00-0,00-1,00	0,00-0,50-1,00	0,00-1,00-1,75	0,25-1,00-2,75
	Minor	20,75-48,00-73,50	11,75-42,40-65,75	29,25-43,50-55,75	36,75-45,50-59,00	20,00-35,00-58,75	24,00-25,50-35,00
	Niet comp	0,00-0,00-0,00	0,00-0,00-0,00	0,00-0,50-1,00	0,00-2,00-3,00	1,25-2,00-3,75	0,25-2,50-4,00
	Ambigu	0,00-0,00-0,00	0,00-0,00-0,00	0,00-0,00-0,00	0,00-0,00-0,00	0,00-0,00-0,00	0,00-0,00-0,00
	Zelfherh	0,50-8,50-22,75	6,25-9,50-24,25	3,25-5,50-10,75	0,00-1,00-3,00	0,00-1,50-5,75	1,25-3,00-4,50
B	Aant uit ana	100	100	100	100	100	100
	MLU	1,00-1,00-1,18	1,10-1,30-1,78	2,23-2,45-2,88	3,05-3,65-4,28	3,95-4,40-4,78	3,78-4,25-4,93
	MLUL	1,00-1,20-2,55	2,00-2,50-3,90	4,40-5,60-6,60	6,75-7,80-8,95	9,85-10,40-10,95	8,60-9,50-11,40
	Total uit	198,0-230,00-292,0	167,5-182,0-238,8	156,5-169,5-198,3	151,5-163,5-178,0	142,5-150,5-182,0	136,5-143,0-150,3
I	N	29,25-53,50-76,00	24,75-40,50-53,25	7,25-16,50-22,25	3,25-4,50-9,50	1,25-3,00-9,50	3,00-4,00-5,00
	V	0,00-14,00-45,75	3,25-5,50-9,75	1,50-3,00-7,25	1,00-2,00-4,25	0,00-1,00-2,00	0,00-1,00-2,00
	Rest	13,75-25,00-32,00	12,50-25,00-42,25	12,25-16,50-17,75	6,50-9,00-13,25	5,25-9,00-11,00	4,00-9,50-12,75
II	SA		0,00-1,00-6,25	2,00-4,00-8,00	3,00-4,00-6,50	1,00-1,50-3,75	2,25-4,00-5,75
	SV		0,00-1,50-4,00	2,00-2,50-5,50	1,00-3,00-4,00	1,00-2,00-3,75	1,50-4,00-5,75
	AV		0,00-1,50-4,75	3,25-6,00-7,00	1,25-3,00-8,25	0,25-1,50-3,00	1,00-2,50-3,75
	dem		2,50-10,50-15,25	7,50-9,50-14,00	11,25-16,00-20,50	7,25-18,00-22,75	12,00-19,50-21,00
	detN		0,00-1,00-6,25	3,25-9,00-13,75	8,50-13,00-18,00	10,25-18,00-20,75	14,00-19,00-23,50
	pers		0,00-1,00-3,00	1,75-12,50-22,00	20,25-30,50-40,75	29,25-36,00-55,00	35,25-39,50-54,75
	dim		0,00-2,50-11,00	6,25-9,00-14,25	4,50-7,50-12,00	4,00-10,00-15,25	4,25-7,50-11,75
	2e/3e enk		0,50-4,00-9,50	11,00-17,50-26,50	25,25-30,00-37,00	29,00-35,50-42,50	29,75-34,00-41,50
III	VX			0,00-1,00-1,00	0,00-1,00-1,75	0,25-1,00-2,00	0,00-1,00-3,75
	VSX			0,00-1,00-3,75	0,00-0,50-1,75	0,00-1,50-2,00	0,25-2,00-3,00

Table 6.2 continued

	I	II	III	IV	V	VI
OV			2,00-3,00-4,75	0,00-1,00-2,00	0,00-1,00-1,00	0,00-0,00-1,00
SC			0,00-1,00-4,00	0,00-0,00-1,75	0,00-0,00-0,75	0,00-0,00-0,75
SVA			4,00-5,50-8,50	9,00-10,50-13,50	8,25-11,00-12,75	7,00-9,00-12,25
AA			0,00-1,00-1,75	0,00-1,00-5,00	0,00-0,00-1,75	0,00-2,00-2,00
SAA			0,00-1,00-2,00	0,00-1,00-2,00	0,00-0,00-1,75	0,00-0,00-1,00
OAV			0,00-1,00-2,75	0,00-1,00-1,75	0,00-0,00-1,00	0,00-1,00-2,00
SVC			0,00-1,50-3,75	3,00-4,50-7,75	4,50-7,00-8,75	2,00-5,00-12,50
SVO			1,00-2,00-3,75	1,25-3,00-5,25	2,50-5,50-7,00	3,00-4,00-8,00
SVAA			0,25-1,00-2,00	1,25-4,50-7,75	2,25-7,00-12,50	2,00-7,00-9,50
SVAO			0,00-1,00-3,75	1,75-4,50-6,75	4,00-8,00-9,75	3,25-6,50-11,00
copula			0,25-3,00-7,25	5,00-9,00-10,75	5,50-9,50-14,75	6,00-6,50-19,50
aux			2,25-6,00-12,50	6,50-14,00-17,00	10,50-13,50-15,75	11,00-16,50-25,75
adjN			0,25-2,00-4,75	1,00-4,50-7,75	3,00-4,50-6,00	1,00-3,00-3,75
prepdetN			0,25-1,50-4,50	2,25-4,00-8,25	5,50-7,00-8,75	3,25-5,50-13,25
prepN			0,00-1,50-5,00	2,25-4,00-4,75	1,25-2,50-5,00	1,25-2,50-5,25
-s/-en			2,00-2,50-11,25	4,00-5,50-11,75	4,00-6,00-10,75	3,25-5,00-8,25
1e enk			1,00-4,50-8,00	7,50-14,00-19,00	8,25-14,00-19,50	11,25-14,50-21,50
adj-e			1,00-2,00-3,75	1,00-2,50-6,00	1,00-5,50-9,00	3,00-5,50-8,75
volt dw			0,25-1,00-1,75	0,25-1,50-4,50	2,00-2,00-2,75	1,00-3,00-6,00
IV QXY				0,25-2,00-3,00	0,00-2,00-5,25	0,25-1,50-3,75
VC				0,00-1,00-2,00	0,00-0,50-1,00	0,00-0,00-1,50
En				0,25-2,00-4,00	3,00-8,00-15,50	3,00-5,50-11,75
OA				0,00-1,00-1,75	0,00-1,50-3,00	0,25-1,00-1,00

Table 6.2 continued

	I	II	III	IV	V	VI
AAV				0,25-1,00-1,75	0,25-1,00-1,75	0,00-0,00-1,00
SVAC				1,00-1,00-3,00	0,25-3,00-4,75	1,25-2,00-3,00
4+				1,00-2,00-7,00	3,25-7,00-10,00	3,00-7,00-9,50
possN				0,00-1,00-3,50	1,00-1,00-2,75	1,25-2,50-5,00
appositie				1,00-2,00-3,75	1,00-1,00-2,00	0,25-3,00-6,75
detadjN				0,00-1,00-1,75	0,25-2,00-3,00	0,25-2,00-2,75
inter				0,00-1,00-2,75	0,00-1,50-5,50	1,00-3,00-9,25
preppers				0,25-1,00-3,75	0,00-1,00-2,00	0,00-1,00-2,00
advadv				0,00-1,00-1,00	0,00-0,50-1,75	0,00-0,00-2,00
ovt				0,00-1,00-2,75	0,25-2,50-4,75	1,25-3,50-6,75
V QXYZ					0,00-1,00-2,00	0,00-0,50-2,50
Subord					1,00-1,00-2,75	1,00-1,50-4,00
Coörd					0,25-3,00-4,00	1,25-3,50-5,75
advadj					0,00-1,00-2,00	0,00-0,50-2,00
indef					0,00-1,00-2,00	0,00-1,00-3,00
VI VSXY						0,00-1,50-2,00
preppossN						1,00-1,00-2,00
er						0,00-1,00-2,00

comprehension problems might have been due to these difficulties. On the Reynell Developmental Language Scales, his score on language comprehension was 56, which corresponds to the language comprehension level of a typically developing child aged 4;6 (S.D. −1.9). There were no other (physical) disorders that could account for his language problems, although he was never submitted to neurophysiological research. Psychological research revealed a huge fear of failure at linguistic tasks. Mark was very aware of his language difficulties, which could explain his emotional problems. The speech therapist saw no reason to assume that the emotional problems might have been the cause of his language problems. Mark's hearing abilities were also researched frequently over the years, without any problems being detected.

Mark's spontaneous speech was recorded in the room of his speech therapist, while playing with a Playmobil circus, with lions and cages, and the various dolls and animals belonging to it. The recording was transcribed orthographically and the transcript divided into 100 analysable utterances. Within this number of analysable utterances, there were utterances that were incomplete, unintelligible, minor utterances, or deviant utterances. The utterances ($N = 46$) that were not analysable were noted in Section A of the profile chart (see Figure 6.2). In the profile chart an overview is given of all frequencies of the structures in Mark's spontaneous speech.

Mark's MLU in morphemes and his MLU of the five longest utterances (MLUL, also counted in morphemes) correspond with the MLU(L) of typically developing children of Stage VI, aged 3;6 to 4;0 years. Therefore, the frequencies of the morphosyntactic structures produced by Mark are to be compared with the frequencies of the same structures produced by typically developing children from Stage VI. In this comparison, only structures that are outside the range of the first and the third quartile are subject to further investigation in order to determine possible goals for intervention, so the discussion below is limited to these structures or categories.

An overview of all the frequencies of Mark's morphosyntactic structures compared to the production of the structures by the typically developing children of Stage VI is given in Table 6.3. In this table an asterisk indicates Mark's frequency. The asterisks are noted in one of the seven columns in the table under Percentiles. An asterisk in the leftmost column indicates a frequency that is below the 25th percentile of the normally developing children. An asterisk in the column headed 25th, in front of the number given in the column, indicates the number of times that Mark produced that structure (e.g. Mark produces a structure consisting of a Subject and an Adverb (SA) on two occasions). An asterisk in the column between the 25th and the 50th percentile indicates that Mark produces a structure with a frequency between that of the first and second quartile of the frequencies produced by the typically developing children at Stage VI, and

Table 6.3 Mark's scores for the structures at Stage VI

	Stage VI Structure	Percentiles 25th	50th	75th
A	Unintelligible	4	8	15 *
	Deviant	0	*1	3
	Minor	* 24	26	35
	Incomplete	0	*3	4
	Ambiguous	0	*0	0
	Repetitions	* 1	3	5
B	Anal. utt.	100	100	100
	MLU	3,58	4,25	* 4,93
	MLUL	8,60	* 9,50	11,40
	Total # utt.	137	143	* 150
I	N	* 3	4	5
	V	0	1	* 5
	Other	4	* 10	13
II	SA	*2	4	6
	SV	2	4	*6
	AV	1	* 3	4
	dem	* 12	20	21
	detN	14	19	*24
	pers	* 35	40	55
	dim	* 4	8	12
	2/3 sing	30	34	* 42
III	VX	0	1	*4
	VSX	*0	2	3
	OV	0	0	1 *
	SC	0	0	1 *
	SVA	7	9	12 *
	AA	0	2	2 *
	SAA	0	*0	1
	OAV	0	*1	2
	SVC	* 2	5	13
	SVO	3	4	* 8
	SVAA	2	7	*10
	SVAO	* 3	7	11
	copula	* 6	7	20
	aux	11	17	* 26
	adjN	1	3	*4
	prepdetN	3	*6	13
	prepN	* 1	3	5
	plurN	3	5	*8
	1 sing	* 11	14	22
	adj –e	* 3	6	9
	past part	1	3	6 *

Table 6.3 continued

	Structure	Stage VI Percentiles 25th		50th		75th	
IV	QXY	0		*2		4	
	VC	0		*0		2	
	En	3	*	6		12	
	OA	*0		1		1	
	AAV	0		0		*1	
	SVAC	*1		2		3	
	4+	*3		7		10	
	possN	*	1	3		5	
	postmodification	0	*	3		7	
	detadjN	0	*	2		3	
	inter	1		3	*	9	
	preppers	*0		1		2	
	advadv	0		0	*	2	
	past tense	1		4		7	*
V	QXYZ	0		1		*3	
	Subord	*	1	2		4	
	Co-ord	*	1	4		6	
	advadj	*0		1		2	
	indef	0		1		*3	
VI	VSXY	*0		2		2	
	preppossN	*	1	1		2	
	er	0		*1		2	

so on. In the table, the rounded numbers are given for all structures or categories, except for MLU and MLUL.

There are 19 utterances that are unintelligible, which is above the 75th percentile of the scores of typically developing children at Stage VI, and this can be explained by Mark's articulation problems. Minor utterances, like *yes, no,* and *bye,* are not often found in his spontaneous speech, contrary to what is expected for children with SLI in a conversation. As a result of the small number of Minors, the total number of utterances is 146, which is within the interquartile ranges. Usually, children with language problems need to use far more utterances than typically developing children to reach the total of 100 analysable utterances that is needed for a GRAMAT analysis.

In Stage I there are no particularities: Mark uses few one-word utterances. Given the fact that the number of one-word utterances has to decrease in the normal course of language development, this can be regarded as a positive aspect of his spontaneous speech.

Name: Mark
Date of birth:
Date of recording:
Age: 5;11

Therapist:
Remarks:

A. Unanalysed 46		
Unintelligible 19		Incomplete 3
Deviant 1		Ambiguous
Minor 23		Repetitions

B. Analysed utterances 100	Total number of utterances 146
MLU 4,4	MLUL 9,2

Stage I 1;0 - 1;6	Noun 1		Verb 2	Other 7	
Stage II 1;6 - 2;0	*Clause*			*Phrase*	*Morphology*
	Imper.	Inter.	Statement		
			SA 2	demonstr. pronoun 6	Diminutive 3
			SV 6	determiner + Noun 24	2/3 singular 39
			AV 2	personal pronoun 27	
Stage III 2;0 - 2;6	VX 4	VSX	OV 6	copula 1	plural of Nouns 8
			SC 2	auxiliary 24	1 singular 6
			SVA 29	adjective + Noun 4	adjective –e 2
			AA 4	prep. + det. + Noun 6	past participle 7
			SAA	prep. + Noun	
			OAV 1		
			SVC 1		
			SVO 6		
			SVAA 10		
			SVAO		
Stage IV 2;6 - 3;0		QXY 2	VC	poss. pron. + Noun	past tense 14
			And 5	postmodification 2	
			OA	det. + adj. + Noun 1	
			AAV 1	interrog. pronoun 4	
			SVAC 1	prep. + pers. pronoun	
			4+ 3	adverb + adverb 1	
Stage V 3;0 - 3;6		QXYZ 3	Subordination	adverb + adjective	
			Co-ordination	indefinite pronoun 3	
Stage VI 3;6 - 4;0		VSXY		prep. + poss.pron + Noun	
				repl./part. "er" 1	
	Other	3		other 4	other

Figure 6.2 Mark's profile chart

What is remarkable in Mark's production of structures at clause level are the low frequencies of SA (Stage II), VSX, SVAO (Stage III), no production of Subordination and Coordination, and high frequencies of OV and SC (Stage III). This corresponds to what is known of the language production of Dutch children with SLI (Bol & Kuiken, 1988). In general, problems are seen in producing structures containing a subject and a predicate. Structures containing adverbial adjuncts (SVA, AA, SVAA in Stage III) are less problematic for Mark, although SVAO is not produced at all. Striking is the adequate number of longer utterances (4+). Mark has no problems formulating clauses that start with a question word (QXY and QXYZ).

At phrase level, Mark shows problems in producing pronouns. Demonstrative pronouns and personal pronouns are produced much less frequently than the typically developing children he is compared to on the basis of his MLU(L). Possessive pronouns also appear to be produced rather infrequently, but typically developing children of Stage VI do not produce these forms very often either. Mark produces a small number of copulas, which goes together with the high number of SC structures, like *doggy sweet*, where the copula is omitted.

At word level, Mark's use of diminutives is small, as well as the use of the first person singular of the verb. Contrary to what is known in general of children with SLI, Mark's use of other verb conjugations (2nd and 3rd person present tense and past tense) are produced sufficiently, compared to normal children aged 3;6 to 4;0. It might be the case that the setting of the conversation, in the room of Mark's speech therapist, playing with the Playmobil circus, prevented Mark from using many 1st person singular verb conjugations.

In sum, Mark's production of morphosyntactic structures shows many inadequacies. Concerning the structures of the profile chart that show a frequency not outside the interquartile ranges, one has to consider that Mark is matched on MLU(L) to children of 3;6 to 4;0 years, while he is six years of age. He has a language delay of at least two years, while some structures are more difficult for him than an overall delay indicates. Considering his language production compared to his language comprehension, one can conclude that Mark's language problem shows more severe problems in production. There is a discrepancy of about one year between what he can understand and what he can produce.

Therapy Based on a Language Analysis by the Profiling Method

Spontaneous language analysis by means of the profiling method has a number of advantages over language testing. This does not mean that the outcome of a language test is less useful than the results of a spontaneous language analysis, but there are differences. One of the most important characteristics of such an analysis is that the speech therapist not only gets an overview of the structures that have to be part of the intervention programme (i.e. those with which children have difficulties) but also gets information where they lie on the developmental path, and this serves as a guideline for intervention. This path – the order of production of morphosyntactic structures that are most frequently used by typically developing children – is outlined in the stages of the profile chart and in the structures that are part of the stages, from Stage I to Stage VI. Moreover, the speech therapist not only obtains detailed information about the categories that have to be part of the intervention programme (i.e. the disabilities of the child), but also about their linguistic abilities. The latter is invaluable, because it gives the speech therapist the option of starting the intervention at the appropriate linguistic level for the child.

For Mark, this would indicate that the intervention programme should start with structures that are produced rather infrequently (except for the unintelligible utterances). In the first place, the pronominal system is difficult for him. So, one should start by training demonstrative and personal pronouns (Stage II). Later, possessive pronouns (Stage IV and VI) can be part of the intervention programme. Structures containing a verb (V) and a complement (C) could be the next intervention goal, given the small number of copulas in his spontaneous speech (and the correspondingly high number of SC structures). The next goal could be SVAO, a structure totally absent in his spontaneous speech, followed by utterances with subordination and coordination. Subsequent goals of intervention would be the use of prepositions, diminutives, first person singular of the verb, and adjectives.

These intervention goals do not in themselves provide information on the *way* intervention should be carried out. That is primarily the decision of the speech therapist. The ten principles for grammar facilitation for children with SLI (Fey et al., 2003) could be a guideline for therapists who treat children with language disorders after having performed a spontaneous language analysis by means of a profiling method.

Acknowledgements

The author wishes to thank Folkert Kuiken, not only for the years of working together on GRAMAT, but also for being a good friend to the present day.

References

Bol, G.W. and Kuiken, F. (1988) *Grammaticale Analyse van Taalontwikkelings stoornissen*. Dissertation: University of Amsterdam.

Bol, G.W. and Kuiken, F. (1990) Grammatical analysis of developmental language disorders: a study of the morphosyntax of children with specific language disorders, children with hearing impairment and children with Down's syndrome. *Clinical Linguistics and Phonetics* 4 (1), 77–86.

Fey, M.E., Long, S.H. and Finestack, L.H. (2003) Ten principles of grammar facilitation for children with specific language impairments. *American Journal of Speech-Language Pathology* 12, 3–15.

Geerts G., Haeseryn W., Rooij, J. de and Toorn, M.C. van den (1984) *Algemene Nederlandse Spraakkunst*. Groningen: Wolters-Noordhoff.
Hunt, K.W. (1970) Syntactic maturity in school children and adults. *Monograph of the Society for Research in Child Development* 134, 35 (1).
Klooster, W.G., Verkuyl, H.J. and Luif, J.H.J. (1974) *Inleiding tot de Syntaxis, Praktische Zinsleer van het Nederlands*. Culemborg: Stam/Robijns.
Pollmann, T. and Sturm, A. (1980) *Over Zinnen Gesproken, Termen en Begrippen van de Traditionele Grammatica*. Culemborg: Tjeenk Willink/Noorduijn.
Toorn, M.C. van den (1979) *Nederlandse Grammatica*. Groningen: Wolters-Noordhoff.
Wells, G. (1985) *Language Development in the Pre-School Years*. Cambridge: Cambridge University Press.

Appendix 6.1 The Dutch profile chart

naam: GRAMAT geboortedatum: datum opname: leeftijd: naam therapeut: opmerkingen:						
A. Niet te analyseren Onbegrijpelijk/onverstaanbaar Afwijkend Minor			Niet compleet Ambigu Zelfherhalingen			
B. Te analyseren uitingen MLU			Totaal aantal uitingen MLUL			
Fase I 1;0–1;6	N	V	Rest			
Fase II 1;6–2;0	Clause				Phrase	Morfologie
	Imper	Inter	Affirmatief			
			SA SV AV		dem detN ers	dim 2^e/3^e enk
Fase III 2;0–2;6	VX	VSX	OV SC SVA AA SAA OAV SVC SVO SVAA SVAO		copula aux ajdN prepdetN prepN	-s/-en 1^e enk adj-e volt dw
Fase IV 2;6–3;0		QXY	VC En OA AAV SVAC 4+		possN appositie detadjN inter preppers advadv	ovt
Fase V 3;0–3;6		QXYZ	Subord Coörd		advadj indef	
Fase VI 3;6–4;0		VSXY			preppossN er	
	Rest				rest	rest

7 LLARSP: A Grammatical Profile for Welsh[1]

Martin J. Ball and Enlli Môn Thomas

Introduction

Although LARSP, and other profiles (see Crystal, 1982, and Chapters 1 and 2, this volume) exist for English, relatively little work has been done for the other languages of Britain. That Britain is indeed a multilingual country can be seen, for example, in Britain (2007). The increased interest in bilingualism and speech pathology is reflected in Hua and Dodd (2006) and McLeod (2007) among many others. Bringing these two developments together has motivated a grammatical profile for Welsh.

The first author previously discussed the desirability of a Welsh version of LARSP (Ball, 1979, 1981, 1982), and this chapter is an attempt to provide this, and is an expansion of Ball (1988a). The Welsh version of LARSP has been christened LLARSP (pronounced [ɬarsp]). This is obviously designed as a humorous 'Welsh' adaptation of LARSP. For those who like their acronyms to stand for something, we suggest *Llawn Asesiad o Ramadeg Siaradwyr â Phroblemau* ('Full Assessment of the Grammar of Speakers with Problems').[2]

The following sections describe how LLARSP was designed, and what the various forms cover. As this chapter is intended for a wide audience, mostly non-Welsh speaking, we have kept examples to a minimum, and not included any sample transcripts or full analyses of data. No discussion is given on sampling procedures for LLARSP, or transcription and scanning of the data, as no changes are necessary in these respects to the guidelines provided in Crystal *et al.* (1976), with the exception of an extra scan in order to analyse mutation information (see below). We begin, however, with a consideration of the bilingual language acquisition situation in Wales.

The Nature of Welsh-English Bilinguals in Wales

Bilinguals are by nature heterogeneous (Grosjean, 1998; Wei, 2000; Romaine, 1995). *Simultaneous bilinguals* (McLaughlin, 1978; also referred to as *early bilinguals* – cf. *bilingual first language acquisition* – De Houwer, 1990) develop their two linguistic systems in close temporal proximity, usually before the age of three, whilst *successive bilinguals* (McLaughlin, 1978; also referred to as *consecutive bilinguals*[3]) typically learn a second language sometime after the development of the first. Whilst most bilinguals in Wales are successive bilinguals exposed to English at home and Welsh at school, there remains a core sample of L1 Welsh-speaking children who are developing bilingually with English as their 'other' L1 or as an L2.

The extent to which bilinguals gain native-like proficiency in their two languages varies from one individual to the next, depending on their linguistic experiences (Gathercole, 1986, 2002a, 2002b, 2002c; Oller, 2005; Oller & Eilers, 2002; Grosjean, 1998, 2000; Li, 1996), age of acquisition (Johnson & Newport, 1989; Mayberry, 2007), language dominance in the community (Gathercole & Thomas, 2009; Paradis, 2010), and a whole host of other socio- and psychological variables (see e.g. Baker (2006) for a review). In Wales, variations in children's linguistic performance across the simultaneous-successive bilingual continuum are largely influenced by exposure patterns (Gathercole & Thomas, 2009) and language use (Morris, 2010). To illustrate, the amount of time Welsh-speaking bilinguals spend hearing and speaking Welsh is related to their success with certain linguistic forms in the language (Gathercole *et al.,* 2001; Gathercole & Thomas, 2005, 2009; Gathercole, 2007a). For example, Gathercole and Thomas (2005) revealed differences in performance on the interpretation of 'distant' gender markers in relation to human antecedents across various 'types' of Welsh-English bilinguals. Children from only Welsh- and mixed Welsh- and English-speaking homes performed well by age five, whilst children from only English-speaking homes performed well by age seven. Moreover, when the (homonymic) possessive adjective *ei* 'his/her/its' was in reference to a feminine human antecedent, children from only Welsh-speaking homes performed well by age five, those from mixed Welsh and English homes performed well by age seven, whereas those from only English-speaking homes showed no progression with age, and performed poorly in general on this construct.

Such delays in certain types of bilinguals' performance are not indicative of a language problem per se. Bilinguals are able to achieve native-like competence with particular structures, albeit at a later stage, once they receive the appropriate 'critical mass of exposure' (Marchman & Bates, 1994) that may be necessary in order to gain native-like command of those structures (Oller & Eilers, 2002; Gathercole, 2007a). This has been demonstrated for vocabulary (e.g. Cobo-Lewis *et al.,* 2002a, 2002b) and certain aspects of morphosyntax (e.g. Gathercole, 2002c). However, when structures are complex, even for L1 speakers, due to opaque form-function mappings, such gains in command are not guaranteed (Gathercole, 2007b; Gathercole *et al.,* 2001; Gathercole & Thomas, 2005; Gathercole & Thomas, 2009; Thomas, 2001; Thomas & Gathercole, 2005, 2007). When aiming to develop tools for the purpose of testing bilingual speaker competence, then, knowledge of the typical developmental patterns of various structures is crucial in order to be able to match a given child's linguistic profile to that which is typical of same age peers. More crucially, however, is the need to match that child to same age peers receiving similar types of exposure to each language (Gathercole *et al.*, 2008; Oller, 2005). Unless such profiles are available, one can easily underestimate children's performance, leading to incorrect diagnosis and interpretations of the results. The next section outlines some of the known developmental patterns relating to bilingual children's acquisition of Welsh.

Acquisition Patterns

Cross-linguistic studies have demonstrated that early verbal morphology, among other grammatical constructs, is acquired in a piecemeal fashion (e.g. Gathercole *et al.*, 1999; Braine, 1976; Bloom *et al.*, 1980; Clark, 1982; Pizzuto & Caselli, 1992, 1993, 1994; Tomasello, 1992, 2000a, 2000b; Pine & Lieven, 1993, 1997; Shirai & Andersen, 1995; Lieven *et al.*, 1997; Pine *et al.*, 1998; Rubino & Pine, 1998). For example, verbs are treated as individual lexical items whose behaviour must be learned one by one; early uses lack a more abstract syntactic argument structure (Tomasello, 2000a). Likewise, with determiners, Pine and Lieven (1997) found that two- to three-year-olds used *a* and *the* with almost completely different sets of nouns. Such findings suggest that early language knowledge does not consist of broad linguistic categories (i.e. the children in Pine and Lieven's study did not possess a general abstract category for determiner that included both *a* and *the*). Rather, children are constructing their own knowledge, learning individual uses of various nouns in combination with a determiner and various uses of verbs on an item-by-item basis. Although little work has been conducted on the acquisition of Welsh, recent studies of children's acquisition of grammatical gender seem to support these cross-linguistic findings.

All nouns in Welsh (animate and inanimate) are either masculine or feminine.[4] The gender of a noun cannot be inferred from the basis of noun form, and the assignment of a noun to a particular gender is often arbitrary. Both Soft Mutation (SM) and Aspirate Mutation (AM) play a crucial role in the way gender is marked in the language.[5] A noun's gender is indicated as follows.

Feminine singular nouns with mutatable onsets undergo SM after the definite article *y(r)* [6] 'the' and after the numeral *un* 'one' – *y gath* < *cath* 'the cat' (fem.), vs. *y ci* < *ci* 'the dog' (masc.). This applies also to adjectives that are used nominally in place of feminine singular nouns (*y fechan* < *bechan* 'the little (girl)') (Tallerman, 1987). When modifying feminine singular nouns, adjectives (or nouns behaving adjectivally) also undergo SM: *cath ddu* < *du* 'black cat' vs. *ci du* < *du* 'black dog'. This applies to all adjectives that occur in a sequence (*cath fawr ddu* < *mawr, du* 'big black cat' vs. *ci mawr du* 'big black dog'). A noun's form provides no indication of its gender (although it is reported that there are some regularities in the endings of some abstract nouns, see Surridge (1989)), but there are small sets of quantifiers and adjectives that have marked feminine forms that do agree with the gender of the co-occurring noun. However, the use of these feminine forms is minimal, even in literary Welsh (Watkins, 1993).

Distant marked elements, in the choice of pronouns and possessives, must also agree with the gender of the antecedent noun. For example, the (homonymic) possessive adjective *ei* 'his/her/its' denotes feminine possession when marked by AM on the modified word (*Mae'r gath wedi brifo ei phen* < *pen* 'The cat has hurt her/its head', *ei thrwyn* < *trwyn* 'her/its nose', *ei choes* < *coes* 'her/its leg'). Masculine possession, in this same context, is marked by SM on the modified word (e.g. *Mae'r ci wedi brifo ei ben* < *pen* 'The dog has hurt his/its head', *ei drwyn* < *trwyn* 'his/its nose', *ei goes* < *coes* 'his/its leg'). Note that SM is used here to mark masculine gender, whereas after the definite article and on modifying adjectives, SM is used to denote feminine gender. Whilst these distant agreement patterns are applicable equally to animate and inanimate nouns alike, the extent to which speakers mark inanimate nouns for gender in this way is unclear (see e.g. Jones (1993) and Jones (1998) for Welsh; Dorian (1976) for Scottish Gaelic).

Beyond the incongruous marking of gender in colloquial speech, and the contradictory association of SM with feminine vs. masculine gender across the two contexts, there are additional features that make the gender system even less transparent (see Gathercole *et al.,* 2001; Thomas & Gathercole, 2007):

(i) There is no one-to-one correspondence between form and function (i.e. SM does not 'mean' any type of gender; other triggering environments also trigger SM).
(ii) There are gaps in the system (e.g. plural feminine nouns do not undergo mutation, not even in the contexts where singular feminine nouns do).
(iii) There are cases in which there is no overt marker of gender – namely words beginning with non-mutatable word-initial consonants (e.g. /v/-, /l/-, /h/-, /s/-initial words).

In relation to children's productive knowledge of the system, results from Gathercole and Thomas's (2005) study demonstrate clearly that children are building up their knowledge of the system around individual items. Children learned to mark masculine before feminine forms and performed better on real than on novel nouns, on nouns with human referents than on nouns with animal or inanimate referents, and on native than on borrowed vocabulary. In relation to their receptive knowledge of long-distant gender constructs, performance was better with pronouns than with the (homonymic) possessive adjective *ei* 'his/her/its', with children exposed to Welsh in the home acquiring masculine and feminine pronouns denoting humans by age five and those exposed to Welsh at school acquiring these forms by age seven. Other parts of the system – for instance, feminine *ei* 'her/its' – seemed to create particular difficulty for children exposed to Welsh at school at all ages, whilst inanimate forms seemed to cause difficulty for *all* children even at age nine. Whether children ever achieve adult-like competence with the system is unclear, especially given that (feminine) gender is marked inconsistently in the input (Jones, 1998; Thomas & Gathercole, 2005). As a consequence, any 'late' development or apparent 'lack' of receptive or productive knowledge of such a system may not necessarily signify language disorder. Instead, such performance may be attributable to the complexity of the system, in combination with the quality and/or quantity of exposure. A similar pattern can be seen for mutation. Thomas and Gathercole (2007) (also reported in Thomas, 2001, 2007) found a continual progression across age (4;6 – 9 years) in relation to children's productive command of Soft Mutation (SM) after selected triggering prepositions, but no progression in relation to Aspirate Mutation (AM) after selected triggering conjunctives. Although they were yet to reach the adult norm with SM, even at age nine, the fact that they were 'approaching' the adult norm is indicative of continual learning. With AM, on the other hand, although the adults outperformed the children, the lack of continual progression across age, coupled with the low performance among the adults (see also Ball, 1984), is indicative of structural change. Profiling children's use of SM is thus more useful than profiling their use of AM, especially for assessment purposes.

Other, equally complex structures may provide good exemplars for a language test. For example, recent exploration of adults' naturalistic speech (Thomas & Schiemenz, in preparation) suggests that Welsh plural morphology is marked appropriately in most cases. Errors are infrequent, with the overextension of the English *–(ie)s* ending being the most common alternative form. Profiling children's use of the plural form over time would help highlight certain difficulties should a child make specific errors with particular items.

Other useful indicators of the linguistic achievements of bilinguals would be those items that all children acquire by a certain age, regardless of their linguistic background. In relation to children's interpretation of sentential arguments in Welsh, Gathercole *et al.* (2005) found an increase in performance across age, with most children (bar those with the least amount of input in Welsh) performing equally well at age nine. In terms of language exposure, when a given sentence involved a verb-noun-noun construction (mirroring the possible VSO word-order pattern of Welsh), children from Welsh-speaking homes interpreted the first noun as the subject more often than children from mixed Welsh- and English-speaking homes, who, in turn, interpreted the first noun as the subject more often than children from English-speaking homes. However, when a given sentence involved a noun-verb-noun construction (mirroring the dominant SVO word order of English), children from mixed Welsh- and English-speaking homes attending bilingual schools tended to interpret the first noun as the subject more often than children from Welsh-speaking or English-speaking homes, even as early as age five. This result is indicative of cross-linguistic acceleration across commonalities in structure, which differs from transfer – the 'incorporation of a grammatical property into one language from the other' (Paradis & Genesee, 1996: 3) – which is a common property among young bilinguals in particular. An essential component of linguistic transfer has to do with the identification of 'systemic' vs. 'episodic' incorporation of a foreign grammar. In order to demonstrate true transfer, one must first demonstrate that the influence is pervasive – 'sustained over a period of time' (Paradis & Genesee, 1996: 3) – not resulting from temporary performance effects (e.g. random instances of code-mixing). Moreover, as a consequence of true transfer, bilinguals' developing grammars will differ necessarily from those of monolinguals, at least temporarily. In order to demonstrate true transfer, therefore, one must also demonstrate differences in bilinguals' patterns of development as compared to those of monolinguals (or near-monolinguals) learning the same language. Since the ultimate goal of an assessment tool is to identify typical vs. atypical language development, the ability to distinguish between instances of transfer and those of true deviance is crucial for a valid assessment of bilinguals.

Design of LLARSP

The adaptation of the LARSP profile for Welsh naturally presented several problems. Perhaps the most important of these is the lack of comprehensive developmental data concerning grammatical development in children's acquisition of Welsh (though see Jones (1980), the important advances in Jones (1986), and the preceding section of this chapter). Further, as noted above, differential types of bilingualism result in different ages at which language structures are acquired. By leaving ages off the chart, we can accommodate children acquiring Welsh from different linguistic backgrounds.

So, even without this information, certain predictions can be made about language development, as work on language universals has distinguished between universal and language-specific characteristics of acquisition in many cases. We can therefore be reasonably certain that the LARSP distinctions between one-word and two-element stages, for example, will hold also for Welsh, as will a stage involving the acquisition of recursion, and so forth.

Many Welsh grammatical patterns are similar to their English counterparts, and can therefore be expected to develop in a similar way. However, there are both clause-level and phrase-level structures, not to mention complex patterns of inflectional morphology and morphophonology, that cannot be related to English equivalents. In the case of these patterns in the syntax, a tentative developmental classification has been attempted. Although this is only tentative, it can naturally be viewed as a developmental hypothesis: a starting-point for further research. In the case of morphology, no developmental metric has been introduced. This is similar to LARSP, where the designers note that detailed information about the normal order of the development of English inflectional endings is lacking, and that the order they propose must be adopted with caution. Because of these factors, the stages of syntax development cannot be so strictly associated with age ranges; therefore, as mentioned, while the stage numbering is retained, the LLARSP-C chart does not show age ranges.

Another problem concerns the inflectional morphology of Welsh. Particularly in respect of the verb, the inflectional morphology of Welsh is much richer than that of English. For this reason, the word-level analysis of the LARSP chart is removed from the Welsh equivalent, LLARSP-C (C = *cystrawen*, 'syntax'), which becomes purely syntactic. Instead, a new morphology chart has been designed: LLARSP-M (M= *morffoleg*, 'morphology'). This contains a maximum amount of morphological information, and in due course it may prove possible to simplify this somewhat. This, however, will depend on feedback from users, and on information regarding developmental morphology. As noted previously, LLARSP-M has no developmental metric, and it is possible this could be added in the future should more research of the type described earlier be undertaken.

The final LLARSP chart, LLARSP-T (T = *treigladau*, 'mutations'), is for recording word-initial consonant mutations (see Ball & Müller, 1992). While these are phonological realizations, they are triggered by morphological and syntactic conditions. Again, due to lack of detailed information, developmental aspects are ignored on this chart. However, an attempt has been made to incorporate sociolinguistic information (see Ball, 1984) on the use of these mutations. Therefore, only those environments that commonly trigger mutations in spoken Welsh (as opposed to literary Welsh; see Price (1984) for discussion of these terms) are included. Furthermore, the layout of the chart avoids an overly simplistic error analysis approach here, containing instead the facility to mark which mutation, if any, was used by the patient. Analysis of the actual usage can then be undertaken with community norms of usage in mind.

A final problem that presented itself concerned the language of the charts and grammatical category labelling. Being a profile of Welsh, there is a strong social argument for LLARSP to be presented in Welsh. The version shown here has not been so presented, however. One reason for this is to aid readers of this chapter. However, potential users of LLARSP will also be familiar with the English LARSP, and will not have to learn a new set of terminology, which, even for the Welsh speaker, might well be unfamiliar. A final point in this respect concerns abbreviations for grammatical categories. The single letter clause level abbreviations of English – S, V, O, C, A – cannot be copied in Welsh, as both 'subject' and 'object' start with the same letter: *goddrych*, 'subject', *gwrthrych*, 'object'. Certain new categories are found at the phrase level (for example, aspect, complementizer), but these are not exclusively Welsh, the English terms having a wide currency. It may indeed be felt necessary in due course to translate headings and so forth into Welsh, but there are strong arguments for keeping the grammatical labels as at present. In general, theoretical labels are not translated: Noun Phrase is NP in English, French, and German. The size of the profiling charts would probably preclude a bilingual presentation as too confusing and difficult to read. Appendix 1 lists the Welsh equivalents of the headings found in LARSP.

LLARSP-C

The same initial sections (A-D) as are found on the LARSP chart were included here (the changes to Section A are discussed under 'Code-switching' below). These are not language specific and are as relevant for Welsh as for English. The Minor/Major sentence distinction is retained for the same reason, as are the distinctions between Command, Question, and Statement, and Connectivity, Clause and Phrase, and the developmental Stages I-VII. The LLARSP-C chart is shown in Figure 7.1.

The structures to be recorded at Stage I of development are so simple (be they Minor or Major) that no differences need be shown here between LARSP and LLARSP-C.

At Stage II the first main differences between the charts emerge. Under Command, the VX category *is* retained, for utterances such as *Dere 'ma, Tyd 'ma,* 'Come here', and so forth. However, an extra category, *paid* X, is included. This is the negative form of the imperative, and is given a separate category as it does not show negative in the same way as other structures. *Paid* (and the less intimate *peidiwch,* which is also included in this category) literally mean 'cease, stop', and may be followed by *â*, but this is not given separate status on the form: *paid â* forms being entered also as Stage II other, phrasal. A one word *paid* command is not differentiated from other one-word commands however. *Cer!* 'Go', and *paid!* are both classed as Stage I Command, V.

The Question column is identical in the two charts; thus QX could stand for *Ble Tada?* 'Where Daddy?', and so on.

The clause level shows only one change, but one that is reflected throughout the chart: SV of LARSP is replaced by VS. Welsh is traditionally termed a VSO language in that, in normal sentences, some part of the verb phrase occurs first. In inflected tenses, this is straightforward:

118 Assessing Grammar

A	**Unanalysed** 1 Unintelligible 2 Symbolic 3 Deviant Noise			**Problematic** 1 Incomplete	2 Ambiguous	3 Stereotypes	
	Codeswitching 1 Sentence 2 Clause 3 Element 4 Phrasal						

			Normal Response				Abnormal	
B	**Responses**	Repetitions	Major				Structural	Problems
			Elliptical			Full	Minor	
	Stimulus type Totals		1	2	3+	Reduced		
	Questions							
	Others							
C	**Spontaneous**							

			General	Structural		Other	Problems
D	**Reactions**						

Stage I
Minor	Responses		Vocatives		Other		Problems
Major	Comm	Quest		Statement			
	'V'	'Q'	'V'	'N'	other	problems	

Stage II
Conn	Clause				Phrase		
	VX	QX	VS	AX	DN	VV	
			SO	VO	NAdj	Vpart	
			SC	VC	NN	IntX	
	paid X		NegX	Other	PrN	Aspyn	
					Cp.yn	Other	

Stage III
X+S:NP	X+V:VP	X+C:NP		X+O:NP		X+A:AP	
VXY	QXY	VSO	VcSC	VOA	DNAdj		DND
		VSA	CVcS	VCA	NAdjAdj	Pron ^p_o	Cop
paid XY	VS(X)	VSC	VcSA		PrDN	Aux ^b_l	Asp
		NegXY		other	NDN		other
gad XY							

Stage IV
XY+S:NP	XY+V:VP	XY+C:NP		XY+O:NP		XY+A:AP	
VXY+	QXY+	VSAA	VcSXY		NPPrNP	VNeg	
	VSX(Y+)	VSOA	CVcSA		PrDNAdj	NegX	
paid		VSOC			NPDNP	2Aux	
XY+	tag	VSCA			cX		
		AAXY		other	XcX		other

Stage V
a	Coord	Coord	Coord	1	1+	Postmod	1	1+
c	other	other	SubordA	1	1+	clause		
s			S	C	O	Postmod	1+	
other			Comparative			phrase		

Stage VI
	(+)					(-)		
NP	VP	Clause		Conn	Clause	Phrase		
Initiator		cael			Element	NP	VP	
	complex	passive		a		D Pr Pron	Aux^b	Aux^l
coord.				c	↔	D Pr	Asp	
		complem.		s	Concord	D↔ Pr↔		
						Gen Cp.yn	Aux^b	Aux
		exclam.					Cop	
Other						Ambiguous		

Stage VII
Discourse			Syntactic Comprehension	
A connectivity	empty mae'n			
Comment Clause	empty mae'na		Style	
Emphatic order	other			

Total no.	Mean No. Sentences	Mean Sentence
Sentence	Per Turn	Length

©D. Crystal, P. Fletcher, M. Garman, 1981 revision, University of Reading.
© Martin J. Ball, Welsh version

Figure 7.1 The LLARSP-C chart

(1) *Dangosodd Siôn y llyfr i Mair*
    'Showed Siôn the book to Mair' >
    'Siôn showed the book to Mair'

However, in periphrastic constructions, the verb phrase is split, with the auxiliary occurring before the Subject, and the rest of the verb phrase (aspect marker and main verb) following it:

(2) *Roedd Siôn yn dangos y llyfr i Mair*
    'Was Siôn aspect show the book to Mair' >
    'Siôn was showing the book to Mair'

Theoretical accounts of Welsh syntax (for example Jones & Thomas, 1977) have proposed various ways of describing this problem. One is to assume an underlying SVO structure, with a transformational rule fronting an AUX (or tense-bearing) category; though equally possible is a VSO structure with uninflected verb structures being moved beyond the Subject NP by a transformation. In analysing sentences for LLARSP, it is suggested that sentences like (1) and (2) above are not differentiated at Clause level, both being assigned a structure of VSOA. The use of auxiliaries can be shown at Phrase level.

(3) *Dangosodd Siôn y llyfr i Mair*
    V   S   O   A
(4) *Roedd Siôn yn dangos y llyfr i Mair*
    V-   S   -V   O   A

At Stage II, VS can stand for adult-like utterances (with an intransitive verb) as well as for shortened immature, or elliptical utterances. The other categories can only be reduced or elliptical utterances.

We need to note, of course, that SV of LARSP and VS of LLARSP-C are simply a conventional ordering of symbols reflecting the unmarked order of elements. Other arrangements of these (and other elements) are naturally encountered. So, VSO, SVO, SOV, VOS, and so on will all be classed as VSO on LLARSP-C, with additional information as to the reason for the marked order (emphatic order, element order, error, etc.) being entered as well.

As in LARSP, NegX is used for non-adult type negation of the entire clause, and should not be confused with phrasal negation. The difference can be seen below:

(5) *Mam dim*
    'Mummy not' > 'That's not Mummy', 'Mummy's not going', etc. Clausal.
(6) *Mam ddim yn mynd*
    'Mummy not aspect + go' > 'Mummy's not going'. Phrasal.

It is often difficult to differentiate between Clausal and Phrasal negation. In English, the presence of the *do* auxiliary with the negative *not* is often taken as a sign of phrasal negation. In Welsh we would suggest that, as in (6) above, the presence of the aspectual marker following the negative in periphrastic verb phrases may be seen as an equivalent. In ambiguous contexts, the general level of the patient's language will aid the decision, though underestimating ability is preferred to overestimating (Crystal, personal communication).

At phrase level, a word-order difference can again be noticed, in that adjectives in Welsh generally follow the noun, though naturally NAdj would cover examples of preceding adjectives as well. IntX is kept, although some intensifiers follow the word they are qualifying (e.g. *hapus iawn*, literally 'happy very'). Two new categories are Asp.*yn* and Cp.*yn*. These concern the connective function of the particle *yn*. As an aspect marker before verbs it indicates progressive aspect: *yn mynd*, 'going'. As a complementizer before nouns and adjectives, it functions as a link between intensive verbs and their complements: *Mae e'n hapus* ('Is he cp. happy' > 'He's happy'): see (7).

(7) *Mae e'n hapus*
    V S C
    cop Pron^P cp.*yn* Adj

These two uses of *yn* cause different mutations,[7] and prepositional *yn* causes yet another mutation condition (Asp.*yn* causes no mutation; Cp.*yn* causes soft mutation; prepositional *yn* causes nasal mutation). For this reason alone a separate classification is justified. It is assumed that the particle uses of *yn* may well begin at this stage, though they may not become widespread until later. For this reason, the other aspect markers are not listed until Stage III.

VPart is retained because, although this is a relatively rare Welsh construction, it has become widespread due to the adoption of calques from English. Thus we get *dechrau lan*, 'start up', and *troi off*, 'turn off'. Blends between Stages II and III, and III and IV are as for LARSP, and need no further comment.

At Stage III further differences are noticeable. In the Command column we have again included the *paid* form. Also we have *gad* (which includes the more formal *gadewch* as well) as the equivalent of *let*, though no ready equivalent of the *do* XY structure presents itself.

The Question column does not differ from LARSP, but VS in the Question column does present a potential confusion with VS in the Statement column. Unlike in English, where word order is an important factor in distinguishing question forms from statements, questions in modern spoken Welsh do not depend on word order. Rather the form of the auxiliary verb *bod,* 'to be', is an important distinguisher (see the section on morphology below). If no auxiliary is present, as in non-periphrastic constructions, intonation is the only sure guide (the claim that initial consonant mutations play a part here does not hold up for many dialects). These two factors must be borne in mind, then, when assigning VS structures (and VS+) to Question or Statement.

At Clause level, all the LARSP structures are repeated (though Verb first), except VOdOi. The indirect object structure does not occur, a preposition always being necessary. Therefore these would be classified as Adverbial. Three new structures are present, all using the symbol Vc. This is used to indicate the copula, as various special sentence patterns are found with the copula at this level. The three indicated on the chart are illustrated below:

(8) VcSC: Mae Llinos yn athrawes
             'is Llinos cp. teacher' >
             'Llinos is a teacher'
(9) CVcS: *Athrawes ydy Llinos*
             'teacher is Llinos' >
             'Llinos is a teacher'
(10) VcSA: *Mae Llinos yng Nghaerdydd*
             'Is Ll. in Cardiff' >
             'Llinos is in Cardiff'

Not only are two of these special structures (because of the word-ordering of CVcS, and because in VcSA the copula is the only intensive verb allowing A as a part compulsory element, though several extensive verbs do), but the copula itself is so morphologically complex that there is a strong argument for it to be pointed out separately at this level.

At Phrase level, many of the classifications are equivalent to those on LARSP. NDN is a new structure, standing for the Welsh genitive structure. This is illustrated below:

(11) *llyfr yr athro*
     'book the teacher' >
     'the teacher's book'

Simpler genitives, not requiring the determiner, are also found, as:

(12) *Tŷ Mr Jones*
     'house Mr Jones' >
     'Mr Jones's house'

These would be classed as NN at Stage II, and it is hypothesized that they are similar developmentally to English NN structures, with reversed word order.

Another new structure at Stage III Phrase level is Asp. This includes the perfective aspect marker, seen in:

(13) *Mae Caryl wedi mynd*
 'is   C.   asp go' >
 'Caryl has gone'

The remaining aspect markers are mostly prepositional in form. These include *ar,* 'about to', *newydd,* 'just' (time), *am,* 'wanting to' and *gan,* 'while', and are all classified here. Complex forms such as *wedi bod yn,* 'have been -ing' are classified as 2Aux. Observation suggests that these aspect markers develop later than the *yn* continuous aspect marker. It may be that the prepositional types, too, develop later than the more basic *wedi.* This is another area where feedback from users is required.

The division of the Aux category also differs from LARSP. Following Jones and Thomas (1977), we have set up a category of Aux^b (b = *bod,* 'to be'). This auxiliary is used with all aspect markers, and to a great extent is the equivalent of Aux^o of LARSP. Aux^l stands for lexical auxiliaries, which cover various modal meanings, though two of these can also be used as simple tense-carrying auxiliaries (*gwneud* and *darfod*). The list of Aux^l is: *gwneud,* 'do', *darfod,* 'happen', *cael,* 'receive (permission, etc.); have', *gallu, medru,* 'to be able', *dylu,* 'to be likely, ought'. Following Jones and Thomas (1977), other similar constructions will be classed as VV, for example *Rwi 'n moyn mynd,* 'I want to go'.

DND represents the common Welsh feature of dividing parts of determiners into pre- and post-noun position. Examples include *y dyn hwn,* 'the man this' > 'this man', and *ei gath e,* 'his cat he' > 'his cat'. Abbreviated forms of the latter example, *gath e/cath e,* should be classed as DN. The possessive determiners also occur with verbs, representing object pronouns in periphrastic verb phrases:

(14) *Mae Pam yn fy ngweld i*
 'Is Pam asp *my* see' >
 'Pam is seeing me/Pam sees me'

This usage appears to be acquired later than with nouns. We have not established a separate category for it, however, and suggest Stage III Other, though this may need to be changed in the future. Abbreviated forms of this usage, for example *mae Pam yn gweld i,* should have the *i* recorded simply as Pron^p. A problem arises in both noun and verb cases if the possessive in pre-noun/verb position is absent, but the mutation is present. This is tackled in LLARSP by recording the mutation in the relevant position on LLARSP-T, but ignoring it on LLARSP-C.

In Stage IV Commands, the LARSP +S category is omitted as inappropriate to Welsh. In the Question column the QVS category is also omitted for, as noted above, word order is not a distinguishing feature of Welsh questions. Following Jones and Thomas (1977), the VSAA structure is differentiated from other AA+ structures in the Statement Clause column. This is to account for verbs like *cwyno .. am .. wrth,* 'complain .. about .. to', and *cytuno .. am .. gyda,* 'agree .. about .. with', which require two adverbial elements. This separate VSAA category may not prove necessary in the long-term. Expanded versions of the Vc structures of Stage III are also found at Stage IV.

Stage IV Phrase level contains one structure different from LARSP: NPDNP allows the classification of more complex genitive structures. VNeg is used rather than NegV, because in spoken Welsh the negative element (often *dim/dddim*) usually follows the verb. Pre-verbal negative particles are rarely heard in modern spoken Welsh, but see below for a discussion of all the pre-verbal particles.

Stage V is virtually identical to LARSP Stage V. It should be noted that spoken Welsh usually omits relativizers, relying on mutation to mark different types of relative clauses. In such cases, the mutation will be marked on LLARSP-T, and no subordinator will be marked.

Stage VI is similar to LARSP Stage VI in its marking of categories not previously identified in Stages I-V, and errors. The categories in the (+) box are mostly the same, although slightly different names are adopted in some instances. The equivalents of English initiators structure differently in Welsh in some cases, in that, while some are pre-determiners, others follow the noun. Examples like *rhai o,* 'some of' are classed as initiators, as is *i gyd,* 'all', even though it follows the noun it qualifies: *rhai o'r moron,* 'some of the carrots', *y moron i gyd,* 'all the carrots'.

Stage VI NP Coordination is retained for apposition, noun lists, and so forth.

The passive to be marked is the *cael* passive, as the inflected passive (or impersonal) is far less commonly found in speech, even by adults:

(15) *Cafodd Owain ei weld gan Gwen*
    'Got Owain his see by Gwen' >
    'Owain was seen by Gwen' *(cafodd < cael)*

Should the inflected impersonal passive occur, it would be classed in (+) box Other category:

(16) *Gwelwyd Owain gan Gwen*
    'Seen   Owain by Gwen' >
    'Owain was seen by Gwen'

The category Complementation is quite common in Welsh, and apart from covering adjective complementation *(Mae'n hapus i fynd,* 'He's happy to go'), it encompasses many similar constructions, such as *Mae'n bryd i mi fynd,* 'It's time for me to go' and *Mae'n rhaid i mi fynd,* 'I must go'.

The *how* and *what* exclamations of LARSP are simply termed 'exclamations' here. This is usually realized in Welsh by *am* constructions: *Am dywydd!,* 'What weather!'.[8]

Many of the errors, listed under (-), do not differ from those of LARSP. Under NP is included a category for errors in the genitive construction. These could either be of word ordering (for example **John het* for *het John,* 'John's hat'), or through use of the partitive *o,* 'of' (for example **het o John).* Also included is omission of the complementizer *yn.*

Under VP, wrong use or omission of the two classes of Aux can be marked, as can the omission of aspect markers. The omission of the copula use of *bod,* 'to be' is counted as an Element Ø error under Clause. The Cop and Aux[b] categories present totals of wrong forms of the verb *bod,* these being classified more fully on LLARSP-M.

The final Stage, VII, is identical to LLARSP, except that the Welsh forms of empty *it* and empty *there* are given *(mae'n* and *mae 'na* respectively). Particularly common in Welsh is the syntactic device of fronting for emphasis, recorded at this stage under Emphatic Order. Illustrated here are subject fronting and verb phrase fronting, though other types would also be recorded here.

(17) *Llinos sydd yn athrawes* = SVC
 'Llinos is cp. teacher' >
 'Llinos is a teacher/it's Llinos who's a teacher'
(18) *Dysgu yn y coleg ydy Llinos* = VAS
 'Teach in the college is Llinos' >
 'Llinos is teaching in the college.

This account of Welsh syntax has not included pre-verbal particles. In written Welsh these have a major role to play in distinguishing commands, questions, and statements, and positives from negatives. In modern spoken Welsh, however, these have largely been dropped or, in the case of *bod,* 'to be', become integrated into the verb: *roedd < yr oedd,* 'was, were'. The only particles in common use are the emphatic statement particles *fe/mi.* Evidence presented by Jones (1985) suggests these are learnt relatively late. The use of all such pre-verbal particles are to be recorded under Stage VI (+) Other. For the implications of particles in consonant mutation, see LLARSP-T below.

LLARSP-M

The inflectional morphology of Welsh is recorded on the LLARSP-M form. This is divided into four main sections plus a summary. The four sections cover verb phrase, noun phrase, prepositional, and adjectival morphology. For each section errors may be noted, although as yet it is unclear when such errors have developmental status. The LLARSP-M chart is shown in Figure 7.2.

The VP section is divided into four subsections: *bod* ('to be', either as copula or auxiliary), VReg (i.e. regular verb inflections), VIrreg (the morphology of the four common irregular verbs), and Responses, the various ways of saying 'yes' and 'no' in Welsh.

The greatest detail is given to *bod*, the correct usage of this complex verb being important in distinguishing positives and negatives, statements and questions, and definites and indefinites. Following Jones and Thomas (1977), verbal paradigms throughout the VP section are identified by the 3rd person singular form. *Mae* is the 3rd person singular present tense of *bod,* so is found as the first group of paradigms. Unlike other tenses, special forms are found in negatives and questions, with indefinite subjects, and with emphatic order sentences. The phonetic realizations of all these forms differ slightly from dialect to dialect, so are not listed on the form, the conventions of *mae* + neg and *mae* + Q and so on being used instead.

The other tenses of *bod* are *oedd* imperfect, *bu* preterite, *bydd* future, *byddai* conditional, habitual, *buasai* conditional, habitual (there are regional restrictions on these last two, though both may be used in some dialects). Separate question and negative forms are not noted here, and should all be classed together under the relevant tense. *Dyma/dyna* ('here is/there is') are the so-called 'deictic' forms of *bod*.

The VReg subsection contains only the two inflected tenses most likely to occur in speech (though even these are often replaced by periphrastic constructions): the *-ith (-ff* in South Wales) paradigm usually expresses future time, *-odd* (sometimes *-ws* in South Wales) expresses the preterite. Imperative forms can also be marked.

VIrreg marks the future and preterite tenses of the verbs *gwneud,* 'do, make', *cael,* 'have, receive', *mynd,* 'go', and *dod,* 'come'. Again, regional differences of form occur with these verbs.

The Error column for these subsections allows the ticking of the use of the wrong person or tense. An error of 'form' for *bod* is also included for instances when the wrong *mae* paradigm is chosen. For example:

(19) *Mae Glyn ddim yn mynd*
     'Is   Glyn not asp go'

for

(20) *Dydy Glyn ddim yn mynd*
     'Is   Glyn not asp go' >
     'Glyn isn't going'

126 Assessing Grammar

	Morphology					Errors
VP	**BOD**					
	mae 1 2 3 1 2 3	mae + neg 1 2 3 1 2 3	mae + Q 1 2 3 1 2 3	mae + indef: does oes? emphatic: ydy/sydd deictic: dyma/dyna		person form
	oedd 1 2 3 1 2 3	bu 1 2 3 1 2 3	bydd 1 2 3 1 2 3	byddai 1 2 3 1 2 3	buasai 1 2 3 1 2 3	tense
	imperative sing:		plur:		Other	
	V reg					
	-th 1 2 3 1 2 3		-odd 1 2 3 1 2 3	imperative sing: plur: Other		tense person
	V irreg					
	gwneud 1 1 2 2 3 3 1 1 2 2 3 3	cael 1 1 2 2 3 3 1 1 2 2 3 3	mynd 1 1 2 2 3 3 1 1 2 2 3 3	dod 1 1 2 2 3 3 1 1 2 2 3 3 imp.s imp.p		tense person
	Other					
	Responses					
	ydw ydy oes oedd do gwnaf ie other nac nac nac nac maddo na nage					pos/neg type

NP	Plural: -au -iau -ion/on -i -iod
	          V→V V→V-au V→V-iau V→V-ion/on
	          Other
	Sing: -en/yn Det: y yr 'r
						∅
						form
						y→yr
						yr→y

Prep	Class 1 (-o/i) 1 2 3 1 2 3 Class 2 (-ddo/ddi) 1 2 3 1 2 3 gan 1 2 3 1 2 3					∅ person class
Adj	feminine comparison -ach -af			Other		∅ ∅ form
Summary	Total Infl. Morphemes	No. Types	Type: Token ratio	Types/categ. VP NP Prep Adj		Total Errors VP NP Prep Adj

©1987 Martin J. Ball

Figure 7.2 The LLARSP-M chart

The Responses subsection lists the most usual 'yes/no' forms which in Welsh depend on the form of the question. The positive forms are listed below with their usages:

(21) *Ydw*: 1st person singular present.
(22) *Ydy*: 3rd person singular present. This category is also to be used to cover all persons except 1st.
(23) *Oes*: 3rd person singular present, indefinite.
(24) *Oedd*: 3rd person singular imperfect. This category is also to be used to cover all persons.
(25) *Do*: preterite all persons.
(26) *Gwnaf*: 'I will do'. Used here to cover any future tense response.
(27) *Ie*: answer to any non-verb-first question.

The negative responses are shown in shortened form on the chart (apart from *naddo*), the full negative equivalents to (21)–(27) above being: *nac ydw, nac ydy, nac oes, nac oedd, naddo, na wnaf,* and *nage*. Errors in responses involve the wrong 'type' of response (for example *naddo* for *nage*), or the confusion of positive and negative responses.

The NP section mainly concerns the usage of various plural allomorphs. The commonest suffixes are listed, together with an Other category. V→V, and V→V + ending stand for plurals which involve a change of internal vowels. The use of the singular ending that some nouns show can also be marked. The three allomorphs of the determiner can be marked: *yr* before vowels, *'r* after vowels, *y* elsewhere. Errors include zero plural, wrong plural allomorph, and wrong determiner allomorphs.

Prepositions in Welsh, when followed by personal pronouns, display the use of a set of inflectional suffixes. Two main classes exist, depending upon whether the endings are added directly to the root of the preposition, or if an epenthetic consonant is included for 3rd person singular and plural (and often in speech to other persons). This added consonant is usually *dd* (/ð/), though *t* also occurs. The two classes are as follows:

Class I: *amdan-*, 'for', *arn-*, 'on', *at-*, 'towards', *dan-*, 'under', *ohon-*, 'of, from', *wrth-*, 'near'.
Class II: *dros(t)-*, 'over', *heb(dd)-*, 'without', *i(dd)-*, 'to', *rhyng(dd)-*, 'between', *trwy(dd)-*, 'through', *yn(dd)-*, 'in'.

Gan is exceptional, and its forms differ from area to area. Obviously, error markings here will have to take into account these variations. Under Errors, Ø means no ending, rather than no preposition, which would be classed on the LLARSP-C chart.

The next section concerns adjectives. Feminine includes the vowel changes of a small group of adjectives having both masculine and feminine forms. Only those used most commonly in speech are included here: *crwn-cron, dwfn-dofn, llwm-llom, trwm-trom, byr-ber, cryf-cref, gwyn-gwen, gwyrdd-gwerdd, hyll-hell,* ('round', 'deep', 'bare', 'heavy', 'short', 'strong', 'white', 'green', and 'ugly' respectively; masculine first). The change to the initial consonant of the feminine forms (soft mutation) is not marked here, but on the LLARSP-T chart. (This change would normally produce the following feminine forms of the above adjectives: *gron, ddofn, lom, drom, fer, gref, wen, werdd, hell,* this last unmutated.) Therefore, both *merch cref* and *merch gref* ('strong girl') would be marked as correct on LLARSP-M, though *merch cref* would be marked on LLARSP-T as non-usage of soft mutation. The remaining adjective features are the suffixes *-ach,* comparative, and *-af* (or *-a* often in speech), superlative. The *-ed,* equative, is not common in speech, and like plural forms of adjectives (also unusual in speech) it is classed under Other.

The final section of LLARSP-M is a summary of inflected morpheme usage. The difference between the total number of morphemes used (here taken to include allomorphs in the plurals section, etc.) and the number of different types utilized is expressed in the type: token ratio box. A categorization of types used and errors made is also available. The diagnostic capacity of this summary is, as yet, unclear.

LLARSP-T

This chart is for recording the use of initial consonant mutations. These are three classes of phonological changes, which are triggered by syntactic factors rather than phonological. Awbery (1975) gives a theoretical account of them, and Ball (1984, 1988b) a study of their usage in spoken Welsh, with Ball and Müller (1992) providing a view of mutations from many linguistic perspectives. The LLARSP=T chart is shown in Figure 7.3.

Developmentally, relatively little appears to be known, but Bellin (1984) suggests that the age of five may be important with respect to some of the mutation-triggering environments.

The recording of usage on this chart deliberately avoids an error analysis approach because, as noted above, usage patterns differ regionally and stylistically. The classification does, however, permit the teacher/therapist to introduce sociolinguistically acceptable patterns of usage for the commonest triggers.

The Soft Mutation (lenition) is the most important of the three classes, affecting many consonants, and having the greatest number of triggers. It changes voiceless stops to voiced, voiced stops to voiced fricatives (though /g/→∅, due to loss of Old Welsh [ɣ]), voiceless liquids to voiced, and /m/ to /v/.

The chart contains the commonest triggers of the Soft Mutation, as the marking of mutation by triggers rather than by overall phonological type is recommended following Ball (1984), who showed variable usage of

LLARSP: A Grammatical Profile for Welsh

Name			Age		Sample date		Type	
SM	Context	+SM	Rad		Context	+SM	Rad	
	Pr + N D + Nf Num + N Poss + N/V dyma/dyna +N				Nf + Adj Yn + N/Adj V + O (part) + V Other			
NM	Context	+NM		rad		+SM		
	fy + N/V yn + Nproper yn + N Other							
AM	Context	+AM		rad		+SM		
	ei + N/V a + N Other							
over-mutation	SM							
	NM							
	AM							
Other								

Figure 7.3 The LLARSP-T chart

mutations by trigger. In the following abbreviations, the + sign indicates that the mutation applies to the following category.

(i) Pr + N: the inflected prepositions (except *rhwng,* 'between' and *yn,* 'in', but including *hyd,* 'until') cause SM (Soft Mutation) to a following noun (e.g. *i Fangor,* 'to Bangor').
(ii) D + Nf: feminine nouns mutate following the definite article *y* (e.g. *merch, y ferch,* 'girl, the girl').

(iii) Num + N: certain numerals cause SM to following nouns (e.g. *dau/ dwy,* 'two, masc / fem' to all nouns; *un,* 'one' to feminine nouns).

(iv) Poss + N: the possessive determiners *dy* 'your', *ei,* 'his' cause SM. This is also shown + V, as are possessives in the other two mutations. Research has shown (Ball, 1984; Thomas, 1984) that possessives preceding verb-nouns in periphrastic constructions containing an object pronoun do not cause mutation as regularly as when preceding nouns. However, the category of non-mutation usage with possessives should not be used if the possessive is omitted altogether (for example *cath fi,* 'cat me'). If the mutation is present but the possessive is omitted, it should be marked as if normal, as this is a common feature of Welsh speech (for example *nghath i,* '(my) cat me').

(v) *Dyma/dyna*: the 'here is /there is' form of the copula causes SM to a following word (e.g. *Dyna ferch dda,* 'There's a good girl').

(vi) Nf+Adj: adjectives mutate if following a feminine noun (e.g. *bachgen da,* 'good boy', *merch dda,* 'good girl').

(vii) Yn + N/Adj: the complementizer *yn* causes SM, the aspect marker does not (e.g. *mae Bethan yn dal,* 'Bethan is tall' *(dal < tal): mae Bethan yn mynd,* 'Bethan is going').

(viii) V+O: the direct object of an *inflected* verb undergoes mutation (e.g. *Gwelodd Dafydd gathod,* 'Dafydd saw [some] cats' *(gathod < cathod)).*

(ix) (part) + V: clause-initial verbs if preceded by various particles indicating emphasis, questions, and so on, undergo mutation (see the discussion on these earlier). In practice, these are omitted in speech in the great majority of cases, but often the SM remains (e.g. *(A) welodd Siôn y cathod?,* 'Did Siôn see the cats?'; *welodd < gwelodd*). As noted, the only particles regularly appearing are the 'emphatics', *fe* or *mi.*

All the Soft Mutation triggers can be marked + SM to show the mutation was used, or 'rad' (= radical) to show that no change occurred. Due to the variable nature of mutation usage in adult spoken Welsh, however, this should not be considered an error analysis exercise in terms of literary norms.

The Nasal Mutation (NM) converts fortis and lenis plosives to homorganic fortis and lenis nasals. The contexts triggering this include *fy,* 'my', *yn,* 'in' (prepositional usage only), and a set of fossilized time expressions included under Other – for instance *pum mlynedd, pum mlwydd oed, pum niwrnod,* 'five years', 'five years old', 'five days', from *blynedd, blwydd* and *diwrnod* respectively. It should be noted that the *yn* trigger has two contexts: with or without a proper noun (i.e. place names). With place names the mutation is often not used, or is replaced by SM. In filling in the form, usage of the nasal mutation, soft mutation, or no mutation can be noted.

The Aspirate Mutation (AM) converts voiceless plosives to voiceless fricatives. It has a fairly large number of triggers, but in spoken Welsh the only two retained with any degree of frequency are *ei,* 'her' and *a,* 'and'. Again scoring allows the three options of AM, SM, or no mutation. AM following other triggers should be marked under Other, and a full list of those triggers found in literary Welsh can be found in traditional grammars such as Williams (1980).

The final sections of LLARSP-T allow the therapist to note any examples where the mutations are over-extended (i.e. used where neither spoken nor literary Welsh would allow them). The Other category allows the marking of such features as reanalysis. This occurs when an already non-mutated word is re-analysed as being mutated, so that a new radical is provided. An example might be if the word *drws,* 'door', is re-analysed as **trws,* with *drws* being considered a soft mutated form (for the source of this example see Ascott & Ball, 1987).

Finally, we must consider the interplay between phonological development and mutation usage. There is, of course, no point in classing an utterance as non-use of SM, for example, if the distinction between + / − [voice] or + /- [continuant] has not been firmly established by the speaker in word-initial position. The effectiveness of LLARSP-T, then, relies to a great extent on an advanced state of phonological development.

An interesting problem arises if a speaker uses a phonological unit produced by mutation, but does not use it in other environments. For example, a client who can say /v/ in *y ferch,* 'the girl', but not in *'fory,* 'tomorrow'. This should be classed as correct mutation usage, but the special aspect of the usage noted under Other.

Borrowing and Code-switching

One point we have not yet discussed is the problem of profiling borrowing and code-switching. Wales is a bilingual country, and as Bellin (1984) points out, the influence of English is pervasive, such that it is difficult to study Welsh without also considering English. It is true that many Welsh-speaking under-fives are almost monolingual, but many are not. After that age, it is almost impossible to avoid the gradual assimilation of English. How should the therapist analyse code-switching: onto a LARSP or LLARSP? To answer this we can examine three scenarios, which we shall call 'borrowing', 'high-level switching', and 'low-level switching'. (We are not of course suggesting that these features need remediation, simply that when they occur they need to be recorded to get a true profile.)

A borrowing is an example where a single lexical item is borrowed from L1 to L2 or vice versa, the rest of the utterance being unaffected. Isolated lexical borrowings from English (sometimes adapted to Welsh morphophonology) are often heard in spoken Welsh:

(28) *Mae'n mynd i weld y headmaster*
    'He's going to see the headmaster'

(29) *Mae hi'n specialiso*
      'She's specializing'

Examples like this should be analysed as Welsh utterances, with the entire utterance entered onto the relevant LLARSP charts. At present, there is nowhere on the chart that is designed to mark amounts of such borrowing, and we feel information of this kind awaits a Welsh PRISM (Crystal, 1982).

The second category, high-level switching, concerns code-switches at major syntactic boundaries. Examples could include:

(30) *He's not coming achos fod e'n sâl*
      'because he's ill'
(31) *I saw Gwilym yesterday and roedd e'n bendant amdano*
      'he was sure about it'

In our opinion these are best analysed on separate profile charts. For (30) we would recommend the following entries on an English LARSP: SVA, Subord A, plus phrase/word information for *he's not coming* only. Onto Welsh LLARSP-C would be entered VSC, s, plus phrase/word/mutation information for *achos fod e'n sâl* only. We would welcome reaction to this, however.

Low-level switching involves switches at more minor syntactic boundaries, but including more than just single-word borrowings. Examples might include the following:

(32) *I saw y dyn newydd yesterday*
      'the new man'
(33) *Mae 'nhad yn dod to see us tomorrow*
      'My father is coming'

These examples certainly present problems to the analyst. One solution is to assign the utterance to that language which is used for most of the utterance. However, as in (32), this is not always easy to ascertain. Another solution is to include such utterances on profiles for both languages; alternatively they could be excluded altogether.

The revised Section A at the top of the LLARSP-C is an initial attempt to deal with code-switching. It is designed to briefly show the syntactic boundaries at which the code-switching took place (between Sentences, at Clause boundaries, between Clause elements, and between Phrase units). The problem still remains as to whether the utterance, or parts of it, should be analysed onto the rest of LLARSP. Crystal (personal communication) raises the possibility of a superordinate chart of both languages to deal with code-switching, with its own developmental norms. He further suggests that monolingual utterances only should be recorded on LARSP and LLARSP.

Another argument put forward by Crystal is that the teaching tradition is generally not happy about code-switching, and would not teach the use of this feature. However, it is often a strong feature, and can be stylistically useful in bilingual speech communities, and perhaps should not be ignored. We are also unsure about the practicalities of superordinate charts.

To conclude, then, we feel that high-level switches should be dealt with as described above, and suggest that low-level switches should be assigned to whichever chart appears to be the main language of the utterance (though naturally phrase/word level information may need to be transferred to the other chart for parts of the utterance). Again, we will be interested to receive feedback on this issue.

Acknowledgements

We would like to thank David Crystal and Glyn Jones for valuable comments on an earlier version of this chapter. Needless to say, all remaining errors are our responsibility.

Notes

(1) An earlier version of this chapter was published in the journal *Clinical Linguistics and Phonetics*. This revised and expanded version is published with the permission of Informa PLC.
(2) We realize that this should properly be abbreviated to LIARSPh, but beg a little latitude in this regard!
(3) See Wei (2000) for a comprehensive list of the various labels that have been coined in the literature to classify bilinguals into various 'types'.
(4) However, there are some nouns that can be masculine and feminine – e.g. *nyth* 'nest' – often depending on dialect or on gender-marked context. See Thomas (2001) for examples.
(5) Mutations are phonological changes to word initial consonants triggered by grammatical contexts. They are returned to in more detail later in the chapter.
(6) There are three allomorphs of the Welsh definite article: *yr*, *y*, and *'r*. In what follows, *y* will be used wherever there is mention of the definite article (according to Watkins (1993: 313): 'despite being chronologically the most recent variant to emerge, *y* is regarded as the citation form').
(7) We return to mutations below.
(8) Constructions with *dyna* 'there is/are' are also common: *Dyna dywydd iti* 'There's weather for you'.

References

Ascott, F. and Ball, M.J. (1987) Measuring language proficiency in bilingual children: A preliminary study from Welsh. *Cardiff Working Papers in Welsh Linguistics* 5, 29–41.
Awbery, G.M. (1975) Welsh mutations–syntax or phonology? *Archivum Linguisticum* (New Series) 6, 14–25.
Baker, C.R. (2006) *Foundations of Bilingual Education and Bilingualism*. Clevedon: Multilingual Matters.
Ball, M.J. (1979) LLARSP? Paper read at the Oxford meeting of the Welsh Dialectology Circle.

Ball, M.J. (1981) Iaith dan brawf. *Barn,* 221.
Ball, M.J. (1982) Asesu iaith. *Y Gwyddonydd* 20, 126–30.
Ball, M.J. (1984) *Sociolinguistic Aspects of the Welsh Mutation System*. Unpublished PhD thesis: University of Wales.
Ball, M.J. (1988a) LARSP to LLARSP. Designing a Welsh grammatical profile. *Clinical Linguistics and Phonetics* 2, 55–73.
Ball, M.J. (1988b) Variation in the use of initial consonant mutations. In M.J. Ball (ed.) *The Use of Welsh (pp. 70–81)*. Clevedon: Multilingual Matters.
Ball, M.J. and Müller, N. (1992) *Mutation in Welsh*. London: Routledge.
Bellin, W. (1984) Welsh phonology in acquisition. In M.J. Ball and G.E. Jones (eds) *Welsh Phonology: Selected Readings*. Cardiff: University of Wales Press.
Bloom, L., Lifter, K. and Hafitz, J. (1980) Semantics of the verbs and the development of verb inflection in child language. *Language* 56, 366–412.
Braine, M. (1976) Children's first word combinations. *Monographs of the Society for Research in Child Development* 41.
Britain, D. (ed.) (2007) *Language in the British Isles*. Cambridge: Cambridge University Press.
Clark, E. (1982) Theory and method in child-language research: are we assuming too much? In S. Kuczaj (ed.) *Language Development (Vol. 1)*. Hillsdale, NJ: Lawrence Erlbaum.
Cobo-Lewis, A., Pearson, B., Eilers, R. and Umbel, V. (2002a) Effects of bilingualism and bilingual education on oral and written Spanish skills: a multifactor study of standardized test outcomes. In D.K. Oller and R. Eilers (eds) *Language and Literacy in Bilingual Children* (pp. 98–117). Clevedon: Multilingual Matters.
Cobo-Lewis, A., Pearson, B., Eilers, R. and Umbel, V. (2002b) Effects of bilingualism and bilingual education on oral and written English skills: a multifactor study of standardized test outcomes. In D.K. Oller and R. Eilers (eds) *Language and Literacy in Bilingual Children* (pp. 64–67). Clevedon: Multilingual Matters.
Crystal, D. (1982) *Profiling Linguistic Disability*. London: Edward Arnold.
Crystal, D., Fletcher, P. and Garman, M. (1976) *The Grammatical Analysis of Language Disability*. London: Edward Arnold.
De Houwer, A. (1990) *The Acquisition of Two Languages from Birth: A Case Study*. Cambridge: Cambridge University Press.
Dorian, N. (1976) Gender in a terminal Gaelic dialect. *Scottish Gaelic Studies* 12, 279–82.
Gathercole, V.C. (1986) The acquisition of the present perfect: Explaining differences in the speech of Scottish and American children. *Journal of Child Language* 13, 537–560.
Gathercole, V.C. (2002a) Command of the mass / count distinction in bilingual and monolingual children: An English morphosyntactic distinction. *Language and literacy in bilingual children,* 175–206.
Gathercole, V.C. (2002b) Grammatical gender in bilingual and monolingual children: Spanish morphosyntactic distinction. *Language and Literacy in Bilingual Children,* 207–19.
Gathercole, V.C. (2002c) Monolingual and bilingual acquisition: Learning different treatments of *that*-trace phenomena in English and Spanish. *Language and Literacy in Bilingual Children,* 220–54.
Gathercole, V.C. (2007a) *Language Transmission in Bilingual Families in Wales*. Welsh Language Board Consultation Document.
Gathercole, V.C. (2007b) Miami and North Wales, so far and yet so near: Constructivist account of morpho-syntactic development in bilingual children. *The International Journal of Bilingual Education and Bilingualism* 10 (3), 224–47.
Gathercole. V.C.M., Laporte, N.I. and Thomas, E.M. (2005) Differentiation, carry-over, and the distributed characteristic in bilinguals: Structural 'mixing' of the two languages? In J. Cohen, K.T. McAlister, K. Rolstad and J. MacSwan (eds) *Proceedings of the 4th International Symposium on Bilingualism*. Somerville, MA: Cascadilla Press.

Gathercole, V.C.M., Sebastián, E. and Soto, P. (1999) The early acquisition of Spanish verbal morphology: across-the-board or piecemeal knowledge? *International Journal of Bilingualism* 3 (2–3), 133–182.

Gathercole, V.C.M. and Thomas, E.M. (2005) Minority language survival: Input factors influencing the acquisition of Welsh. In J. Cohen, K.T. McAlister, K. Rolstad and J. MacSwan (eds) *Proceedings of the 4th International Symposium on Bilingualism.* Somerville, MA: Cascadilla Press.

Gathercole, V.C.M. and Thomas, E.M. (2009) Bilingual first language development: Dominant language takeover, threatened language take-up. *Bilingualism: Language and Cognition* 12, 213–237.

Gathercole, V.C.M., Thomas, E.M. and Hughes, E.K. (2008) Designing a normed receptive vocabulary test for bilingual populations: A model from Welsh. *International Journal of Bilingual Education and Bilingualism* 11 (6), 678–720.

Gathercole, V.C.M., Thomas, E.M. and Laporte, N.I. (2001) The acquisition of grammatical gender in Welsh. *Journal of Celtic Language Learning* 6, 53–87.

Grosjean, F. 1998 Studying bilinguals: Methodological and conceptual issues. *Bilingualism: Language and Cognition* 1, 131–49.

Grosjean, F. 2000 *Life with Two Languages: An Introduction to Bilingualism.* Harvard: Harvard University Press.

Hua, Z. and Dodd, B. (eds) (2006) *Phonological Development and Disorders in Children: A Multilingual Perspective.* Clevedon: Multilingual Matters.

Johnson, J.S. and Newport, E.L. (1989) Critical period effects in second language learning: The influence of maturational state on the acquisition of English as a second language. *Cognitive Psychology* 21, 60–99.

Jones, B.M. (1993) *Ar lafar ac ar bapur: cyflwyniad i'r berthynas rhwng yr iaith lafar a'r iaith ysgrifenedig.* Y Ganolfan Astudiaethau Addysg: Aberystwyth.

Jones, J.M. (1980) *Cymraeg fel Mamiaith.* Unpublished MEd thesis: University of Wales.

Jones. M.C. (1998) *Language Obsolescence and Revitalization: Linguistic Change in Two Sociolinguistically Contrasting Welsh Communities.* Oxford: Clarendon Press.

Jones, R.M. (1985) Iaith plant – gwallau? Paper read at the Welsh Linguistics Conference, Gregynog.

Jones, R.M. (1986) *Agweddau ar Ystyrau a Phatryman iaith Plant Pump Oed.* Unpublished manuscript: Coleg Prifysgol Aberystwyth.

Jones, R.M. and Thomas, A.R. (1977) *The Welsh Language: Studies in its Syntax and Semantics.* Cardiff: University of Wales Press.

Li, D.C.S. (1996) *Issues in Bilingualism and Biculturalism: A Hong Kong Case Study.* New York: Peter Lang.

Lieven, E., Pine, J. and Baldwin, G. (1997) Lexically-based learning and early grammatical development. *Journal of Child Language* 24, 187–220.

Marchman, V.A. and Bates, E. (1994) Continuity in lexical and morphological development: a test of the critical mass hypothesis. *Journal of Child Language* 21, 339–66.

Mayberry, R. I. (2007) When timing is everything: age of first-language acquisition effects on second-language learning. *Applied Psycholinguistics* 28, 537–49.

McLeod, S. (ed.) (2007) *The International Guide to Speech Acquisition.* San Diego: Delmar-Thomson.

McLaughlin, B. (1978) *Second-Language Acquisition in Childhood.* Hillsdale NJ: Lawrence Erlbaum.

Morris, D. (2010) Young people and their use of the Welsh language. In D. Morris (ed.) *Welsh in the Twenty-First Century* (pp. 80–98). Cardiff: Cardiff University Press.

Oller, D.K. (2005) The distributed characteristic in bilingual learning. In J. Cohen, K.T. McAlister, K. Rolstad and J. MacSwan (eds) *Proceedings of the 4th International Symposium on Bilingualism* (pp. 1744–9). Somerville: Cascadilla Press.

Oller, D.K. and Eilers, R.E. (2002) *Language and Literacy in Bilingual Children.* Clevedon: Multilingual Matters.

Paradis, J. (2010) The interface between bilingual development and specific language impairment. *Applied Psycholinguistics* 31, 227–52.
Paradis, J. and Genesee, F. (1996) Syntactic acquisition in bilingual children: Autonomous or interdependent? *Studies in Second Language Acquisition* 18, 1–25.
Pine, J. and Lieven, E. (1993) Reanalysing rote-learned phrases: Individual differences in the transition to multi-word speech. *Journal of Child Language* 20, 551–71.
Pine, J. and Lieven, E. (1997) Slot and frame patterns and the development of the determiner category. *Applied Psycholinguistics* 18, 123–38.
Pine, J., Lieven, E. and Rowland, C.F. (1998) Comparing different models of the development of the English verb category. *Linguistics* 36, 781–806.
Pizzuto, E. and Caselli, M.C. (1992) The acquisition of Italian morphology: Implications for models of language development *Journal of Child Language* 19, 491–557.
Pizzuto, E. and Caselli, M.C. (1993) The acquisition of Italian morphology: A reply to Hyams. *Journal of Child Language* 20, 707–12.
Pizzuto, E. and Caselli, M.C. (1994) The acquisition of Italian verb morphology in a crosslinguistic perspective. In Y. Levy (ed.) *Other Children, Other Languages: Issues in the Theory of Language Acquisition*. Hillsdale, NJ: Lawrence Erlbaum.
Price, G. (1984) Welsh as a literary, standard and official language. In M.J. Ball and G.E. Jones (eds) *Welsh Phonology: Selected Readings*. Cardiff: University of Wales Press.
Romaine, S. (1995) *Bilingualism*. London: Blackwell.
Rubino, R. and Pine, J. (1998) Subject-verb agreement in Brazilian Portuguese: What low error rates hide. *Journal of Child Language* 25, 35–60.
Shirai, Y. and Andersen, R.W. (1995) The acquisition of tense-aspect morphology: A prototype account. *Language* 71, 743–62.
Surridge, M. (1989) Factors in the assignment of grammatical gender in Welsh. *Etudes Celtiques* 26, 187–209.
Tallerman, M. (1987) *Mutation and the Syntactic Structure of Modern Colloquial Welsh*. Unpublished PhD dissertation: University of Wales.
Thomas, E.M. (2001) *Aspects of Gender Mutation in Welsh*. Unpublished PhD dissertation: University of Wales.
Thomas, E.M. (2007) Natur prosesau caffael iaith gan blant: marcio cenedl enwau yn y Gymraeg. *Gwerddon* 1, 58–94.
Thomas, E.M. and Gathercole, V.C.M. (2005) Obsolescence or survival for Welsh in the face of English dominance? In J. Cohen, K.T. McAlister, K. Rolstad and J. MacSwan (eds) *Proceedings of the 4th International Symposium on Bilingualism*. Somerville: Cascadilla Press.
Thomas, E.M. and Gathercole, V.C.M. (2007) Children's productive command of grammatical gender and mutation in Welsh: An alternative to rule-based learning. *First Language* 27 (3), 251–78.
Thomas, E.M. and Schiemenz, S. (in preparation) *Acquiring Welsh in a bilingual setting: Stage 1 – exploring speakers' use of plural and responsive*. Funded by a Development Fund Grant awarded by the ESRC Centre for Research on Bilingualism in Theory and Practice: Bangor University, Wales, UK.
Thomas, P.W. (1984) Variation in South Glamorgan consonant mutation. In M.J. Ball and G.E. Jones (eds) *Welsh Phonology: Selected Readings*. Cardiff: University of Wales Press.
Tomasello, M. (1992) *First Verbs: A Case Study of Early Grammatical Development*. Cambridge: Cambridge University Press.
Tomasello, M. (2000a) The item-based nature of children's early syntactic development. *Trends in Cognitive Sciences* 4 (4), 156–63.
Tomasello, M. (2000b) Do young children have adult syntactic competence? *Cognition* 74, 209–53.
Watkins, T.A. (1993) Welsh. In M.J. Ball and J.Fife (eds) *The Celtic Languages*. London: Routledge.
Wei, L. (2000) *The Bilingualism Reader*. London: Routledge.
Williams, S.J. (1980) *A Welsh Grammar*, Cardiff: University of Wales Press.

Appendix I Welsh terms for some LLARSP headings

Unanalysed	nis dadansoddwyd
Problematic	problematig
Code-switching	codgroesi, newid cod
Responses	atebion
Repetitions	ailadroddiadau
Elliptical	eliptig
Reduced	gostyngiad
Full	llawn
Major	prif
Minor	llai
Structural	cyfluniadol
Problems	problemau
Normal	normal
Abnormal	annormal
Spontaneous	digymell
Reactions	ymatebion
Command	gorchymyn
Question	cwestiwn
Statement	gosodiad
Connectivity	cysylltiad
Clause	cymal
Phrase	ymadrodd
Stage	cam
Other	arall

Appendix II

This appendix contains a sample analysis of a simple and a complex sentence. The levels of analysis below each sentence are Clause, Phrase, Morphology and Mutation (shown as C1, Ph, M and T respectively).

Example sentences:

(i) *Welais i'r ferch fach sy'n byw drws nesaf ond doedd hi ddim yn 'ngweld i achos bod ei brawd hi yn y ffordd.*
'I saw the little girl who lives next door but she didn't see me because her brother was in the way'.

(ii) *Roedd y dyn yn y parc yn bwyta rhai o'i frechdanau.*
'The man in the park was eating some of his sandwiches'.

Analysis

(1)

```
       Welais i' r ferch fach sy'n byw drws nesaf
Cl     V      S  O       _____  _____
                          s  V      A
Ph     Pronᴾ D N Adj Auxᵇ Aspyn N Adj
M      -odd|s 'r        sydd
T      (part)+V D+Nf Nf + Adj
       ond doedd hi ddim yn ngweld i achos bod ei brawd hi yn y ffordd
Cl     c    V-   S   -V       O   _____A_____
                     s  Vc    S            A
Ph     Auxᵇ Pronᴾ neg V Aspyn Pronᴾ  Cop D N D Pr D N
M      oedd3s                         bod Other
T                    fy+V
```

(ii)

```
       Roedd y dyn yn y parc yn bwyta rhai o'i frechdanau
Cl     V-    S        -V              O
Ph     Auxᵇ  D N  Pr D N Aspyn  Init. D N
                  (= NPPrNP)
M      oedd3s                         – au
T                                     Poss + N
```

8 An Investigation of Syntax in Children of Bengali (Sylheti)-Speaking Families

Jane Stokes

Introduction

This chapter draws on work done during the 1980s in East London as part of a research project investigating the stages of language development in children under five years of age, speaking Bengali (Sylheti) at home (Stokes in Duncan, 1989). The purpose of the latter project was to develop an assessment procedure for children referred to speech and language therapy from the Bengali-speaking population. Language data was collected from 30 children between the ages of 18 months and four years. A framework for analysing the language data collected was devised which examined syntactic, semantic, and lexical features. The information collected has contributed to knowledge about the stages of language development of Bengali children growing up in the UK and is presented here as background information for researchers and clinicians working with this community.

Information on Bengali

Bengali is the national language of Bangladesh, and is also spoken in West Bengal, the part of India that borders Bangladesh and of which Calcutta is the capital. Bengali is the written language used in the whole of Bangladesh and is taught in the schools. Sylheti is the regional variety spoken by people from the Sylhet region and is generally not written. There are considerable differences in syntax (e.g. in word endings), lexicon, and phonology between Bengali and Sylheti, but many of the words are the same. Differing views exist on whether standard Bengali and Sylheti are mutually intelligible: in general it seems that Sylheti speakers can understand standard Bengali, but that Bengali speakers unfamiliar with Sylheti have some difficulty in understanding it. There is a recognition in East London that Sylheti should be regarded as a language in its own right (Kershen, 2005).

Main Syntactic and Morphological Features of Bengali

Bengali is an Indo-European language deriving from Sanskrit. It shares many grammatical features with other North Indian languages (e.g. Gujarati, Hindi) but differs from the Dravidian languages spoken in southern India (e.g. Tamil and Malayalam). The basic word order is subject-object-verb, compared to subject-verb-object in English. The verb comes at the end of the sentence (e.g. **dada ʧɪps anbo**, granddad chips will bring, 'granddad will bring chips').[1] Adverbials tend to precede the verb: /**fari:da gari:t gesʊngi**/ (Farida in the car went 'Farida went in the car'). The negative tends to come at the end of the sentence (e.g. /**gorom na**/, hot not, 'it's not hot'). The copula is often omitted as in /**paki: ʃʊndor**/ (bird beautiful 'the bird is beautiful'). Bengali is a pro-drop language, that is, the subject, which can be inferred from the word ending, is often omitted (e.g. /**ba:t kʰaɪtam**/, rice I will eat, 'I will eat rice'). Here the first person and the future tense is indicated by the ending /**tam**/ so there is no explicit subject. Questions are formed either by intonation alone, /**skulo gese?**/ (to school he has gone⸮ 'has he gone to school⸮') or by the insertion of a question particle, or question word, with no alteration of word order (e.g./**aba koj gesʊn**/, Daddy where he has gone⸮ 'Where has daddy gone⸮') Unlike English, there is no auxiliary 'do' in questions and no inversion of the verb.

Adjectival and nominal morphology are light, but verbs are highly inflected for person and tense and to indicate honorific status, but not for number. Bengali nouns are not assigned gender, so adjectives are not inflected to express this. The 1st, 2nd, and 3rd person pronouns have two forms, ordinary and honorific, /**tʊmi:**/ is second person 'you' (familiar) and /**apni:**/ is second person 'you' (formal) used when speaking to someone older. Both nouns and pronouns are inflected for case. The 3rd person pronoun has no gender distinction – the same word /**taɪ**/ is used for 'he' and 'she'. In most contexts, determiners are not obligatory and there is no equivalent of an indefinite article. Postpositions correspond to prepositions in English and, as the term implies, come after the noun or noun phrase (e.g. /**ʃopo tone**/, shop from, 'from the shop'). Location may be expressed by a word ending rather than by a postposition, for example, /**mati:t**/ (ground-on 'on the ground') where the ending –t indicates 'on'.

Bengali verbs are highly inflected and are conjugated for person and tense. They mostly follow a regular pattern for inflection. Verbs divide into two classes: finite and non-finite. Non-finite verbs have no inflection for tense or person, while finite verbs are fully inflected for person (1st, 2nd, 3rd), tense (present, past, future), aspect (simple, perfect, progressive), and honour (intimate, familiar, formal), but not for number. Conditional, imperative, and other special inflections for mood can replace the tense and aspect suffixes. Compound verbs, including a stem and a suffix, are commonly used in Bengali. These are similar to phrasal verbs or particle verbs in English, such as 'to go shopping' with the main semantic weight being borne by the lexical verb, usually in its root form. The second verb, sometimes termed the formant verb, often changes its original meaning and modifies the main verb (e.g. in expressing the meaning 'bring' two verbs are combined /ana/ 'to bring' and /dawa/ 'to give' to form a compound verb /ana dawa/). Bengali has four simple tenses: present, simple past to indicate recent events, habitual past which is also used as a conditional, and the simple future tense. There are also several compound tenses.

The Project in Whitechapel

As indicated earlier, the work presented here came out of a project carried out in the mid-1980s in Whitechapel, East London. Whitechapel was then, and still is, an area with a large number of families with origins in Sylhet in Bangladesh. There was a clear clinical need to explore language development in the children of this community as about 30% of referrals to speech and language therapy were from children whose first language was Bengali. A project was set up, supported by the King's Fund, to investigate the stages of language development in typically developing children from this community. The project employed a speech and language therapist working half-time over three years, and a Bengali-speaking assistant working half time over eighteen months. The expressive language of 30 children between the ages of 18 months and four years was recorded through visits to the homes. The children were selected randomly from health records but had to meet certain criteria to demonstrate that they were developing typically. They had all passed developmental checks carried out, and neither they nor their siblings had any history of deafness or other disability. All children were exposed only to Bengali at home and the majority were born in England and had not spent any time in Bangladesh. The age range of 18 months to four years was divided into five groups, and six children were selected in each age group (three boys and three girls). The children were visited at home three times for a period of one and half hours each. A minimum of 200 spontaneous utterances for each child was collected using audio tape recordings and transcription at the time by the research assistant. An analysis of the relationship between language structure, mean length of utterance (MLU), and age was carried out in order to provide information about ages and stages of language development in this population.

Syntactic Analysis and Adaptation of LARSP

In constructing a framework for the analysis of syntax, there were some changes made to the LARSP framework to allow for differences between English and Bengali. At clause level, the order of constituents was different to reflect the word order of Bengali, so SVO become SOV. At phrase level,

Post was used to represent postpositions, and Det is not an obligatory category in many contexts. At word level, tense, person, possession, and location are represented by suffixes.

At the one-word level, question words, nouns, verbs, adverbs, and adjectives were recorded. Some of these one-word utterances may be elliptical (e.g. responses to questions) but some will represent immature forms of longer adult utterances (e.g. /dudʰ/, milk, to mean 'give me some milk').

At the two-word level, the major two-word utterances were recorded at clause level as follows: SV, SO/C, O/CV, Adv X, Neg X, Q X. As Bengali is a pro-drop language, it should be noted that O/CV may be a complete adult form of utterance, so /tʃa kʰaɪtam/ (tea drink 'I want to drink some tea').

At phrase level at the two-word level, the following categories were used: VV (to indicate the compound verb), Adj N, Det N (although as the determiner is not obligatory in most contexts this was not found frequently), and N Post (e.g. kʌbɔder bitɔre, cupboard-in inside, 'inside the cupboard').

At the three-word level the following categories from LARSP were used:

SC/V, SAV, C/OAV, Neg XY, Q XY. At phrase level, D Adj N is included, but was rarely found because of the different uses of determiners in Bengali. DN Post was not included as there were no instances of this structure.

At the four-word level the following categories from LARSP were used:

SC/OAV, AA XY, Neg XYZ, Q XYZ, c X, and X c X. At phrase level, N Post P was not used as there were no instances of this structure occurring.

In carrying out the syntactic analysis the stages laid out in the LARSP procedure were not used. The age bands acted as stages, and the framework for analysis was organized on a scale of progressively longer and more complex sentence structure. Children within each age group were compared and syntactic categories used by all children in an age group were compiled as a list of *key features* of that age group. Children were also grouped according to mean length of utterance, and the same process was carried out for each MLU group. There was a strong correlation between age and MLU, so syntactic measures were compared to MLU alone.

The samples of language collected from each child were analysed using the framework for syntactic analysis outlined above. Information emerged from this about the number of times a particular syntactic structure was used on each visit. The number of occurrences of each syntactic structure was recorded and added so that a total was obtained over the three visits. Means, standard variations, and ranges were calculated for each MLU group.

Findings on Stages of Grammatical Development

The results of the analysis will now be presented according to age groups, with an indication of the key features of syntax that occurred. The categories are listed in order of frequency based on mean.[2]

1;6–2;0

N	Adv
V	SO/C
O/CV	Neg X
SV	

At the one-word level all the children were using nouns, verbs, and adverbs. These can be classified as key features of this age group. Question words were only used by two of the children. Five of the children were using adjectives as one-word utterances, but only one child showed more than one instance.

At the two-word level, all children were using SV, SO/C, O/CV, and Neg X. These are key features of this age group. SO/C is the only key feature that appears just once in one child and this is in the sample taken from the youngest child. All the other two-word utterances are fairly widely used by all children at this age. It can be said, therefore, that two-word utterances are typical at this age in this group of children. Most of the children are using Adv X and Q X (only one child did not) so these are clearly categories that are developing at this age. Compound verbs are not yet being used by all children at this age, although one girl at 1;10 showed 44 instances of compound verbs. Adj N, Det N and N Post are not used consistently by all children. Three-word utterances are not widely used by this group. Neg XY is beginning to develop and is used, albeit scarcely, by five of the six children.

2;0–2;6

N	Adv X	S O/C
V	Adv	Neg XY
O/CV	Det N	Adj
SV	Neg X	

At the one-word level all the children were using N, V, Adv and Adj. There is a noticeable increase in the number of adverbs used at this age; two of the children each had more than 20 instances. The number of adjectives used was small; each child showed at least one instance, but two children used an adjective only once.

At the two-word level all the children used SV, SO/C, O/CV, Adv X, Neg X, and Det N. Again the increase in the use of adverbs together with another element is noticeable. Only three out of six children were using questions involving a question word and another element. Compound verbs were used frequently by four of the children but not used by all. Although adjectives are used at the one-word level, they are not used yet in combination with nouns. Determiners are used together with nouns at this stage, although one child uses this structure only once. N Post is used by five out of the six children in the group, so this is a structure that is developing at this age. There is a clear progression of structures such as this, which are used by one age group but not by all children, and which then appear in the data of all children in the next age group and can then be classified as key features. This is true of Neg XY, which was beginning to develop in the age group 1;6–2;0 and is then found in all children at 2;0–2;6. Other three-word utterances are not used consistently by all children, although in some children there are instances of SC/OV, SAV and C/OAV. There are few examples of four-word utterances in this age group, although Neg XYZ is used by three of the children.

2;6–3;0

O/CV	Neg X	SO/C
N	(Adv)	Neg XY
V	SC/OV	N Post
SV	Det N	
VV	Adv X	

At the one-word level there is now a less consistent use of adverbs and adjectives. Not all children are using them in one-word utterances, so they cannot strictly be included as key features. They appear in the final chart in brackets, as they are key features of the younger age group and appeared in the data of five out of six children in this age group. Question words are also not used on their own.

At the two-word level all children are using SV, SO/C, and O/CV. Both SV and O/CV are very frequently used and make up the bulk of the utterances. Many of the verbs used at this stage are compound verbs: this feature is found in all six children in this age group. Several of the children show a wide variety of compound verbs.

Adv X and Neg X are also used by all children. The X in Adv X is either subject or verb in fairly equal distribution. Q X is not used by all six children, nor is Adj N, although five out of six children are using this. Det N is used by all, and N Post is now a key feature, used by all children.

Three-word utterances are becoming more common. SC/OV and SAV are used by all the children, although one child uses them only once, and another child uses SAV only once. Neg XY and Neg XYZ are used by all the children, though Neg XYZ is not used widely. It seems that in each age group the use of negatives is the first example of a longer utterance. When the children are predominantly using two-word utterances, as at age 2;0–2;6, the only instance of a three-word utterance is Neg XY. This is therefore a sign that the child is progressing to longer utterances. Similarly, at this age, the only example of a four-word utterance is Neg XYZ.

3;0–3;6

VV	Adv	SO/C
V	Neg X	C/OAV
O/CV	SC/OV	(Neg XYZ)
N	SAV	(Adj)
SV	Neg XY	SC/OAV
Adv X	N Post	
Det N	Adj N	

At the one-word level, nouns, verbs, and adverbs, but not adjectives, are used on their own. Adjectives, however, are, for the first time, used together with nouns as two-word (Adj N) utterances by all children, although one child uses this only once. Question words are used on their own by four out of six children, and in two-word utterances by five out of six children. The use of questions is clearly determined by context, and it may well be that the data do not truly reflect ability, but usage.

At the two-word level, all children are using SV, SO/C, O/CV, Adv X, Neg X, Adj N, Det N, and N Post. All combinations of two words are used except Q X, and it can therefore be said that the children have mastered two-word utterances and are using them widely at this age.

At the three-word level, there is wider use of SC/OV where the children show many instances (one child of three years showed 19 instances of SC/OV). All children are using SAV and, for the first time, C/OAV and Neg XY are also used by all children; Q XY is used by five out of six. C/OAV is used only once by two children.

At the four-word level, SC/OAV is now used by all children, albeit infrequently; four children use this structure only once. Other four-word utterances are not used regularly by all six children. Neg XYZ, which had emerged at age 2;6–3;0 as a key feature, is now not used by all children. Q XYZ is used by five out of the six and it is noticeable that it is the same child who does not use questions as one-, two-, three-, or four-word utterances. All the other children use Q X, Q XY and Q XYZ.

3;6–4;0

N	SC/OV	Adj N
O/CV	Adv	Q XY
V	Neg XY	Neg XYZ
VV	Neg X	Q
SV	SAV	Adj
Det N	N Post	Q XYZ
SO/C	Q X	(SC/OAV)
Adv X	C/OAV	

By this age most of the structures at the one-, two-, and three-word levels listed in the analysis are used by all children. At the one-word level, for the first time, question words are used by all children. Questions now form an important part of the child's language. At the two-word stage, Q X is now used by all children, although one child uses it only once. Q XY appears in all the children's data at this age, although it is used only once by one child. Adjectives are used by all children, although only once by one child. This is a key feature of the 2;0–2;6 age group, but not in the other groups. At the three-word level, there are examples in each category of analysis except for D Adj N. This is used by two children but is clearly not a frequently used structure.

At the four-word level, all the children except one uses SC/OAV (a key feature of the age group 3;0–3;6), though two children only use it once. There is increasing use of AA XY. Neg XYZ and Q XYZ are used by all children. Five out of the six children at this age are using connectives either as c X or X c X.

Full table of key features

The full set of key features for each age group is shown in Table 8.1. The key features are those common to all children at that age, but which do not appear at the previous age range. Items asterisked appear for the first time at that age. Items bracketed are those that occur in an earlier age group, but not in the next age group. Although these items are used by five out of six children, they cannot be strictly classed as key features.

For the most part, key features that emerge at one age continue to appear in the subsequent age groups. There are a few exceptions to this. Adj and Adv appear in the 2;0–2;6 group but not in the next age group. Adj does not appear in the 3;0–3;6 group, but returns at 3;6–4;0. SC/OAV appears in the 3;0–3;6 group but not in the next one. This is usually because one of the children at a subsequent age is not using these features; five out of six children in an age group are using them, but they cannot be classed as key features unless all six children are using them. It may be an accident of

Table 8.1 Key features

1;6–2;0	2;0–2;6	2;6–3;0	3;0–3;6	3;6–4;0
				Q*
N	N	N	N	N
V	V	V	V	V
Adv	Adv	(Adv)	Adv	Adv
	Adj*	(Adj)	(Adj)	Adj
SV	SV	SV	SV	SV
SO/C	SO/C	SO/C	SO/C	SO/C
O/CV	O/CV	O/CV	O/CV	O/CV
	Adv X*	Adv X	Adv X	Adv X
Neg X	Neg X	Neg X	Neg X	Neg X
				Q X*
		VV*	VV	VV
			AdjN*	AdjN
	DetN*	DetN	DetN	DetN
		NPost*	NPost	NPost
		SC/OV*	SC/OV	SC/OV
		SAV*	SAV	SAV
			C/OAV*	C/OAV
	Neg XY*	Neg XY	Neg XY	Neg XY
				Q XY*
			SC/OAV*	(SCO/AV)
		Neg XYZ*	(Neg XYZ)	Neg XYZ
				Q XYZ*

Items asterisked appear for the first time at that age. Items bracketed are those that occur in an earlier age group, but not in the next age group.

sampling that they are not found in all six children, rather than an indication that children are not yet able to use them at this age, again reflecting the problem of distinguishing actual use from possible use.

Use of this Information in Assessment

The profiles that emerged from this investigation of language development provide a basis for making some decisions about the syntactic categories used by children with a Bengali background. The study examined certain aspects of spontaneous expressive language. By focusing on those features which are used by every child at each age group, the researcher or practising therapist can analyse a sample of spontaneous language, looking specifically for key features. This provides a starting point for identifying those syntactic structures that a child is using and comparing these with the children observed in this study. It is important to point out that the key features can in no way be viewed as norms, but merely as aspects of language seen in these children at these ages. The use of key features would require further investigation to determine reliability and representativeness.

It cannot be claimed that this study provided a Bengali version of LARSP. Rather it was the case that LARSP provided us with the categories to look for, and while there did need to be some adjustment for use with Bengali, it was possible to apply the majority of the structures developed for English. The study has provided preliminary information about the structure of Bengali not previously available and has contributed to the understanding of local speech and language therapy practitioners.

Notes

(1) Examples given in this chapter are in Sylheti rather than standard Bengali and derive from utterances transcribed during the data collection. They are presented in IPA (International Phonetic Alphabet).
(2) In these and later lists the order of frequency is to be read from top to bottom in each column.

References

Kershen, A.J. (2005) *Strangers, Aliens and Asians: Huguenots, Jews and Bangladeshis in Spitalfields, 1660–2000*. London: Routledge.
Stokes, J. in D.M. Duncan (ed.) (1989) *Working with Bilingual Language Disability*. London: Chapman and Hall. http://www.experiencefestival.com/a/Bengali_grammar_-_Verbs/id/4845835

9 ILARSP: A Grammatical Profile of Irish[1]

Tina Hickey

Introduction

This chapter explores the adaptation of LARSP to Irish.[2] The data are from typical L1 acquisition, but this work also contributes to the knowledge base needed in the clinical assessment of Irish in atypical acquisition. At a wider level, the crosslinguistic study of language acquisition contributes to the discrimination of putative universals from language-specific strategies (Slobin, 2006), and the development of grammatical assessment instruments in a range of languages is a critical aspect of such crosslinguistic study. As Ball notes in this volume regarding the construction of a Welsh LARSP, the contrastive analysis possible as a result of the retention of the same basic framework allows the detection of features peculiar to particular languages, as well as those common to them. The successful adaptation of LARSP to a number of other languages such as Dutch, French, Welsh and Hebrew as detailed in other chapters of this book indicates that it is a valuable instrument both for intralinguistic and crosslinguistic analysis.

A profiling method such as LARSP is particularly attractive in examining the acquisition of languages such as Irish, since relatively little is still known about structural development in the language. Irish is designated by the EU both as a 'regional, minority language' and, more recently, as an official language of the EU. It is described as 'the first official language' in the Constitution of the Republic of Ireland, although most citizens are English-speaking. While Irish has significant state support in terms of an established place in the primary school curriculum in the Republic of Ireland, it still lacks a body of research on fundamental aspects of the acquisition, teaching and learning of the language to support it. The second-language acquisition of Irish has received some attention, such as in Owens' (1992) case study of her daughter's early L2 acquisition of Irish, Mhic Mhathúna's (1995) study of early SLA, and Hickey's (1997, 1999, 2001, 2007) studies of children's acquisition of Irish in immersion preschools, while Ó Duibhir (2009) looked at older L2 learners aged 11–12 years. Looking specifically at L1 acquisition, McKenna and Wall (1986) carried out an early study of the acquisition of Irish syntax, and Hickey (1987, 1991) looked at the use of basic measures such as MLU in studies of Irish L1 acquisition, while Hickey (1990a) examined the issue of word order in children's acquisition of this VSO language. Hickey (1993) examined the role of formulas in Irish acquisition data. Goodluck *et al.* (2001, 2006) have examined aspects of Irish syntax from a formal perspective, while Cameron and Hickey (2011) have taken a constructivist approach to a corpus of Irish L1 acquisition. Phonological development in Irish has been examined by Brennan (2004). O'Toole and Fletcher (2008, 2010) have examined lexical development in Irish-dominant children using an Irish adaptation of the Communicative Development Inventory (ICDI). Recent research such as Singleton *et al.* (2000), Hickey and Cameron-Faulkner (2009), Hickey (2009), and O'Toole and Fletcher (2008, 2010) have given explicit consideration to issues of parental language background, language dominance, bilingualism and language mixing, given the now overwhelming influence of English even on young children acquiring Irish as L1.

Despite the modest increase in research on the L1 and L2 acquisition of Irish, the grammatical development in Irish first-language acquisition remains under-researched. A symposium entitled the *Assessment and Profiling of Irish Language Development* in July 2010 found that speech and language therapists who encounter children for whom Irish is the/a primary language of the home are still lacking norms and quick methods of assessment for Irish development (see O'Toole & Hickey, in preparation), though they were aware of the LARSP adaptation to Irish. This adaptation was developed in order to allow monitoring of typical development in samples of output from the same child over time, and between children. An earlier adaptation of LARSP to Irish was constructed by Hayden (1984), but the adaptation reported in this chapter is applied to data from an acquisition study. It was based on data collected in the mid-1980s from four children living in an Irish-speaking district (*Gaeltacht*) in the south-west of Ireland whose acquisition was studied between the ages of 1;4 and 3;6 years. These children were from Irish-speaking homes, and while they had varying levels of exposure to English on television and from visitors, they were Irish dominant, and in fact had very little English at the time of data collection, especially the two younger children.

In this discussion, the adaptation of LARSP to Irish will be referred to as Irish LARSP or ILARSP.[3] The question of whether to use Irish or English on the chart itself was problematic. As a profile of Irish, there is a strong case to be made for presenting the chart in Irish. However, it was thought that retaining the English terms would be helpful for potential users of the chart, since most of them would already be familiar with the English LARSP. In addition, as Ball notes (this volume), there is at present a convention that theoretical labels such as NP are not translated. If it were considered advantageous to translate the chart and its categories into Irish at some time in the future, that would require a change from the single-letter abbreviation(s), since some Irish categories begin with the same letter. A chart with Irish labels might also be confusing to those accustomed to the English chart, since there would be a change in the function represented by some labels. For example, A on an Irish chart would represent the subject (*Ainmní*), and C the object (*Cuspóir*).

This adaptation of LARSP was mainly based on data from three Irish-speaking children at different stages of development (with some data from a fourth, older child included). The examples used here are from the children's data, are provided with a gloss and a translation, and are kept to a minimum in order to make the discussion accessible to non-Irish speakers. Following Ball (1988), there is no discussion here of the transcription or scanning of the data, as the methods used do not differ significantly from the procedure described by Crystal *et al.* (1981). The samples on which ILARSP analyses were based were selected for their representativeness of a full session with each child. The percentage of utterances from Stage II or later was calculated for the transcript of an entire session, and the first 100 major Irish utterances after the 51st, which contained a similar percentage of such utterances (+/-5%), were selected for analysis. This ensured that the sample was representative, and was not, for example, depressed by a concentration of Stage I utterances. Before discussing the design of the ILARSP chart, a brief description of some of the salient characteristics of Irish is given.

Outline of Features of Irish Grammar

Irish is an almost paradigmatic example of a VSO language, according to Greenberg's (1966) universals. The basic order of elements is: Verb + Subject + X, where X can be object, indirect object, adverbial, prepositional phrase, verbal noun and so on. Negatives and interrogatives are marked by the appropriate particle in front of the verb. Stenson (1981: 17) characterized Irish as an 'inflectional language, tending more towards isolating than polysynthetic in general'. There are some 14 irregular verbs in Irish, but apart from these the verb paradigm is highly regular, with tense and person forms based on the root.

The Irish alphabet has only 18 letters, extended by a length mark over vowels, but it has a high phoneme count. While this varies between the three main dialects (Ulster, Munster and Connacht Irish), Greene (1966: 16) noted that it is not likely to be lower than 60 (the difficulties arising from Irish orthography's attempt to represent these are analysed in greater depth by Hickey & Stenson, 2011). A significant feature of Irish is the two series of consonants, traditionally referred to as 'broad' and 'slender'. Broad consonants include velar consonants and velarized labials and dentals. Slender consonants include palatal consonants and palatalized labials and dentals. Examples (1)-(4) show minimal pairs of broad and slender consonants in different word positions, with the palatalized consonant in the right column marked with a following /´/ according to the norms of Irish phonetic transcription.

Broad (velar) consonant   Slender (palatalized) consonant
(1)   *buí*   /bi:/   'yellow'   *bí*   /b´i:/   'be'
(2)   *bó*   /bo:/   'cow'   *beo*   /b´o:/   'alive'
(3)   *bád*   /ba:d/   'boat'   *báid*   /ba:d´/   'boats'
(4)   *teas*   /t'as/   'heat'   *tais*   /tas´/   'damp'

Note that the 'i' in *báid* and *tais* in examples (3) and (4) are not syllabified as /id/ or /is/ but signal palatalisation of the following /d´/ and /ʃ/ (=/s´/).

Another prominent feature of Irish is its initial mutations. The initial consonants of words may change when governed by various particles, among them the definite article, possessives and question and negative particles. These initial mutations, a characteristic feature of Celtic languages, are pervasive in Irish. The initial consonant mutations of the dialect studied here, the Munster dialect, are lenition, eclipsis, and /h/ before initial-position vowels (Ó Sé, 2000). These mutations were originally phonetically conditioned, but now signal various morphological processes. With lenition, stops and the nasal [m] are replaced by fricatives usually at the same place of articulation, and fricatives are treated as follows: [f]→Ø, [s]→[h]. Orthographically this is marked by the letter 'h' following the lenited consonant (e.g. *cóta* 'a coat' *mo chóta* 'my coat'). With eclipsis, a voiced segment becomes nasalized, a voiceless segment voiced, marked orthographically by writing the eclipsing consonant before the eclipsed one (e.g. *gort* 'a field' → *i ngort* 'in a field'). Other features of the language that are notable are the existence of two verbs that correspond to the English copula. They are the copula *is* and the substantive verb *bí*. The copula generally predicates inherent qualities, while the substantive verb predicates more temporal qualities such as location or transient state (Stenson, 1981: 94). There are parallels with *ser* and *estar* in Spanish, although there are also differences in usage.

Design

The LARSP profile is organized structurally as sentence, clause, phrase and word types. There was a precedent for applying this organisation to Irish also in Ward's (1974) description of Munster Irish (also the dialect of this study), where the language was described at sentence, phrase and word level. An exploratory attempt to analyse Irish data with LARSP categories showed that there are many categories common to both languages, as Ball also found in his adaptation to Welsh (see Chapter 7). Of course, the order in many of these categories is inappropriate for Irish as for Welsh; for example, the SV of LARSP needs to be changed to VS on ILARSP, since Irish is a strong VSO language. However, it is not enough to find a general 'fit' between the English LARSP chart and Irish categories, since care must also be taken to ensure that the Irish chart is comprehensive and representative of the structures of the language. Thus, there was need for some adjustment of the chart in order to adapt it to the requirements of the language, and this will be shown below in the description of ILARSP.

Ball (1988) chose to restrict his LLARSP chart for Welsh to clause and phrase- level structures, with a separate comprehensive chart for morphological development (LLARSP-M) and another chart (LLARSP-T) for recording word-initial consonant mutations. In analysing the Irish data, a separate word-level chart was used containing the maximum of information initially, but in the course of using this in data analysis it was possible to whittle it down to a number of categories, now represented in the word-level column. In order to expedite analysis, it is suggested that users of the chart use these general categories in cases where this level is not the focus of assessment. Where this is the case, the most satisfactory method for an in-depth analysis of word-level phenomena is the use of particular subheadings under these general categories. It was considered that the advantage of having a fuller word-level representation on a separate chart was offset by the disadvantage of reducing the range of the language represented on the ILARSP chart and fragmenting the profile. In addition, it was felt that the detail required at this level was not great for about the first three stages, and that the best way to indicate the paucity of word-level phenomena in this period was to maintain the integrity of the chart. At later stages, it is suggested that the user should note in detail the particular structures used at this level using sub-headings under the general headings given.

Ball (1988: 56) noted that even without comprehensive developmental data on grammatical development in a language, 'certain predictions can be made about language development...[such as that] the LARSP distinctions between one-word and two-element stages, for example, will also hold for Welsh'. This is also true in the case of Irish, but in addition to such broad predictions, the allocation of structures to particular stages in ILARSP is based on the acquisition of three participants for most of the stages. However, as the sample is so small, age ranges are not discussed here.

Clause division in ILARSP

The most striking difference between the Irish chart and the LARSP chart is the separation of the Negative column from Statement, and its placement between the Command and Question columns (see Figure 9.1). Irish shows a regularity in the formation of the negative and interrogative which is not seen in English. Given the extreme regularity of the declarative, negative and interrogative systems in Irish, it seems that carrying over the

154 Assessing Grammar

Name	Age		Date			No. of analysed units	
A	Unanalysed			Problematic			
	Unintelligible	Symbolic Noise	Deviant	Incomplete	Ambiguous		Stereotypes

	Codeswitching						
	Sentence	Clause		Element		Phrasal	
B	Responses		Normal Response			Abnormal	
				Major			
	Stimulus type	Totals	Repetition	Elliptical 1 2 3+	Reduced Full	Minor Structural Ø	Problems
	Requests						
	Others						
C	Spontaneous						
D	Reactions		General	Structural	Ø	Other	Problems

	Minor neó			Vocatives	Social	huh?	Other
I	Major	Comm.	Neg.	Quest	Statement	[imitations]	
		'V'	'Neg-V'		'N' 'V' 'Adj'	'Adv' 'Dem'	Other
	Conn				Clause	Phrase	Word
II		VX	No X Neg V Neg-VX	QX	VS VC/O SVn SC/O SA CopX AX DemX Other	DN VV N Adj V Part Pr N NN(ps) NN(-c) Other PVn	tá bhí beidh is ea ní hea Vn Vadj an na Dependent V
			NegVimp-V	(an)V			
	X+S:NP	X+Q:NP	X+A:AP	X+C:NP	X+V:VGp	C-R	Irreg. past Fut.
III		VXY NegVimpX	NegX NoXY NegQV	QVX QXY anVX	VSO VOO VSC CopXY VSA DemXY VSVn SVnX VnOO Other	DNAdj IntX PrDN PrPn NAdjAdj Prons/o Adv(s/d) Cop Other	V+person N pl -i -anna Oth. Reg. past Fut. Dim. emph. reflx
	XY+S:NP	XY+Q:NP	XY+A:AP	XY+C:NP	XY+V:VGp	C-R	AL II N + N
IV		+s VXY+ NegimpXY	NegVX Y NegQVX	OXY+ an VX+	VSOA CopXY+ VSCA AAXY VSVnX VSOO Other	NPPrNP cX PrDNAdj XcX Other	Poss pl + N ND + Npl Other Ní + Adj NNm + Adj
V	agus c s	Coord. Other	Coord. Other	Coord. Other	Coord. 1 1+ Subord. A 1+ S C 0	Post-mod. Cl 1 1+	N + Adjpl Other
	CLAUSE	(NP)		PHRASE	(VGp)	WORD	
VI	*W.O. -Element	*AL *Pron *D *Pr	-Pron -D -Pr -c	*AL *Tns -Tns V	-PVn -cop -Dep	*Pl -Pl *PrPn -PrPn	AL III PrD + N Poss pl + N ND + Npl Other
VII	Discourse A connectivity Comment clause Emphatic Order		empty tá Style	Syntactic comprehension			t- v/s h- v Autonomous Genitive Compar./super.
	Total no. of utterances		Mean no. of utterances per turn		Mean utterance length in words		

©D. Crystal, P. Fletcher, M. Garman, 1981 revision, University of Reading.
© Tina Hickey, Irish Version.

Figure 9.1 ILARSP Chart

practice in LARSP of treating negatives with statements (with questions separate) in the Irish chart would be to impose a framework on the language that ignores one of its basic structural features. In Irish, the interrogative and negative are achieved by the presence of clitics before the verb of the positive declarative sentence, for example:

(5) *Tháinig Sean isteach go luath* 'Came John in early' > 'John came in early'
(6) *Ar tháinig Sean isteach go luath?* 'Q came John in early?' > 'Did John come in early?'
(7) *Níor tháinig Sean isteach go luath* 'Neg came John in early' > 'John did not come in early'
(8) *Nár tháinig Sean isteach go luath?* 'Neg-Q came John in early' > 'Didn't John come in early?'

It could, in fact, be argued that interrogation and negation should be treated at phrase level, since they are achieved in Irish by the presence of clitics in the verb group. There are, however, considerable advantages in treating negation at clause level. It allows representation of the similarity of negative questions and negative statements by collapsing the columns at the appropriate points to allow for this blending of function. Maintaining the communicative distinction drawn by LARSP between statements, questions and commands is reasonable in functional terms, and the additional separation of negatives from statements allows the representation of the overlap not only in syntactic realization between questions and negative, but also the functional blending of interrogative and negative and command and negative. We know that children early on use utterances with the function of commands, negatives, and questions as well as statements, and it appears that the most insightful way to profile Irish acquisition is to display these functions separately.

ILARSP

Sections A-D of the LARSP chart are reproduced on the Irish chart, since they are not language specific. The second part of section A, entitled *code-switching*, is based on Ball's LLARSP chart. While the children studied were from Irish-speaking homes in *Gaeltacht* communities, they were nevertheless exposed to some English from television or from tourists who stayed with the families in the summer months. The participant children had some English words, such as *dirty*, *sweetie*, and *OK*. One child began to attend an Irish-medium pre-school at about 2;4 and quickly acquired some English phrases from monolingual English speakers in the group. In more recent years the extent of exposure to English has increased considerably, and there is significant concern about language attenuation and convergence (Hickey,

2009). Thus, it is important to have a place on the chart where such use of English can be marked. However, it is recommended that if the child's use of English is extensive, then it should be analysed on the LARSP chart. If his or her English use is limited to a number of phrases and words, then the tokens of words and phrase-types should be counted at the bottom of the chart, since this may also give an indication of formulaic use.

Stage I

In analysing data from the ILARSP chart, only Major utterances in Irish were used. Utterances with English phrases or clauses were not included (although those with a commonly used English word, such as *Tabhair dom sweetie* 'Give me a sweet' were). Minor sentences such as *neó* (Ó Siadhail's (1973) spelling of the Irish pronunciation of the English negative using a palatalised 'n'), vocatives, social stereotypes and 'huh'?' (included because of its high frequency in the children tested) were noted under Stage I Minor. The structures listed in LARSP Stage I are extremely simple, but ILARSP lists them in more detail, so that a more comprehensive picture of the one-word stage is gathered. This is particularly useful in studies of normal acquisition, but if this level of detail is not required, the user can simply ignore the categories Adj, Adv, and Dem. The structure Neg-V listed in the Negative column covers the use of *níl* (Neg-be-Pres), the negative of the present tense of the verb 'to be'. This was sometimes used as a general negative reply, although it is only correct in reply to a question containing the present tense of the verb 'to be'. There is no structure listed in the Question column, since it is not possible to use a question clitic alone, and this was never observed in the data. However, children acquiring Irish bilingually in recent years have been noted to use *céard* 'what' as a one-word interrogative, which is possibly the result of convergence with English, and such use could be noted in the Stage I Question column.

Stage II

There are more divergences between LARSP and ILARSP at Stage II. However, the Command column remains the same, with VX for utterances such as *Oscail é* 'Open it' and *Tabhair dom* 'Give me'. A negative imperative is included in the collapsed column between Command and Negative, NegimpV, for utterances such as *Ná déan* 'Don't'. The new structures in the Negative column reflect developmental strategies of expressing negative in Irish. It was found that one of the children's earliest and most frequent negatives was the English *no* (pronounced in Irish as *neó,* with a slender 'n'). Examination of input to the children revealed that adults often preceded a negative utterance to children with a stressed *neó,* before the correct Irish negative. In the children's speech, it was combined with a range of word classes, as in *Neó bainne* 'No milk' or *Neó dul* 'No going'. Neg V was used for the correct Irish negative in, for example, *Ní raibh* 'Not was', or a fairly frequent negative form used by the children *Ní* thit* 'Not fell' (using the general negative particle instead of the past-tense marked *níor*). The last category, Neg-VX, was a development from the Stage-I use of *níl*, the present tense negative of the verb 'to be', and usually occurred with nouns as in *Níl Bran* 'Bran is-not'.

In the Question column, the structure QX represents many open questions in Irish. The children's frequent *Cad é sin?* ('What it that?' > 'What's that?') was analysed as Stage II, as a variant of *cad sin* (which is also well formed but very infrequent), and co-reference was marked at Transitional Stage II-III in the category C-R because the pronoun *é* is co-referential with the subject (the demonstrative *sin* 'that') and the question word. The new structure in Stage-II questions was *(an) V*, which represented *yes/no*-questions such as *an raibh?* (be-Past Questions), or *an bhfuil?* (be-Present-question). The question clitic *an* should be marked as optional on the grounds that it is often elided in adult speech when the following verb is the dependent form of irregular verbs used in questions.

In Stage-II statements, one of the main differences from LARSP is the change in word order. SV has become VS, and this reversal is applied throughout the chart. Irish is a strong VSO language, and the unmarked word order in simple sentences is VSOX, where X includes adverbials of different kinds, prepositional phrases and so on. For example:

(9) *Cheannaigh Máire leabhar do Sheán*
    'Bought   Maire a-book   Prep Seán' >
    'Máire bought a book for Seán'

No clause constituent may intervene between the verb and subject in a simple sentence. However, where aspect is marked by the combination of the verb 'to be' and the verbal noun (rather than by the habitual tenses), the order of such a sentence is:

(10) *Tá mé ag scríobh*
     'Be I   Prt write(Verbal N) '
     'I am writing'

Example (10) would be analysed as VSVn at Stage III of the ILARSP chart. A decision was made to analyse sentences with verbal nouns marking aspect separately from simple sentences, since there was perceived to be a developmental significance in the use of such utterances. In a study of word order in Irish acquisition (Hickey, 1990a), it was found that SVn marked the children's earliest frequent verb use, and analysing it as VS as on Ball's LLARSP chart would obscure both the omission of the auxiliary and the later introduction and comparatively lower frequency of simple verbs. Thus, VS at Stage II can stand for well-formed utterances with an intransitive verb such as *Thit baba* ('Fell baby' > 'Baby fell') or immature or elliptical utterances such as *Tá bó* 'Is cow'.

VSVn utterances are not treated as expansions of VS at the transitional level, in accordance with work by Stenson (1976) and McCloskey (1983), who did not treat this construction as a VP. However, McCloskey did argue convincingly that the progressive construction itself constitutes a surface VP, which he called a ProgP, with the head of this ProgP, the sequence *ag*+ *Vn* (PVn) being the smallest ProgP there is. The main difference between the LARSP procedure on this issue and the ILARSP one is that in the Irish chart there is no Aux category and, therefore, Aux cannot expand a VP. Instead, the Aux equivalent is included explicitly in such categories as VSVn. If we retain the expansions S, C, O, and A, and restrict V expansion to PVn, VnV-part, or VnVn, calling it VGp (verb group rather than VP in order to underline the distinction), then no information is lost and comparability of a sort is retained with the English chart, while at the same time an essential feature of the language is fully represented on the chart.

Structures such as SC, SO, VC, and VO are retained. Subject-initial utterances were found to be frequent in the children's data (see Hickey, 1990a), mainly due to the omission of the verb 'to be'. Thus, many categories in Stage-II Clause represent reduced or elliptical utterances, with the exception of CopX *(is ea,* which is the reply to copular utterances) and Dem X such as *Seo piosa* 'Here's a piece' or *Sin é daidí* 'That's daddy', where the co-referentiality of *é* with the subject and complement is marked at Transitional Stage II-III. Dem X utterances are traditionally analysed as having an implicit copula (i.e. *is eo píosa),* but it was decided to mark them separately in profiling development in order not to overestimate control of the copula at an early stage when such Dem X utterances are common and may be formulaic (see Hickey, 1993).

It is often difficult to decide whether an utterance such as *Mamaí dána* 'Mammy naughty' should be analysed as SC or NAdj. Crystal *et al.* (1981) noted that such utterances are often ambiguous even in English, where normal word order distinguishes them. In Irish this ambiguity is greater, since the normal word order of the full VSC utterance is *tá mamaí dána.* In the children's speech, the verb was often dropped from such utterances. Crystal *et al.* recommended the analysis of stress in attempting to resolve this ambiguity, but this is not helpful in Irish. A conservative policy was adopted here, whereby all noun-adjective combinations occurring alone would be marked on the ILARSP chart as SC, while those which occur as expansions of an element in a 2+ element construction would be marked as NAdj. It is recognized that this is not ideal, but it appears to be preferable to making inconsistent and arbitrary decisions on this matter.

Other differences from the LARSP chart in the marking of Stage-II Phrase categories are the analysis of utterances such as *leaba *mamaí* as NN, but with the possibility of marking the absence of the lenition mutation under the asterisk column next to N + N at word level. The category NN(-c) is included because it was found to be relatively frequent at this stage for utterances such as *Mamaí daidí* 'Daddy [and] mammy'. Int-X was moved to Stage-III Phrase, because, on the basis of the data currently available, it was not used until other Stage-III constructions became frequent. PVn is introduced at Stage-II Phrase in order to indicate the use of the aspect marker *ag* before verbal nouns, as in *ag ithe* ('at eating' > 'eating'). Thus, what McCloskey termed ProgP is marked as a V expansion and as PVn at Stage II Phrase so that its impact on VGp can be distinguished from other V expanders. There is a precedent for such a double marking in that Aux V is marked as a V expansion on LARSP, while Aux is also marked separately at phrase level.

Stage III

In Stage III Commands, the only category is VXY since the *let* and *do* categories are not appropriate for Irish. The NegVX category marks utterances containing negation of verbs other than the verb 'to be' as well as the suppleted form *níl* of that verb. The negative question category NegQV marks utterances such as *Nach bhfuil?* ('Not-QPresent is?' > 'Isn't it?') and *Nár tháinig?* ('Not-Q-Pat come?' > 'Didn't [he] come?'). It may be that Stage III is too early to place productive use of such structures, but some of them were used, at least formulaically, at about this stage. Utterances that appeared to be formulaic were analysed at the stage appropriate to the construction, but were marked with a dagger so that their questionable productivity was clear. In fact, the use of a Stage-III structure by a child whose utterances are mainly Late Stage I/Early Stage II is a pointer that that utterance may not be productive.

The two question categories at this stage, QVX and QXY, distinguish the usual *wh*-questions of the type *Cá bhfuil baa?* 'Where are baa (sheep)?' and another, frequent type, *Cén rud é sin?* ('What thing that?' > 'What's that?'). This is an extended form *(Cad é an rud é sin)* of *Cad é sin?* 'What's that?', and the decision was made to mark it separately at a later stage (marking co-reference on the transitional line), since its use began later. An VX marks more complex *yes/no*-questions that those in Stage II, such as *(An gcíonn tú?* 'You see?' and *(An) bhfuil seacláid?* ('Q is chocolate?' > 'Do [you] have chocolate?')). Such utterances may still be reduced or elliptical.

New categories at State-III clause level are mainly extensions of new categories introduced in the previous stage. The CopXY category represents utterances such as *Is liomsa é* ('Cop with-me-emphatic it' > 'It's mine') as well as **Mise garsúinín maith* ('[Be] I a-little-boy good' > 'I'm a good little boy'). It was decided to analyse the latter as CopXY rather than as the simpler SC at Stage II because there appeared to be evidence of a developmental split between the early SC pattern, already discussed, and the later copular SC pattern which is a copular identification sentence (the more normal order for such a sentence would be *garsúinín maith mise*). The CopXY category also covers identification sentences which are common in this dialect, such as:

(11) *Capall is   ea   é*   'It's a horse'
     C1   Cop C2 S

Ó Sé (personal communication) points out that in this case what he calls the indefinite ('neuter') pronoun *ea* refers not only to the Complement *capall* 'horse' but is also coreferential with the Subject *é*. The word order of such copular sentences warrants their representation by separate categories on the ILARSP chart.

New categories at Stage-III phrase level are Adv, which comprises static and dynamic adverbs such as *amuigh* 'outside – static' and *anuas* 'down from – dynamic'. It was found that such adverbs were used quite frequently by the children, and their use was obscured if they were marked only as an A component of a clause structure. Thus *Daidí amuigh* 'Daddy outside' was analysed as SA, with static/dynamic adverbs (Adv(s/d)) marked at Stage III Phrase level, while *Baby istigh sa chotaí* 'baby inside in the cot' was marked as:

(12) *Baby istigh sa chotaí* ('Baby inside in-the cot' > 'Baby in the cot'
      S   A   A   Stage III Clause
           Adv   Pr-D N
           Stg III Phr   Stg III Phr

It was found useful to mark dynamic adverbs of this type as a subscript and static ones as a superscript after the Adv category. A similar method was used with the Pron category: Subject pronouns were marked as superscripts while object pronouns were marked as subscripts. PrPn represents the category of Prepositional Pronouns which are a feature of Irish.

Stage IV

Stage-IV commands do not differ markedly from the LARSP chart. The question categories are extensions of those in the earlier stages. There is no tag category, since such questions are covered by the earlier question structures, and seem to appear earlier than Stage IV, although it is not clear if they are fully productive then. It may be necessary to add a separate tag category in Stage IV, so that such questions can be discriminated from earlier immature forms. NegQVX covers utterances such as *Nach bhfaca tú?* (Neg-Q V S) 'Didn't you see?' Other Stage-IV clause structures are extensions of those discussed earlier.

Stage-IV phrase structures such as NP Pr NP *(cailín le mála mór* 'a girl with a big bag'), Pr D N Adj *(go dtí an siopa nua* 'to the new shop'), and CX and XcX are the same as the English Stage-IV categories. However, the Neg and Aux categories on the English chart at this stage are omitted as inappropriate.

Stage V

Stages V and VI in this version of the chart are not based on data from children acquiring the language, as the children studied did not reach these levels. Therefore they are provisional, and must await further data. The LARSP categories at Stage-V command level are appropriate to Irish, with the substitution of a*gus* for *and*.

Stage V is the stage of recursion in LARSP, and this is marked similarly on ILARSP. Coordination and subordination are marked for statements, commands, negatives and questions. Differences at Stage-V Phrase level are the omission of the category 'Post-modifying phrase 1+'. Utterances of this type seem quite implausible in Irish (as well as extremely stilted in English) and thus the category is omitted.

Stage VI

Stage VI in ILARSP, as in LARSP, looks at what the child cannot do, since at this point of development that is a more economical strategy than looking at what he or she can do. However, the ILARSP Stage VI is structured differently to LARSP's. It focuses mainly on the omission of, or incorrect use of, phrase or word-level structures. The most frequent errors noticed among the children are listed here, but need to be extended by data from children who are more than about four years old. *W.O. under 'Clause' indicates incorrect word order, while '-Element' indicates the omission of a clause element. This convention, whereby * indicates an incorrect form, and '-' its omission is used throughout the stage. It is suggested that using this stage (or an amplified version of it) might be a useful first strategy for SLTs dealing with Irish-dominant children referred for assessment in order to get a picture of the areas causing them difficulty.

Stage VII

Stage VII ILARSP is almost identical with LARSP's, covering aspects of sentence connection, topicalization, syntactic comprehension and style. The notation *empty tá* is used to clarify the function which in LARSP is marked as *it* and *there*. The other categories are suitable for Irish and are retained.

Word Level

Crystal *et al.* (1981) consider that, in English, inflections are used systematically from about Stage III, and base the inflections at word level in their chart on Brown's 14 morphemes. Irish is far more complex at word level, and the first difficulty is in deciding on the degree of comprehensiveness to be aimed at. It would be possible to compose a word level which would take up more space than clause and phrase, on the lines of Ball's LLARSP-M or -T charts. A similarly detailed word-level chart was initially used in the analysis of the acquisition of the three children studied by Hickey (1987), but it was found that this level of detail was unnecessary up to the age of three years at least. As already noted, such a separate chart has the disadvantage of fragmenting the profile, and this level of detail may not be required in every case. Instead, it seems preferable in the case of Irish to present a reasonably general word level which can then be elaborated upon if this level is to be focused on because the evidence indicates that this is warranted. The ILARSP word level has, however, been extended somewhat since the initial study, so that it is more easily interpretable alone, without the use of the detailed chart.

It must be pointed out that, while there is an attempt to represent a developmental order at word level, this will require further data on development later than Stage IV. The ILARSP word level begins with the three earliest tensed forms of the verb 'to be' used by the children studied. The development of this verb appears to have special significance in the acquisition of Irish, and thus it is presented in more detail than other verbs on the chart. Underneath it are the affirmative and negative response forms of the copula, which may be overgeneralized as general responses equivalent to 'yes' and 'no'. Vn and VAdj refer to verbal nouns and verbal adjectives, respectively, and these also begin to be used quite early, around Stage II. The singular article *an* and the plural article *na* follow next, although there appears to be a developmental lag between them, so that it may be preferable to place *na* later in the chart if further studies substantiate this.

Irregular verbs have 'dependent forms' when used in questions and negatives in some tenses, and this is marked as Dependent V. The irregular past and future tense categories are then given. Next to noun plural (N pl), two of the most common plural suffixes are listed, since these are the first to be used productively, and were overgeneralized by the older children. However, as the means of marking the plural in Irish are extremely varied (with up to 13 categories of plural formation as identified by Ó Sé, 1983), it is suggested that other plurals be noted down separately if further detail of this development is required. The regular past and future marking is listed next. *Dim, emph,* and *rflx* refer to diminutive and emphatic particles and to reflexive pronouns. These seem to appear quite early in the children's speech, although they may not be fully productive until some time later.

It was necessary to represent the children's development of the system of initial mutations as it applies to nouns and adjectives. This is represented in the next part of the chart under AL II (Allomorph) and AL III. Allomorph II is the notation for the lenition mutation, whereby consonants are systematically weakened. Orthographically this is marked by the insertion of an 'h' after the initial consonant. Allomorph III represents eclipsis, whereby a voice segment becomes nasalized or a voiceless segment voiced. This is marked orthographically by the addition of the appropriate item from the list: *b, m, d, n, q, g* or *bh* to the eclipsed consonant. Strictly speaking, these mutations are phrasally determined, but it was thought that the most convenient place to represent them in some detail on the chart was at word level, though with some effort to indicate their dependence on their environment. The categories listed under each of these AL II and AL III headings are only a sample of the environments of these mutations, but they are selected as being among the most likely to appear in child language. If this level of detail is not required, then the heading AL II or AL III only may be marked.

N + N indicates the lenition of the second noun in possessive constructions such as *Leaba mhamaí* 'Mammy's bed', and Poss + N covers the lenition that follows after first, second and third masculine singular possessives such as *mo dhaidí* 'my daddy' or *a dhinnéar* 'his dinner'. Pr + N indicates that lenition occurs after simple prepositions such as *do Sheán* 'for Seán'. D + Nf refers to the lenition of feminine nouns following the article (e.g. *an bhean* 'the woman'), while Nf + Adj indicates that adjectives following a feminine noun are also lenited (e.g. *bean mhór* 'a big woman'). ND + Nm indicates that masculine nouns in the genitive are lenited, as in *hata an fhir* 'the man's hat'. N + Adjpl refers to the lenition of plural adjectives if they follow a masculine noun ending in a slender consonant (e.g. *fir mhóra)*. The category 'Other' covers a range of other environments for lenition. Such is the complexity of the mutation system in Irish, it is suggested that the full acquisition of this system is not complete until after the age of five years and possibly even later into the school years, as has been shown with regard to aspects of Welsh (Thomas & Gathercole, 2007). They argue that children's development of productive command of grammatical gender and mutations in Welsh point to item-based rather than rule-based learning.

The categories listed under Allomorph III or eclipsis begin with PrD + N. This is placed first in this section because eclipsis occurs in this environment in the Munster and Connacht dialects, whereas lenition is used instead in the Ulster dialect. Plural possessives (Posspl + N) eclipse the following noun (e.g. *ár bpáistí* 'our children'). ND + Npl indicates that plural nouns in the genitive are eclipsed, as in *scoil na gcailíní* 'the girls' school'. The mutation which inserts a *t-* before masculine nouns beginning with a vowel, or before *sl-, sn-,* or *sr-* feminine nouns in the nominative and dative singular, and masculine nouns in the genitive singular, is indicated on the chart by 't- v/s'. The insertion of a *h*-mutation before singular feminine nouns in the genitive and plural masculine nouns in the nominative and dative is indicated by the category 'h- v'.

It was decided to have a special error column next to the initial mutation categories at word level in order to allow for the collection of information on this complex aspect of acquisition without having to develop a separate chart for the mutations. Errors in other categories are covered at Stage VI, but the notation of mutation errors at word level is a means of saving space on the chart, without forfeiting details. This mutations column allows for the marking of substitution (*) or omission (-) of the correct mutation, but the same caution must be used in marking such errors as is urged by Crystal *et al.* concerning the marking of errors in LARSP Stage VI. It is suggested that this column should only be used when there is evidence that the child is using at least some of the environments for the mutations productively. An example of mutation error is the overgeneralization by one of the older children of an eclipsed form *an *mbord* 'the table' as the base form of *bord* 'table'; such an error would be marked under * at word level next to AL III.

The remaining categories at word level are Autonomous, which refers to an impersonal form of the verb that does not specify the subject. An example of this form is *Dúnadh an doras* '(Somebody) closed the door'. Genitive refers to the different marking of the genitive case on nouns, which varies between noun conjugations. Finally, there is a category for comparative and superlative, which use the same adjective form, but are preceded by a different particle.

Conclusion

The use of this adaptation of LARSP in a study of the acquisition of Irish as mother-tongue by three children aged between 1;4 and 3 years shows that ILARSP can adequately and comprehensively represent the L1 acquisition of Irish, allowing useful comparisons between the same child's language at different ages, and between different children of the same age. Basing this adaptation of the LARSP chart on typical Irish acquisition and testing the adaptation against normal longitudinal data are important steps towards the development of an instrument which can be used both in crosslinguistic research and to assess language impairment. It is hoped to extend the base of information on normal development by using data collected more recently, so that the later stages of the chart can be fully tested and so that age norms can be developed for Irish acquisition.

Acknowledgements

The author wishes to thank Michael Garman, Paul Fletcher, Con Ó Cléirigh, Diarmuid Ó Sé and Martin Ball for their help and comments.

Notes

(1) An earlier version of this chapter was published in the journal *Clinical Linguistics and Phonetics*. This revised and expanded version is published with the permission of Informa PLC.
(2) In Irish, the language is referred to as Gaeilge, and the term 'Gaelic' is derived from this. However, the term 'Irish' is preferred in Ireland in referring in English to the language, in order to distinguish it from (Scottish) Gaelic.
(3) Irish postposes adjectives, so in Irish the name would be *LARSP na Gaeilge* yielding the unpronounceable LARSPG. Since the name LARSP is itself an English acronym, it was decided to use the English term of Irish in the title of the adaptation, ILARSP.

References

Ball, M. (1988) LARSP to LLARSP: The design of a grammatical profile for Welsh. *Clinical Linguistics & Phonetics* 2, 55–73.
Brennan, S. (2004) *First Steps: Early Development of Irish as a Primary Language: Focus on Phonology*. Dublin: Comhdháil Náisiúnta na Gaeilge. http://d1375888.gdm64.gravitate.ie/downloads/Na_Chead_Cheimeanna_Leagan_Bearla.PDF
Cameron, T. and Hickey, T.M. (2011) Form and function in Irish child directed speech. *Cognitive Linguistics* 22, 569–594.
Crystal, D., Fletcher, P. and Garman, M. (1981) *The Grammatical Analysis of Language Disability: A Procedure for Assessment and Remediation* (2nd edn). London: Cole & Whurr (Original work published 1989).
Goodluck, H., Guilfoyle, E. and Harrington, S. (2001) Acquiring subject and object relatives: evidence from Irish. *Journal of Celtic Language Learning* Vol. 6: First Language Learning, 21–33.
Goodluck, H., Guilfoyle, E. and Harrington, S. (2006) Merge and binding in child relative clauses: The case of Irish. *Journal of Linguistics* 42, 629–61.
Greenberg, J. (1966) *Universals of Language* (2nd edn). Cambridge, MA: MIT Press.
Greene, D. (1966) *The Irish Language*, Dublin: The Three Candles.
Hayden, C. (1984) *An Adaptation to Irish of LARSP*. Unpublished MA thesis: Trinity College Dublin.
Hickey, T. (1987) The Early Acquisition of Irish: Grammatical Patterns and the Role of Formulas. Unpublished PhD dissertation: University of Reading.
Hickey, T. (1990a) The acquisition of Irish: A study of word order development. *Journal of Child Language* 17, 17–41.
Hickey, T. (1990b) ILARSP: A grammatical profile of Irish. *Clinical Linguistics & Phonetics* 4, 363–76.
Hickey, T. (1991) Mean length of utterance and the acquisition of Irish. *Journal of Child Language* 18, 553–69.
Hickey, T. (1993) Identifying formulas in first language acquisition. *Journal of Child Language* 20 (1), 27–42.
Hickey, T. (1997) *Early immersion education in Ireland: Na Naíonraí/An Luath-Thumadh in Éirinn: Na Naíonraí*. Baile Átha Cliath: ITÉ. http://www.eric.ed.gov/ERICDocs/data/ericdocs2sql/content_storage_01/0000019b/80/15/65/86.pdf
Hickey, T. (1999) *Luathoideacheas trí Ghaeilge sa Ghaeltacht* ('Early education through Irish in the Gaeltacht). Baile Átha Cliath: Údarás na Gaeltachta & ITÉ.
Hickey, T. (2001) Mixing beginners and native speakers in Irish immersion: Who is immersing whom? *Canadian Modern Language Review* 57 (3), 443–74.
Hickey, T. (2007) Children's language networks in minority language immersion: What goes in may not come out. *Language and Education* 21, 46–65. http://www.multilingual-matters.net/le/021/1/default.htm

Hickey, T. (2009) Codeswitching and borrowing in Irish. *Journal of Sociolinguistics* 13, 670–88.
Hickey, T.M. and Cameron-Faulkner, T. (2009) Contact induced change in the Irish negation system: Rebels without a clause? Paper presented at the *International Symposium on Bilingualism 7*: University of Utrecht.
Hickey, T.M. and Stenson, M. (2011) Irish orthography: What do teachers and learners need to know about it, and why? *Language, Culture and Curriculum 24 (1), 23–46*.
McCloskey, J. (1983) A VP in the VSO language? In G. Gazdar, E. Klein and G. Pullum (eds) *Order, Concord and Constituency*. Dordrecht: Foris.
McKenna, A. and Wall, E. (1986) *Our First Language*. Dublin: The Glendale Press.
Mhic Mhathúna, M. (1995) SLA before ABC: Factors facilitating second language acquisition in Irish-medium playgroups. *Teanga* 15, 127–36.
Ó Duibhir, P. (2009) The Spoken Irish of Sixth-Class Pupils in Irish Immersion Schools. Unpublished PhD dissertation: Trinity College Dublin.
Ó Sé, D. (2000) *Gaeilge Chorca Dhuibhne*. Baile Átha Cliath: Institiúid Teangeolaíochta Éireann.
Ó Siadhail, M. (1973) Abairtí freagartha agus míreanna freagartha sa NuaGhaeilge. *Ériú* 24, 134–59.
O'Toole, C. and Hickey, T. (in preparation) Assessing and diagnosing language impairment in bilingual children: A minority language study.
O'Toole, C., and Fletcher, P. (2008) Developing assessment tools for bilingual and minority language acquisition. *Journal of Clinical Speech and Language Studies* 16, 12–27.
O'Toole, C., and Fletcher, P. (2010) Validity of a parent report instrument for Irish-speaking toddlers. *First Language* 30 (2), 199–217.
Owens, M. (1992) *The Acquisition of Irish: A Case Study*. Clevedon: Multilingual Matters.
Singleton, D., Harrington, S. and Henry, A. (2000) At the sharp end of language revival: English-speaking parents raising Irish-speaking children. *CLCS Occasional Paper* 57, Trinity College Dublin.
Slobin, D. (2006) Cross-linguistic comparative approaches to language acquisition. In K. Brown (ed.) *Encyclopaedia of Language and Linguistics* (pp. 299–301) (2nd edn). London: Elsevier.
Stenson, N. (1976) Topics in Irish Syntax and Semantics. Unpublished PhD dissertation: University of California, San Diego.
Stenson, N. (1981) *Studies in Irish Syntax*. Tubingen: Narr.
Thomas, E. and Gathercole, V. (2007) Children's productive command of grammatical gender and mutation in Welsh: An alternative to rule-based learning. *First Language* 27 (3), 251–78.
Ward, A. (1974) The Grammatical Structure of Munster Irish. Unpublished PhD dissertation: University College Dublin.

10 Persian: Devising the P-LARSP[1]
Habibeh Samadi and Mick Perkins

Introduction

This chapter describes P-LARSP, an adaptation of the LARSP profile for Persian. It is based on data collected as part of a longitudinal study of three monolingual Persian-speaking children between the ages of 1;8 and 3;0, 2;2 and 3;2, and 2;4 and 3;4 (Samadi, 1996), and the resulting profile chart represents the full range of grammatical structures produced by these children. As well as providing the first published overview of the acquisition of Persian syntax and morphology, the profile also constitutes an outline description of contemporary spoken Persian, a pro-drop, inflectional, and mostly verb-final language which has been very little studied. In addition, the P-LARSP profile is also the first formal procedure devised for assessing language impairment in Persian, and can be used to compare the language of different children as well as the same child's language at different stages of development.

The primary motivation for developing a Persian version of LARSP was to provide Iranian speech and language therapists and other language professionals with a general language assessment and remediation procedure, which has hitherto been lacking. A further motivation was to provide a framework which would encourage the collection of data and facilitate research on the acquisition of Persian. Although a few scholarly articles and pedagogical texts on Persian grammar have been published since the research on which this chapter is based was carried out, there is still no comprehensive and authoritative Persian grammar available to provide information about the varieties of structural patterns in this language. The structure of Persian, however, is of considerable interest, since it shares a number of features with other pro-drop languages, and linguistic profiling of such a group of languages should be able to throw new light on language acquisition in general. The only developmental study of Persian grammar to date that we are aware of is Doroudian (1979), who investigated the acquisition of Persian and English in her bilingual child. Her primary focus, however, is on the acquisition of English rather than Persian. Samadi's (1996) work, on which P-LARSP is based, therefore constitutes an important landmark in the study of Persian language acquisition.

The Corpus

The first step towards adapting LARSP for Persian consisted of the collection of a corpus of normative data from three monolingual Iranian children aged between 1;8 and 2;4, 2;2 and 3;2, and 2;4 and 3;4 who were living temporarily in England but in a totally Persian-speaking environment. The children were videotaped for between 30 and 45 minutes every month while interacting with a parent. The recordings were transcribed orthographically and occasionally phonetically immediately after each session. A total of 32 samples were collected. The first 100 utterances after the 51st utterance in each sample were analysed morphologically and syntactically, thus providing an analysed corpus of 3200 utterances, which is available on the CHILDES database. The transcript and grammatical analysis were coded using the CHAT system (MacWhinney, 1995) and structures at clause, phrase, and word level were recorded in accordance with the LARSP procedure. The following short extract provides an illustration.

@Begin @Participants: FAA Faeze child, DAD father
@date: 22-JUN- 93
@Age of FAA: 2;8
@Filename: FAEZE. CHA
@Situation: free talk
*FAA: xodet.
         'yourself'
%mor: proreflex|xod-INF|et&2s.
%syn: elliptical.
*DAD: xodam barda:ram?
         'pick (it) up myself?'
*FAA: ha:n
         'yes'
%syn: minor.
*DAD: ma:sha:la: xob beya: pa:ein barda:r dige.
         'Great, well get down, pick (it) up like this'
*FAA: in dorost nisht
         (this right not is)
         'this is not right'
%mor: pro|in adj|dorost neg|ni#cop|st&pres_3s.
%syn: <SCV>.
*DAD: che tori doroste?
         'How is it right?'
*FAA: yeba:r dige ba:zi bekonam?
         (once more play do-I)
         'Do I play once more?'
%mor: adv|yeba:r adv|dige n|ba:zi be#v|kon&pres-INF|am&1s.
%syn: <X CompVI>.[DNN]. XY+A:AP.

```
*DAD:   ina: beza:r pa:ein. beza: pa:ei ina:reo.
        (these put down)
        'Put these down'.
*FAA:   na.
        'no'
%syn:   minor.
*DAD:   rixtesh mixa:st ruye miz xalvat ba:she betune una:ro bechine. chi
        shode?
        'It smashed. She wanted the table to be cleared so she can set those
        up. What happened?'
*FAA:   ekast.
        (broke it)
        'it broke'
%mor:   v|shekast&past_3s.
&syn:   <V>.
@End.
```

Before discussing the P-LARSP profile, a brief description of some of the salient features of Persian grammar will be helpful.

A brief Outline of Persian Grammar

The objective of this section is to familiarize readers with some specific features of Persian grammar, which are included in the P-LARSP profile but not discussed fully elsewhere. These include nouns and noun phrases, definite and indefinite nouns, *ezafe* and *ma:l,* pronouns, verbs, negation, questions, the object marker *ro/o,* the past participle *-e,* auxiliaries and modals.

The language analysed in this study is modern colloquial Persian, which is spoken as a first language in Iran, Afghanistan, Tajikistan and to some extent in Pakistan and India. In Iran, Persian, known as Farsi, is spoken by half the population. Modern Persian is a member of the Indo-Iranian language group, which belongs to the Indo-European family. It has a relatively 'rudimentary' inflectional system (Windfuhr, 1979) and studies by traditional grammarians, as well as recent works in the field of linguistics, have described modern Persian as a mostly verb-final language (for example, Bateni, 1970b; Farrokhpey, 1979; Dabir-Moghadam, 1982; Samiian, 1983; Karimi, 1989). Persian is also considered a pro-drop language (i.e. pronominal subjects may be omitted, and in such cases the subject appears only as a verb suffix. For example, *raft-am* ('went-I' > 'I went')). In addition, some prepositional phrases, according to their function, can also be considered as adverbials, as Quirk *et al.* (1985) have suggested for English, and Ball and Thomas (this volume) for Welsh (e.g. *Be-de be man* 'imp-give to me' > 'Give me', where 'me' is an indirect object).

Nouns and noun phrases

The simple noun phrase in Persian may include: the plural marker *ha:/a:,* the definite marker *e,* the indefinite marker *i,* some prepositions, the object marker *ro/o* and the demonstratives *in* 'this' and *a:n* 'that'. All nouns in Persian are assumed to be countable; the subdivision of nouns into countable and uncountable does not exist for this language (Bateni, 1976).

Definite and indefinite nouns

Generic and specific definite nouns are not marked as such in Persian. All Persian nouns are identified as definite except when marked with the indefinite suffix *i.* Bateni (1970a) presents the following table for Persian definite and indefinite nouns:

[P = plural   S = singular   0 = zero = definite marker]
generic (0 + S)
definite (0 + S; 0 + P) rarely *(an + P/S; S + e)*
indefinite (S/P + *i; yek* +S + *i*)

As seen above, there is usually no definite marker in Persian.

Ezafe

A common non-verbal construction in Persian is *ezafe,* which literally means 'addition', specified by the occurrence of a morpheme *e* before the phrasal complement and a modifier following the head. The *ezafe* construction occurs in all non-verbal phrase categories: the adjective phrase, the noun phrase and the prepositional phrase. Modifiers in Persian follow their head nouns and *ezafe* is placed between the modifier and the head (e.g. *pesar e xub* ('boy good' > 'the good boy')). The order of all non-verbal phrase categories except prepositional phrases is the opposite of their English counterparts (e.g. *keta:b e pesar* ('book boy' > 'the boy's book')). *Ezafe* is also used in forming prepositional phrases (e.g. *zir e a:b* ('under water' > 'under the water')).

Ma:l

Ma:l 'the property of' is followed by the genitive noun phrase and pronouns to express possession (e.g. *ma:l e hassan* ('the property *of* hassan' > 'the property of Hassan'); *ma:l e man* ('the property *of* me' > 'mine')).

Pronouns

Persian pronouns have neither gender distinctions nor different grammatical forms (i.e. Persian subject, object, and possessive pronouns are the same). However, the subject pronouns in the form of inflections are different from their object and possessive counterparts. These inflections are attached to verbs as well as to adjectives, nouns and pronouns. Object inflections either appear as a verb suffix in the 3rd person singular, past tense (e.g. *Gerft-mun* ('Caught-us' > 'She/he caught us')) or they are used after the subject inflections (e.g. *Gerft-am-et* ('Caught-I-you' > 'I caught you')). On the other hand, possessives in the form of inflections are attached to nouns (e.g. *ota:q-am* ('room-my' > 'my room')).

Verbs

Most researchers agree that there are two independent roots of the present and past as the basic forms for the formation of all verbal categories in modern Persian. Infinitives are formed by attaching *-an* to the past root. However, infinitives as well as bare roots are rarely used in Persian. For example, the present root always appears with the prefix *mi-* or *be-/bi-/biy-*, and the past root is always inflected except in cases where there is no specific ending for 3rd person singular. The following illustrates the infinitive, past root, present root, present and past tense of the verb *xord-an* 'to eat':

Infinitive	**Past root**	**Present root**
xord-an	*xord*	*xor*
'to eat'	'ate'	'eat'

Present tense

mi-xor-am	(pres-eat-I) 'I eat'	*mi-xor-im*	(pres-eat-we) 'we eat'
mi-xor-i	(pres-eat-you) 'you eat'	*mi-xor-id*	(pres-eat-you) 'you eat'
mi-xor-e	(pres-eat-he) 'she, he, it eats'	*mi-xor-an*	(pres-eat-they) 'they eat'

Past tense

xord-am	(ate-I) 'I ate'	*xord-im*	(ate-we) 'we ate'
xord-i	(ate-you) 'you ate'	*xord-id*	(ate-you) 'you ate'
xord	(ate-he) 'she, he, it ate'	*xord-an*	(ate-they) 'they ate'

In addition, the majority of Persian verbs are compounds consisting mostly of Adj + Verb and N + Verb (e.g. *sohbat kurd-an* ('speech do' > 'to speak')).

According to Mirhassani (1989), the verb *bud-an* 'to be', like all the other verbs, is regular with present roots *ba:sh* and *hast* and past root *bud*. The present copula *bud-an* 'to be' in inflected form is formed by attaching the person suffixes to adjectives, nouns and pronouns (e.g. *Sard-e* ('Cold-is' > 'It is cold'); *Da:neshju-am* ('Student-am' > 'I am a student'); *Ma:-im* ('We-are' > 'We are')). It should be borne in mind that subject + complement (e.g. *Mahdi bad* 'Mahdi bad'), is not grammatical in Persian, and such sentences cannot appear without subject inflections. For example, the correct structure for the above utterance is *Mahdi bad-e* ('Mahdi bad-is' > 'Mahdi is bad') and the negative form appears with the copula (e.g. *Mahdi bad ni-st* ('Mahdi bad neg-is' > 'Mahdi is not bad')). Therefore it seems plausible to consider the person suffixes as copular in these structures.

Negation and questions

In Persian, the prefix *na* or *ne* is attached to the beginning of main verbs or modal auxiliaries to indicate negation (e.g. *raft* (he/she/it went), *na-raft* (he/she/it did not go)). The only way of forming *yes/no*-questions in the language is to change the intonation of affirmative sentences. *Wh*-questions also have rising intonation (e.g. *key raft?* (when did he/she/it go?)).

Object marker *o/ro*

The suffix *o/ro* is usually added to an object in Persian, *ro* occurring post-vocalically (e.g. *Hassan-o did-am* ('Hassan-Omarker saw-I' > 'I saw Hassan'); *Shoma:-ro daʔvat kard-an* ('You-Omarker invite did-they' > 'They have invited you')).

Past participle *-e*

The suffix *-e* is added to the past root and forms the past participle of the verb. An auxiliary usually follows the past participle form of the verb; for example, *Nevesht-e bud* ('Wrote-PP aux' > 'She/he had written').

Auxiliaries and modals

Farrokhpey (1979) suggests that there are three auxiliaries in Persian:

- *bud-an* 'to be' (e.g. *Raft-e bud* 'Went-PP aux' > 'She/he has gone')
- *shod-an* 'to become' (e.g. *Bast-e shod* 'Closed-PP become' > 'It was closed')
- *xa:st-an* 'to want' (e.g. *Xa:had raft* 'aux went' > 'She/he will go' (this form is rarely used in colloquial Persian); *Mi-xa:-m be-r-am* ('Pres-want-I subj-go-I' > 'I want to go')). The latter form mostly satisfies the criteria for modal auxiliaries rather than auxiliaries. In the present study both forms are regarded as auxiliaries.

Ferrokhpey also suggests three modals:

- *momken bud-an* 'may' = colloquial *mishe* (e.g. *Mishe be-r-am* 'modal auxiliary subj-go-I' > 'May I go')

- *tava:nest-an* 'can' (e.g. *Mi-tun-am be-nevis-am* 'pres-can-I subj-write-I' > 'I can write')
- *ba:yest-an* 'must' (e.g. *Ba:yad be-r-e* 'must subj-go-she/he' > 'She/he must go').

In addition, Windfuhr (1979) has noted an 'aspectual auxiliary' in Persian: *da:r* 'have' with three imperfective forms *(da:r* 'have', *da:sht* 'had', and *da:sht-e* 'has had'), which is used to express progressive aspect. This auxiliary precedes the main verb and takes the same inflections as the main verb. However, in contrast to modal auxiliaries, it does not bear any prefixes (e.g. *Da:r-e shena: mi-kon-e* ('Have she/he swim pres-do-she/he' > 'She/he is swimming')).

P-LARSP

Overall design of the profile chart

Since sections A-D of the LARSP chart are not language-specific, these same sections have been retained in the P-LARSP profile chart (see Figure 10.1). Likewise with the rest of the chart, the Minor/Major sentence distinction is retained, as are the distinctions between Command, Question and Statement; Connectivity, Clause, Phrase and Word; and the developmental Stages I-VII. Owing to the relatively small amount of child language data available for Persian, the age column is not reproduced on the Persian chart. Ball and Thomas (this volume) and Hickey (this volume) omit age equivalents for each stage of their Welsh and Irish profiles for the same reason. It is hoped that the age norms can be established by collecting more data from children in different age groups in the near future. An attempt to analyse Persian data using LARSP categories has shown that there are many constructions and categories common to both languages, although there are a number of categories unique to Persian (Samadi, 1996). As with the English version, constructions have been assigned to different stages of the P-LARSP chart based mainly on the number of constituent morphemes. Ball and Thomas (this volume) and Hickey (this volume) likewise note that LARSP distinctions such as that between one-word and two-word stages also hold for Welsh and Irish.

In assigning patterns to Clause, Phrase, and Word levels, the following criteria were used. Persian is a pro-drop language, and inflections play both syntactic and morphological roles. They are therefore listed not only in the Word column, but in the Command and Statement columns as well. On the other hand, prefixes function morphologically in Persian and are placed only in the Word column. Due to the late acquisition of compound verbs in the Iranian children's data, this category without any inflections is placed in the Clause column at Stage II and analysed as N/AdjV at Stage II Phrase level.

174 Assessing Grammar

Name			Age		Sample date			Type		

A Unanalysed			Problematic		3 Stereo-
1 Unintelligible	2 Symbolic Noise	3 Deviant	1 Incomplete	2 Ambiguous	types

B Responses				Normal Response					Abnormal		
			Repet-	Major							Prob-
			itions	Elliptical			Red		Struc	Ø	lems
Stimulus Type		Totals		1	2	3	uced	Full	Minor tural		
	Questions										
	Others										

C Spontaneous

D Reaction			General	Structural	Ø	Other	Problems

	Minor			Responses		Vocative		Other		Problems
Stage I	Major	Comm.	Quest.	Statement						
		'V'	'Q'	'NegV'	'V'		'N'	Other		Problems
	Conn.			Clause				Phrase		Word
Stage II		VX	ɑX	SV	OV	CompV	DN/Pro	NAdj	Pron	V/C +
				C(V)	VI	VV	NN	IntX	Aux/I	Person
		CompV		SO	SC		PrN/Pron		Adj/NV	Poss/O
				XA	XNeg	Other		Other	Obj/O/ro	
		X + S:NP		X + V:VP	X + C:NP		X + O:NP		X + A:AP	be-/bo-/
Stage III		VXY		XVI	SVA	Other	Adj/NVI		mal Cop	biy- na-/ne-
		CompVX		VIsIo	XC(V)		DNAdj			pl
				SOV	XCompV		PrDN/Pron			Obj/-o
				CompVI					Other	mi-
		XY +S: NP		XY + V:VP	XY + C:NP		XY+ O:NP		XY + A:AP	ezafe/
Stage IV		+ S		SOVI		Complex	Adj/NIVI		Aux/ M	e/ey
		VXY+		AOVI		SVIsIo	PrDNAdj		O	def/ -e
		CompVXY		XCompVI		Other	cX		Other	indef/
				SAVI			XcX			-i
	dige	Coord.		Coord.	1	1+	Postmod. 1	1+		aux/PP
Stage V	badan						clause			-e
	c	Other		Subord.A+	1	1+	Postmod.	1+		-tar
	s			S	C	O	phrase			-tarin
	Other					Comparative				

	(+)					(-)				
	NP	VP	Clause	Conn.	Clause		Phrase			Word
Stage VI	Initiator	Complex+		dige	Ø		D Ø			Poss/O Ø
				adan			Pr		CompV	ezafe V
	Coord			c	Concord		P			reg
				s						Ø
		Other						Ambiguous		

	Discourse				Syntactic Comprehension	
Stage VII	A Connectivity		Emphatic Order			
	Comment		Other		Style	

Total No. Sentences	Mean No. Sentences Per Turn	Mean Sentence Length

Figure 10.1 The P-LARSP chart

The object marker *o/ro* is placed in Stage II Phrase and Word columns. In the case of negative utterances, which have a simple structure in Persian and are acquired after Stage II, the negative prefix *na-/ne-* is placed in the Word column, and the rest of the utterance, like any other Statement utterances, in the Clause column. Auxiliaries in the form of inflections are placed at Phrase and Word levels. The Persian chart, like LARSP, is presented on a single page because, firstly, unlike in the case of Welsh (Ball & Thomas, this volume) the number of inflections is insufficient to require a separate chart, and secondly, one of the aims of designing P-LARSP has been to facilitate the work of assessment for Iranian speech and language therapists, not to make it more complicated.

Detailed description of the P-LARSP chart

In the following description of the P-LARSP chart, examples have been kept to a minimum so as to be accessible to non-Persian speakers. Those who are interested in the detailed explanation of the chart and examples are referred to Samadi (1996). The examples are mostly transcribed orthographically and occasionally phonetically. The vowel system of Persian is relatively simple, and vowels are transcribed phonetically with *a:* representing a long mid-back vowel. Consonants are also transcribed phonetically with *q* representing a voiceless uvular plosive, *x* a voiceless uvular fricative and *ʔ* a glottal plosive.

Stage I

The structures listed at Stage I are the same as those on the English LARSP chart with the exception of Neg-V, which is added at this stage in the Statement column to account for the use of *nist* (Neg-be-Pres). It is clear that *nist* is a formula at this stage (since no novel combinations were observed). As with LARSP, negatives are grouped with statements. As explained before, the reason for this is that the negative system is not complicated and the prefix *ne* – or *na* – is added to the beginning of both modal auxiliaries and main verbs.

Apart from the emergence of negative *nist* at this stage, the other difference between the Persian and English LARSP charts is the two-element command system in Persian. The presence of prefix *be-/bo-/biy-* in Persian commands is observed from the early stages of language acquisition in the children's data (e.g. *be-de* 'give' and *be-ya:* 'come'), since simple verb command forms always appear with a prefix in Persian.

Similar to LARSP, the inverted commas around the terms reflect the controversy in the literature as to whether utterances at Stage I can be called 'sentences' (see Crystal *et al.,* 1989). Question utterances such as *ku,* 'where', are listed in the Question column. In P-LARSP, since *yes/no*-questions do not have a specific structure they are treated like affirmative sentences and are placed at clause level.

Any uninflected verb is included under 'V' in the Statement column. In Persian, uninflected verbs have the form of simple past 3rd person singular – for example, *gerft* 'caught' and *zad* 'beat'. Utterances such as *ma:ma:, ba:ba:* 'Mum', 'Dad', are listed under 'N'. P-LARSP lists words like *ax,* 'bad / dirty' and *bad,* 'bad' under the Other category, since they are used for functions other than the identification of objects and actions. P-LARSP Problems includes any ambiguous utterances (e.g. a form which could either be the past root or 3rd person singular and past tense).

Stage II

There are more divergences between LARSP and P-LARSP at this stage (see Figure 10.1). Under Command, the Compound V such as *Pa:sho* or *Boland sho,* 'Get up', constitutes the first main difference between the charts. The *be-/bo-/biy-* VX category for utterances such as *Be-de man* 'Give me' is shown in this column. The Question column is identical in the two charts at this stage. The structure QX represents the children's frequent use of *Xa: le ku* ('Aunt where' > 'Where is aunt') or *Ku amu* ('Where uncle' > 'Where is uncle').

At Stage II Statements, one of the main differences from LARSP is the change in word order. VO, AX, VC, and NegX have become OV, XA, C(V), and XNeg because the canonical word order in Persian is (S)(O)VI (where VI = 'verb + inflection'). The development of negation in Persian-speaking children at this stage accords with Bellugi's (1967) first stage, in which the child produces negatives external to the sentence. Negation in Persian has a simple construction and is present in Iranian children's utterances after this stage. Hence the negative prefix is placed in the Word column and the rest of the sentence analysed like affirmative utterances after Stage II. Other differences from the LARSP chart are firstly, as indicated above, that V appears in the form (V) in the C(V) category. The reason for this is that, in Persian, 'verbless'-type utterances in the present tense occurring after the complement are in fact the most commonly-encountered form, as in this example:

```
ax-e        sard-e
bad (is) it  cold (is) it
C   (V) S   C    (V) S
```

Windfuhr (1979) observed that these kinds of sentences, C + person agreement, indicate a colloquial tendency of the verb to be in the present tense (e.g. *Am* 'It is me'). In the following example, the first person agreement is regarded by Windfuhr as the copula 'am':

```
man irani    (hast) am
I    Iranian       (am)
'I am Iranian'
```

The new categories VI and CompV are also included in the Clause column at this stage. In the case of VI, it was found that the emergence of the inflections *-am* and *-i* is relatively frequent for utterances such as *Raft-am* 'Went I' > 'I went' and *Did-i* 'Saw you' > 'You saw'. Since pronominal subjects may be omitted in Persian it is necessary to list inflections at both syntactic and morphological levels of the P-LARSP chart. It should be borne in mind that the C(V) and VI categories are morphologically specified in Persian and they should not be regarded as being similar to English *-ing* and *–ed*, where the suffixes are part of a purely morphological paradigm. CompV is also listed in this column. At this stage, Iranian children use Adj/N + simple verb, past tense, 3rd person singular (the only verb construction that has 'zero' inflection). This category was placed at Stage II due to its later emergence than Stage I categories in the Iranian children's data. The following is an example:

Qat kard
(cut did)
'She/he disconnected'
Comp V

N   V

The VV category is listed at Clause instead of Phrase level since, in contrast to English, Persian is a pro-drop language and verbs do not appear as bare roots (see Hyams, 1992); that is, the VV category is produced in utterances such as *raft xa:bid* ('She/he went slept' > 'She/he went to sleep'). Such utterances are grammatically complete and well formed in Persian.

Other differences from the LARSP chart are seen in the Stage-II phrase categories AdjN, NN and possessive pronoun determiners, which appear in a different order from LARSP.

To economize the P-LARSP chart and avoid repetition, the categories which are different in the order of their constituent elements are placed under one category. For example DN/Pron or ND is listed under DN/Pron. The auxiliary *budan* 'to be' in the form of 3rd person singular present tense for utterances such as *Raft-e ba:la:* ('Went-aux&3s up' > 'Has gone upstairs') was more frequent than the other auxiliaries in the children's data. This form has the least complex structure among Persian auxiliaries and, generally, the inflection *-e* (present 3rd person singular) after the past root is regarded as having an auxiliary role. The present 3rd person singular form of auxiliary *budan, hast,* is usually omitted in colloquial Persian. This inflected auxiliary (Aux/I) is placed in both the Statement and the Word columns. The other new categories, the object marker *ro/o* for utterances such as *In-o be-de* ('This-Omarker imp-give' > 'Give this') and Adj/NV for the utterance

Xara:b kard ('Ruin did' > 'She/he broke'), are also included in this column.

Pronouns in Persian have a very simple structure – there is no difference between subject, object and possessive pronouns when they are not in the form of inflections. Therefore, unlike LARSP, which makes a distinction between personal pronouns (P) and other sorts of pronouns (O), P-LARSP lists them under Pronouns only. Figure 10.1 shows that the LARSP phrase categories are retained in P-LARSP too. However, the Vpart structures such as *dar ovord* 'took off' are placed under Other since they are rare in Persian. Subject, object, and possessive pronouns are listed at Stage II Phrase level.

Transitional Stage II-Stage III: expansions

At the transition between Stage II and Stage III, three-word utterances begin to emerge. For example, at clause level *Adam + hit* and *hit + ball* can now be combined into *Adam + hit + ball* (Brown, 1973: 183). At phrase level *hit + ball* may now be expanded to *hit + Adam ball* (Peters, 1986: 318). This is also the case in Persian, as illustrated in the following examples:

Stage II   Clause level   Phrase level
                 Man-e   *Ma:shin man*   'It is mine' 'My car'
                 (mine-is)   (car   my)
                 C (V)   N   D

Stage II-Stage III transition
C/expansion   *Mashin man-e*   'It is my car'
               (car   my-is)
                 C   (V)
                 ―――――――――
                 N   D

The expansions also include noun phrases, adverbial phrases and verb phrases.

Stage III

At Stage III (see Fig. 10.1) the command *be-/bo -/biy-*/VXY category – for example, *Potqa:l man be-de* ('Orange me imp-give' > 'Give me an orange') – is similar to LARSP, and the prefix *be-/bo-/biy-* is listed in the Word column. There is no verb equivalent of 'let' in Persian. This notion is indicated by adding the prefix *bo-/be-/biy-* to the present root, plus inflections at the end. Sometimes it appears in compound verbs without the prefix. Such utterances are distinguished from statements by intonation. For example, the utterance *A:da:ms be-xor-im* can be interpreted as SVI 'We eat chewing gum' or 'Let's eat chewing gum'. Since P-LARSP, like LARSP, does not take intonation into consideration, these utterances are listed under Statement only.

At this stage the 'do' category is not appropriate for Persian. The CompVX category is also included in this column, for example:

Pa:ra-sh kon
(tear it do)
Comp X V

Adj I	V

'Tear it'

There are no complex question structures in Persian, and *wh*-questions correspond to the adult model at this stage.

New categories at Stage III clause level are mainly extensions of the categories introduced in the previous stage. Some of these extensions are in the form of inflections. For instance, the XVI category represents utterances such as *Mi-shkan- e* ('This pres-break-it' > 'This breaks') (SVI); *Unja: raft-am* ('There went-I' > 'I went there') (A VI); and *Sham xord-am* ('Dinner ate-I' > 'I ate dinner') (OVI). The COMPVI category for utterances such as *Harf mi-zan-im* ('Talk pres-be at-we' > 'We are talking' as well as the VIsIo (verb + subject inflection + object inflection) category for utterances such as *Gereft-am-esh* ('Caught-I-it' > 'I caught it') are also listed here.

The SVA category such as *Mahdi raft Iran* 'Mahdi went to Iran' also includes utterances with an indirect object; since this structure is not distinct in Persian, a preposition is always necessary. Ball and Thomas (this volume) also classify comparable structures in Welsh as adverbials. In Persian most adverbials, as well as those which cover indirect object structures, appear after the subject or at the beginning of a sentence in null-subject utterances. However, as seen above, the adverbial of place usually appears after verbs in spoken Persian.

XC(V) is another construction which differs from LARSP. It is the extension of C (V) from the previous stage. This is seen in:

In ma:shin-e
(this car is)
S   C (V)
'This is a car'

The SOV category is used for utterances such as *ma:ma:ni dastma: l bast* ('Mum scarf fastened' > 'Mum fastened a scarf').

PrDN/Pron and DNAdj are listed as Stage III phrase categories. The copula *budan* 'to be', particularly *hast/-st* 'is' (3rd person singular form, present), for utterances such as *Pa:-m bala:-st* ('Foot-my up-is' > 'My foot is up') and the genitive marker *ma:l* as in *Mal man-e* ('gen mine-is' > 'It is mine') are also listed here, as is the new category Adj/NVI for utterances such as *Xara:b kardam* ('Ruin did I' > 'I broke down').

Stage IV

At Stage IV (see Figure 10.1), commands +S such as *Bacha: beya:n tu* 'Children come in' and *be-/bo- /biy-*XYV + categories for utterances such as *In-o bara:m be-xun -esh* ('This- object marker for- me imp -read-it' > 'Read these for me') are retained and the prefix *be-/bo-/biy-* is listed in the Word column, as mentioned earlier. The CompXYV+ category as in *Chasb-o pa: ra-sh kon* ('Tape-object marker tear-it do' > 'Tear the tape') is listed in this column. There are no tag questions in Persian. The nearest equivalents are expressions like *mish-e* ('possible is' > 'is it possible?') and *mage na* ('so no' > 'isn't it?'). These tag-like questions are rare but their structures are similar to the Statement categories. Therefore they are listed under Other at this level.

At Stage IV Statement again one of the main differences from LARSP is the presence of inflections. At this level, the (SVIsIo) category for sentences such as *Man mi-bin-am-et* ('I pres-see-I-you' > 'I see you') contains both subject and object inflections and is the expansion of VIsIo of the previous stage. In this structure the object pronoun only appears in inflected form and is attached to the subject inflection. In Persian, object pronouns either appear before verbs or as a verb suffix after the subject inflection. The new category Complex is for utterances with an auxiliary or modal auxiliary such as *Mi-xa-m be-bor-am* ('pres-want-I subj-cut-I' > 'I want to cut'). Most modal auxiliaries and auxiliaries in Persian take the same inflections as main verbs and, in fact, may be seen as incorporating an embedded object clause. However, since these utterances contained four elements, and they emerged simultaneously with other four-element structures in the children's data, they are listed under Complex at this level.

Stage IV Phrase categories are mainly the expansions of the categories introduced at the previous stage. The Adj/NIVI category represents utterances such as *Xara:b-esh kard-am* ('Ruin it did I' > 'I knocked it down').

The phrase structures PrDNAdj (e.g. *az un-a: gerda:lu sejid* 'of that-pl round white' > 'of those round white') and cX (e.g. *dige man nusha:be* 'also me drink') and XcX (e.g. *dust o surat* 'hand and face'; *mohammad va mahdi* 'Mohammad and Mahdi') are the same as the English Stage IV categories. However, the NPPrNP and Neg X categories were rarely used by the children investigated, and are therefore assigned to the Other category. The 2Aux category on the English chart is omitted as inappropriate; that is, two auxiliaries rarely appear in one construction in Persian.

The new categories, modal auxiliaries (Aux/M) and other auxiliaries (Aux/O), are listed at this level. Modal auxiliaries such as *momken budan* 'may' = colloquial *mishe* (e.g. *Mishe be-za:r-am?* 'May sub-put-I' > 'May I put?') are included in the phrase column at this stage.

Auxiliaries are not common in Persian. At this stage of Iranian children's language development the main verb forms of *xa:stan* 'to want' emerged in utterances such as *Mi-xa:-m peyda: kon-am* ('pres-want-I finding do-I' > 'I want to find'), and are listed under Complex in the clause column.

Stage V

Crystal *et al.* (1989) labelled this stage as 'recursion', referring to the extension of sentence patterns by the repeated application of a single rule. This is the same in Persian. The first recursive process that emerges at clause level is the use of coordinating words, (c), such as *dige* 'also' and *badan/ badesh* 'then' corresponding to the function of 'and' in English (see Fig. 10.1). These two conjunctions are used frequently by Iranian children to link clause elements. They are therefore listed separately from the other coordinating conjunctions (e.g. *va*). The following example was selected from the data of one of the children when he was 3;0. He is telling a story similar to *Little Red Riding Hood*.

Leba:se-esh pushlid dar bast   badan   raft bara:-sh ma:shin be-xar-e
(dress-her put on door closed   then   went for-her car subj-buy-she)
    Clause   Ø   Clause   *badan*   Clause
'She put on her dress, shut the door, and went to buy a toy car for him'

Stage V commands do not differ markedly from those in LARSP. Utterances such as *Bacha: beya:in man ta:b bedin* ('Children come push me') are noted under Coord, and imperative constructions with more than four elements are listed under Other.

At Stage V Clause level Coord 1, two clauses are linked by *badan/badesh* or *dige*, Ø, or conjunctions, (c), as in the following:

Ba:yad qaza:-sh-o bo-xor-e badesh be-r-e madrese
Clause   *badesh*   Clause
(should food-his-Omarker subj-eat-he then subj-go-he school)
'He should eat his food then go to school.'

In Coord 1+ more than two clauses are linked by *badan*, (c), or Ø, as in the example given above. Subord A1 covers a clause containing an adverbial which is itself a clause:

Unja:ei ke raft-e bud-im   mashid am omad-e bud
        A   S   V
─────────────────
    s   AUX VI
(where that went-PP marker were-we Mashid too come-PP marker was)
'Where we had gone Mashid had come, too.'

Subord A1 + represents a clause containing at least two adverbial clauses:

182 Assessing Grammar

Ke kojolu bud-am das be sar-am mi-zad-am inja: dard gerft
                          A   A   CompV
_____
 s   C   VI   A comp VI
(that small child was-I hand at head-my past cont-put-I here hurt it)
'When I was a young child (when) I was touching my head it hurt here'

Subord S represents a clause containing a subject that is itself a clause. This structure was rare in the data examined and the only example is shown below:

Tush hamuni did-i mi-xun-e
    S   VI
_____
 A   0   VI
(inside that one saw-you pres-sing-it)
'Inside the one you saw sings' [that you saw inside = radio]

Subord C represents a clause containing a complement element which is itself a clause, as in the following description of chewing gum:

Adams-e   sefid gerda:lu-e
  C   (V)   C
         _____
          C   (V)
(chewing gum-is white round-is)
'It is chewing gum which is round and white'

Subord O represents a clause that contains an object element which is itself a clause:

Be-hetgoft-am ke-tiger-e
  A   VI   O
              _____
               s C(V)
(to-you said-I that tiger-is)
'I told you that it is a tiger'

Subord O was the most common structure in the children's data at this stage.

In LARSP, Comparative refers to a clause containing a grammatical marker of comparison in English. This does not occur in Persian. The comparative suffix *-tar* is added to adjectives, nouns and adverbs, being used in utterances such as *In bo zorg-tar-e* ('This big-er is' > 'This is bigger').

Postmodifying clauses and phrases in P-LARSP are mostly identical to those in LARSP; that is, a small range of clauses or phrases may be introduced as part of a noun phrase structure as one means of postmodifying the head noun. For example, one of the children produced a postmodifying clause when she was concluding her story, as illustrated below:

A:dam ke mi-r-e ba:yad bach-a-sh-o negah da:r-e
  S   O   Comp VI

S   s   VI

(person who pres-go-she should children-pl-her-Omarker care have-she)
'A person who goes away should take care of her children'

Postmod phrase 1+ was rarely found in the children's data, but was included to give a general picture of this stage. The only example was produced by one of the children when she was 2;8:

Az un-a: ke   gerda:lu   sefid-e
(of that-pl that round   white-def)
'Those that are round and white'

Stage VI

Stages VI and VII are not based on data from children acquiring Persian, as the children studied did not reach these levels. These still need further research.

The LARSP Stage VI chart (+) mostly corresponds to the Persian chart, while the P-LARSP chart (-) is largely different from its English counterpart (see Fig. 10.1). Initiators in LARSP are those items preceding the determiner in a noun phrase. In P-LARSP this category may be used for utterances such as *hame-ye in bache-ha:* ('all-*ezafe* this child-*pl*' > 'all these children'). In utterances such as *sara/doxtar-e behna:z xa:nom* 'Sara/Behnaz's daughter', labelled as NP Coord, two noun phrases are coordinated without any formal marker of the coordination present. In the centre of the + box in the LARSP chart, Complex+ refers to more complex kinds of verb phrases such as 'he might not go'. In P-LARSP the Complex category may be used for utterances such as:

Dust da:r-am harf be-zan-am
Comp VI   Comp VI

Adj VI   N VI
'I like to talk'

Passive structures rarely occur in Persian; therefore they are omitted from the chart. Complements are not used in the same form as in English, so they are likewise omitted.

P-LARSP (-) is mostly different from the corresponding section in LARSP. For example, in LARSP, pronouns are a frequent source of error. This is not the case in Persian, since Persian pronouns have neither gender distinctions nor different grammatical forms. The pronouns – *man, to, u, ma:, shoma:,* and *una:* – are used as subject, object, and possessive pronouns, and in all cases their form is the same. In addition, generic and specific definite nouns are not marked in Persian and there are no irregular nouns. Regular inflections are not over-generalized to irregular forms, resulting in errors like 'foots' and 'sheeps', so these grammatical forms are not predicted to be areas of error in Persian. On the other hand, compound verbs are a possible source of error at this stage. For example, the child may use a compound verb instead of a simple form of the verb (e.g. *bustash bekon* ('fasten-it do') instead of *beband-esh* ('fasten it') or vice-versa). In the Word column the possessive and object inflections, as well as the *ezafe* marker *e/ey*, are sometimes omitted. Other categories of LARSP Stage VI (-) correspond more or less to those of P-LARSP. DØ stands for a determiner which has been omitted (e.g. *Meda:d be-de* ('Pencil imp-give' > 'Give pencil') instead of *Meda:d-am be-de* ('Meda:d-my imp-give' > 'Give my pencil')). P in the LARSP chart stands for a preposition being in the wrong place and V_{reg} represents the wrong form of a regular verb. These categories are also predicted to be areas of error in Persian. There are two forms of verb root in Persian: present and past. The child may use the present root where the past root should be used. For example, the verb *ka:shtan* 'to plant' has two verb roots: *ka:sht* 'planted' and *kar* 'plant'. The child may produce *Ka:rid-am* 'I planted' instead of *Ka:sht-am*.

Stage VII

Apart from existential 'it' and 'there', which do not exist in Persian, other categories of Stage VII on the LARSP chart are likely to be the same (see Fig. 10.1). Comment Clause refers to a parenthetical clause introduced into connected speech (e.g. *mi-dun-i* 'you know'). Emphatic Order refers to an alteration in the normal word order of a clause for reasons of emphasis – for example, *Ali to be-ya; pish-e man* ('Ali you imp-come to-*eza:fe* marker me' > 'Ali/you come to me'). The category Other is used for any further constructions which have no place elsewhere on the chart. Syntactic Comprehension refers to any cases where syntactic production seems to be in advance of comprehension. Style on the P-LARSP chart refers to alternative grammatical varieties, styles or any special forms that exist in the collected sample.

Word level

The word level inflections on the LARSP chart are based on Brown's 14 grammatical morphemes. Some of these inflections are seen at Stage II, but Crystal *et al.* (1989) consider these to be used systematically from about

Stage III. During Stages III and IV most of these inflections are introduced or established. A similarly detailed word-order chart was used by Hickey (1987) for Irish. In addition, Ball and Thomas (this volume) have devised separate charts (LLARSP-M and LLARSP-T) for recording developmental morphology and word-initial consonant mutations in Welsh. However, Hickey (this volume) revised her chart and presented a general Word level. She found that a detailed word-level analysis was not necessary up to age three, and pointed out that the separate morphological charts in Ball's Welsh version had the disadvantage of fragmenting the profile.

In the case of Persian, the Word level of LARSP was preferred since the number of inflections in Persian is not so great as to necessitate the production of another chart for them. The P-LARSP Word level begins with the present form of the verb *budan* 'to be' used by the children studied (see Fig. 10.1). As explained earlier, copular 'be' is expressed by suffixing the person agreement affixes to the complement. These affixes, which are regarded as copulas, are *-am, -i, -e, -im, -id,* and *-and*. These are used as 1st, 2nd, and 3rd person singulars and plurals respectively. At the early stages of Persian-speaking children's language development most utterances have the C + person agreement structure in which the 3rd person singular agreement, *e*, is the most common form (e.g. *Ha:pu-e* 'Dog is'). In addition, V + person begins to appear for utterances such as *Did-i* ('Saw-you' > 'I saw') and *goft-am* ('Said-I' > 'I said'). These inflections are shown as V/C + Person in the Word column.

The six inflections *-am, -et/t, -esh, -mun, -tun* and *-shun,* which are used for the 1st, 2nd and 3rd person singular and plural respectively, are attached to nouns and pronouns as possessive determiners. Similarly, these suffixes are attached to verbs, or the subject suffixes of the verbs, as object inflections. Poss/O on the charts reflects the above.

The prefix *be-/bo-/biy-* has different functions in Persian. It is added to the present root in order to express either imperative or subjunctive forms of the verb. Verbs after the modal auxiliaries also have this kind of form. It is shown as *be- /bo-/biy-* on the chart.

The prefix *na-/ne-* is attached to the beginning of main verbs or modal auxiliaries to show negation.

Since there is no distinction between countable and mass nouns in Persian, the suffix *(h)a:* marks plurality in both classes. This is shown as *pl* in the Word column.

The prefix *mi-* on the chart is added to the verb root to form the present, present continuous and future tense. The following examples are selected from the children's data:

Present continuous:
Nega: tofang mi-gir-am   unja:
(look gun   pres-point-I there)

'Look I am pointing the gun there'
Present:
Shax mi-zan-e
horn pres-does-it
'It horns'
Future:
Ma:shin mi-gir-am
(car   pres-buy-I)
'I will buy a car'

According to Samiian's (1983) study, *ezafe*, which literally means 'addition', refers to the unstressed morpheme *e/ye*, which appears between the head of the phrase and certain modifiers and complements following the head. The *ezafe* construction occurs in non-verb phrase categories such as the noun phrase, the adjective phrase, and the prepositional phrase. The examples below are selected from the children's data:

Noun phrase:
sar-e ba:ba:
head-*eza:fe* daddy
'daddy's head'
Adjective phrase:
pesar-e xub
boy-*ezafe* good
'good boy'
Prepositional phrase:
zir-e a:b
under-*ezafe* water
'under the water'

This is shown as *ezafe e/ey* on the chart. As illustrated above, modifiers follow their head nouns. However, the order is opposite in the prepositional phrase.

The suffix -*e* is sometimes added to singular nouns to mark them as definite (e.g. *Xa:nom-e am goft inished* ('Lady-def too said finished' > 'The lady also said finished')).

On the chart, the -*i* stands for the indefinite suffix since most Persian nouns appear to be definite except when they are marked with the indefinite suffix -*i* (e.g. *Yek-i elfente dust-am-e* ('One-indef Effente friend-my-is' > 'One is Effente who is my friend')).

The past participle inflection -*e*, which is also regarded as the present 3rd person singular auxiliary, is also used in passive utterances such as *Bast-e shod* 'It was closed'. This is shown as Aux/PP-*e* on the chart.

The comparative suffix *-tar* was used for utterances such as *bozorg-tar* 'bigger' and *zeya:d-tar* 'more'. The superlative inflection *-tarin* did not appear in the children's data. However, in order to give a general picture of the children's development, and since it is anticipated that this suffix will appear later, it was included in the P-LARSP chart.

Conclusion

The P-LARSP profile chart described above provides a means of assessing the level of language development in Persian, and is based on data obtained from a longitudinal study of three monolingual Persian-speaking children aged between 1;8 and 3;4. The resulting chart is able to represent the full range of grammatical structures produced by these children. The profile, which is based on normal language development, provides a preliminary assessment tool that can be used to compare the same child's language at different stages and that of different children at the same stage of language development. Moreover, the profile constitutes the first formal procedure devised for assessing language impairment in Persian. It provides a detailed general picture of normal language development from Stage I towards the end of Stage V. It is hoped that the collection of data from normally developing children can be extended so that the later stages of the chart can be fully tested and plotted.

Acknowledgements

The authors thank Mike Garman, Tina Hickey and John Locke for their comments on an earlier version of P-LARSP.

Note

(1) An earlier version of this chapter was published in the journal *Clinical Linguistics and Phonetics*. This revised and expanded version is published with the permission of Informa PLC.

References

Bateni, M. (1970a) *Zaban va Tafakor* ('Language and Thought'). Tehran: Honar va Andishe.
Bateni, M. (1970b) *Saxteman e Zaban e Farsi* ('The Structure of Persian'). Tehran: Amir Kabir.
Bateni, M. (1976) *Chehar Goftar Darbare ye Zaban* ('Four Articles about Language'). Tehran: Entesharat e Agah.
Bellugi, U. (1967) *The Acquisition of Negation*. Unpublished PhD dissertation: Harvard University.
Brown, R. (1973) *A First Language: The Early Stages*. London: Allen & Unwin.
Crystal, D., Fletcher, P. and Garman, M. (1989) *The Grammatical Analysis of Language Disability* (2nd edn). London: Whurr.

Dabir-Moghadam, M. (1982) Passive in Persian. *Studies in Linguistic Science* 12, 63–90.
Doroudian, M. (1979) The Acquisition of Persian and English Syntax. PhD thesis: University of London.
Farrokhpey, M. (1979) A Syntactic and Semantic Study of Auxiliaries and Modals in Modern Persian. PhD thesis: University of Michigan.
Hickey, T. (1987) The Early Acquisition of Irish: Grammatical Patterns and the Role of Formulas. PhD thesis: University of Reading.
Hyams, N. (1992) Morphosyntactic development in Italian and its relevance to parameter-setting models: Comments on the paper by Pizzuto & Caselli. *Journal of Child Language* 19, 695–709.
Karimi, S. (1989) Aspects of Persian Syntax, Specificity and the Theory of Grammar. PhD thesis: University of Washington.
MacWhinney, B. (1995) *The CHILDES Project: Computational Tools for Analyzing Talk* (2nd edn). Hillsdale, NJ: Lawrence Erlbaum.
Mirhassani, A. (1989) Contrastive analysis of English and Persian verbs. *International Review of Applied Linguistics in Language Teaching* 27, 325–45.
Peters, A.M. (1986) Early syntax. In P. Fletcher and M. Garman (eds) *Language Acquisition*. Cambridge: Cambridge University Press.
Quirk, R., Greenbaum, S., Leech, G. and Svartvik, J. (1985) *A Comprehensive Grammar of the English Language*. London: Longman.
Samadi, H. (1996) The Acquisition of Persian: Grammatically Based Measures for Assessing Normal and Abnormal Persian Language Development. PhD thesis: University of Sheffield.
Samiian, V. (1983) Structure of Phrasal Categories in Persian: An X-bar Analysis. PhD thesis: University of Washington.
Windfuhr, B. (1979) *Persian Grammar: History and State of its Study*. The Hague: Mouton.

11 Frisian TARSP. Based on the Methodology of Dutch TARSP

Jelske Dijkstra and Liesbeth Schlichting

Introduction

This chapter presents the Frisian version of LARSP: Fryske Taal Analyze Remediearring en Screening Proseduere ('Frisian Language Analysis Remediation and Screening Procedure'), or F-TARSP (Dijkstra, 2008). West Frisian, a West Germanic language, is a minority language spoken by approximately 480,000 residents of a northern region of the Netherlands (i.e. the province of Fryslân). It is the mother tongue of almost 50% of its children (Gorter & Jonkman, 1994; Provinsje Fryslân, 2011). Frisian-speaking children are bilingual in that they also acquire the majority language Dutch at a young age.

Frisian grammar shows parallels to Dutch grammar. Due to language contact, interference between Dutch and Frisian has lately increased. Language therapists urgently need diagnostic instruments for Frisian language assessments. The design of the Frisian study was identical to that of one of the two Dutch versions of LARSP: Taal Analyse Remediëring en Screening Procedure ('Language Analysis Remediation and Screening Procedure'), or TARSP (Schlichting, 1987–2009) (for Bol & Kuiken's version see Chapter 6 of this volume).

Grammatical Sketch of Frisian

This section covers aspects of Frisian grammar that are relevant to the Frisian version of LARSP (see Tiersma (1999) for more detailed information on Frisian grammar).

Word order

The 'normal' position of the verb is at the end of the clause (SOV), which we see in subclauses as in *Ik tink dat ik har moarn sjoch* ('I think that I her tomorrow see' > 'I think I will see her tomorrow'). In main clauses the finite verb moves to the second position and the non-finite verbs are in the end position (cf. *Ik sjoch*$_{finite(f)}$ *har moarn* ('I see$_{finite(f)}$ her tomorrow' > 'I'll see her tomorrow') vs. *Ik sil_{finite(f)} har moarn sjen_{non-finite(nf)}* ('I will_{finite(f)} her tomorrow see_{non-finite(nf)}' > 'I will see her tomorrow')).

In verb phrases consisting of a finite verb and two or more non-finite verbs, the main lexical verb (e.g. *sjen* 'to see') is located at the left of the verb cluster (e.g. *Ik sil_f har moarn sjen kinne_{nf}* ('I will_f her tomorrow see can_{nf}' > 'I'll be able to see her tomorrow')). Here, Frisian differs from Dutch, which has the main lexical verb (e.g. *zien* 'to see') in non-finite clusters at the end (e.g. (Dutch) *Ik zal_f haar morgen kunnen zien_{nf}* ('I will_f her tomorrow can see_{nf}' > 'I'll be able to see her tomorrow')).

In main clauses opening with an adverbial adjunct or a complement, there is always inversion of subject and finite verb: $XV_{finite}S(O/A)(V_{non-finite})$ (e.g. *Moarn sil ik har sjen* ('Tomorrow will I her see' > 'I will see her tomorrow')). *Wh*-questions and *yes/no*-questions always have SV-inversion as in *Wa sjoch ik moarn?* ('Who see I tomorrow?' > 'Who will I see tomorrow?') and *Sjoch ik har moarn?* ('See I her tomorrow?' > 'Will I see her tomorrow?'). Tag questions, which are invariable, are placed at the end of statements and ask for confirmation (e.g. *Hy spilet goed, hin?* 'He plays well, doesn't he?'). Intonational questions are statements with a rising pitch at the end of the utterance.

Negation

Negation in Frisian is usually expressed by the word *net* 'not'. For example, *Ik yt dat net* ('I eat that not' > 'I do not eat that').

Verbs and Verb Inflections

Frisian has strong and weak verbs. The strong verbs mark past tense and the past participle by means of a change in the vowel of the stem, also called ablaut, rather than the addition of a suffix (e.g. *rinne* [rɪnə], *rûn* [run], *rûn* [run] 'to walk, walked, walked'). There are two classes of weak verbs: one with infinitives ending in *-e (e.g. bakke* 'to bake'), and one with infinitives ending in *-je (e.g. wurkje* 'to work'). The inflections in simple present and past of both strong and weak verbs are given in Table 11.1. Note that the strong verbs take the same endings as the weak verbs.

Sometimes infinitives get inflected with the suffix *–n* (e.g. *Hy sil te silen* ('He will to sail' > 'He is going to sail')). This inflection occurs when the verb follows *te* 'to', *oan it* 'to', or is accompanied by the verbs *gean* 'to go', *bliuwe* 'to stay', *komme* 'to come', *sjen* 'to see', *hearre* 'to hear' or *fiele* 'to feel' (Tiersma, 1999).

In colloquial Frisian, children as well as adults use modals as lexical verbs (e.g. *De plysje wol dêrhinne* ('The police want there' > 'The police want to go there')).

The perfect is composed of an auxiliary *wêze* 'to be' or *hawwe* 'to have' and a past participle. Compound verbs consist of a verb and a word from

Table 11.1 Inflections of present and past tense of strong verbs and the two types of weak verbs

	Strong verbs rinne 'to walk'		Weak –e-verbs bakke 'to bake'		Weak –je-verbs wurkje 'to work'	
	Present tense					
1sg	stem + ø	rin	stem + ø	bak	stem + je	wurkje
2sg	stem + st	rinst	stem + st	bakst	stem + est	wurkest
3sg	stem + t	rint	stem + t	bakt	stem + et	wurket
pl	stem + e	rinne	stem + e	bakke	stem + je	wurkje
	Past tense					
1sg	past stem + ø	rûn	stem + te / de	bakte	stem + e	wurke
2sg	past stem + st	rûnst	stem + test / dest	baktest	stem + est	wurkest
3sg	past stem + ø	rûn	stem + te / de	bakte	stem + e	wurke
pl	past stem + en	rûnen	stem + ten / den	bakten	stem + en	wurken

another category (e.g. *fuortrinne* ('away-walk' > 'to walk away')). In main clauses the finite forms are often split up as in *De poes rint fuort* 'The cat walks away'.

Nouns and determiners

Nouns are neuter or non-neuter. Determiners relevant to F-TARSP are articles, demonstratives and possessive pronouns. The indefinite article *in* 'a' is used with all singular nouns. The definite article *it* 'the' is used with singular neuter nouns, while *de* 'the' is used with singular non-neuter nouns and all plural nouns. In the same way the demonstratives vary: *dit* 'this' and *dat* 'that' are used with singular neuter nouns, while *dizze* 'this / these' and *dy* 'that / those' are used with singular non-neuter nouns and all plural nouns. The demonstrative pronouns are also used substantively (e.g. *Dy moat yn de kast* ('That-one must in the closet' > 'That one must go into the closet')).

Inflection of nouns and adjectives; compounding

Nouns can be inflected with the diminutive markers –*ke*, –*tsje* or –*je*, and/or plural markers –*s* or –*en*. The adjective before a noun usually gets the suffix –*e*, except when it is placed between the indefinite article *in* and a neuter noun (cf. *it grutte hûs* 'the big house' vs. *in grut hûs* 'a big house'). Compound nouns are noun-noun compounds (e.g. *bistetún* ('animal-garden' > 'zoo')), and verb-noun compounds (e.g. *meanmasine* ('mow-machine' > 'lawn-mower')).

Personal pronouns

Subject pronouns are generally obligatory, except in the 2nd person singular where the pronoun (i.e. *do* 'you (fam.)') may be omitted (cf. *Do ytst in banaan* 'You eat a banana' vs. *Ytst in banaan* '(Ø-You) eat a banana') where the subject pronoun *do* is deleted. When following a finite verb or a subordinating conjunction, the subject pronoun *do* occurs as the clitic *–sto*. In the same positions the clitic *er* is used for the pronoun *hy* 'he' (e.g. *Alle moandeis docht er de wask* ('Every Mondays does he the laundry' > 'Every Monday he does the laundry'), or *Ik tink dat er de wask docht* ('I think that he the laundry does' > 'I think he does the laundry')). People are usually addressed in the 3rd person by their title or name (e.g. *Wol mem my helpe?* ('Want mum me help?' > 'Do you want to help me, mum?')).

Pronominal adverbs

Pronominal adverbs are very common. They are combinations of a locative adverb and one or more prepositions (e.g. *dêrop* ('there-up' > 'up there') and *hjirtuskenyn* ('here-between-in' > 'in between here')). They occur as a single word and in some contexts are split up, as in *Ik doch dêr in bytsje wetter by* ('I do there a bit water by' > 'I add a bit of water').

Adverbs

Spoken Frisian has an abundance of one-word adverbial adjuncts, mostly modality adverbs, sometimes three consecutively in one sentence. For example, *Ik sil dy aanst ek even dwaan* ('I will that-one later also just do' > 'I will also do that one later').

Design of the Study

This section presents the methodology for Frisian TARSP, which was based on the cross-sectional study that led to Dutch TARSP (see further Schlichting, 1996).

Subjects and setting

Spontaneous language samples were taken from 100 children aged between 1;9 and 4;2 years. Most subjects were selected at random by municipal authorities. Their parents received information about the study and they could indicate if they wanted to participate. In initial contact the researcher asked after the languages used by both parents as well as siblings. Only subjects from households where all members spoke (mainly) Frisian to each other were included in the study. Frisian was the main home language in these families. The samples were recorded in the children's homes when playing with both one parent and the researcher.

The age of the subjects is spread across five age groups of 20 in ranges of six months. These age groups allow for two variables per group: sex and two levels of socio-economic status, resulting in four subgroups of five subjects per age group.

Segmentation of the language samples

Language samples were segmented into utterances defined as minimal conversational contributions (Wells, 1985: 60). Up to three main clauses with their subordinate clauses were regarded as one utterance. In every language sample, 200 child utterances were transcribed with the accompanying utterances of the interlocutors. If needed for interpretation, glosses of the utterances were made and non-verbal behaviour was noted. These utterances were analysed as Minor or Major. Minor utterances are stereotyped sentences or non-expandable one-word utterances. The grammatical analysis is performed on the Major utterances. The number of clause elements in an utterance is taken to be an indication of the syntactic level of development.

A special point must be made in this respect concerning the various sentence types. Wells' findings, that interrogative sentences of a certain number of clause elements develop after declarative sentences with the same number of clause elements, suggested that declarative sentences must be distinguished from other sentence types. Theoretically, this is an attractive proposition: producing a question might well be a more complex linguistic act than producing a declarative sentence. This implies that the question is produced later than the declarative sentence and that it will be shorter than the declarative sentences acquired in the same period. Schlichting (1996) assumed that interrogative and imperative sentences of N clause elements are acquired at the same time as declarative sentences containing $N + 1$ clause elements. She carried out a longitudinal study to test the hypotheses concerning the increase in the number of clause elements because Dutch children develop syntactically with the following results:

(a) Emerging Dutch as a first language shows a systematic increase in the number of clause elements (S, V, C and A) in its declarative sentences of up to five clause elements, and in its interrogative and imperative sentences of up to four clause elements.
(b) *Yes/no-* and *wh*-questions and imperatives have one clause element less than the declaratives developed in the same period. The first imperatives emerge at Stage III. The first questions emerge at Stage IV. Six-element declarative structures and complex clauses emerge in the same period, after Stage V, denoted as Stage VI. Declarative two-element structures including negation or a particle do not reach the criterion of acquisition in Stage II, but in Stage III.

Table 11.2 Developmental scale of clause element structure: Stages II–VI

Stage	Statement	Question	Command	Multi-clause
II	2 elements (excluding negation and particle)			
III	3 elements negation + 1 element particle + 1 element		1–2 elements	
IV	4 elements	1–3 elements	3 elements	
V	5 elements	4 elements	4 elements	
VI	6 or more elements	5 elements	5 elements	coordination subordination

On the basis of these results a developmental scale of clause element structure was drawn up, as shown in Table 11.2. This scale was used in the cross-sectional studies of both Dutch and Frisian.

Stratifying the language samples

In both the Dutch and Frisian cross-sectional studies, the 100 spontaneous language samples consisting of 200 utterances each were indexed, or stratified, across the six syntactic stages. The language samples were first analysed into Minors and Majors. The Majors were coded for the various sentence types (statement, question, command, one-clause, multi-clause), and the number of clause elements in these sentences. With the help of these codings the language samples were indexed to the subsequent stages of syntactic ability displayed in Table 11.2. The following frequency criteria were used:

(1) A language sample is indexed on the basis of its longest utterances, 'longest' referring to the maximum number of clause elements.
(2) The criterion for 'maximum number' is that 5% of the majors in a language sample shall contain N clause elements for a language sample to be indexed as Stage N (questions and commands were calculated as having an extra clause element).

The syntactic codings together with these frequency criteria constitute the Clause Element Index (CEI) (Schlichting, 1996) which resulted in the indexation of 96 language samples to the six developmental syntactic stages. The language samples of four of the children were assigned to preliminary Stage VII, based on 5% of the Majors which were coded as Stage VII sentence structures.

Table 11.3 The distribution of the 100 Frisian subjects across the seven syntactic stages

	Stage I	Stage II	Stage III	Stage IV	Stage V	Stage VI	Stage VII
N	0	4	20	27	21	24	4

The indexation of Sjoerd's language sample to Stage IV furnishes an example. In his 200-utterance sample, Sjoerd had 91 Minors and 109 Majors (note that a Major may consist solely of one simple or complex phrase). Sjoerd needed a minimum of five clause structures (5% of 109) in a particular stage for his sample to be indexed to that stage. His language sample was analysed at clause level as follows.

Stage I:	11 clause structures
Stage II:	22 clause structures
Stage III:	31 clause structures
Stage IV:	22 clause structures
Stage V:	3 clause structures
Stage VI:	0 clause structures
Stage VII:	0 clause structures

Sjoerd did not produce sufficient Stage V clause structures to be classified as Stage V; his three Stage-V structures were added to his 22 Stage-IV structures, which resulted in 25 (23%) clause structures of at least Stage-IV level, which is more than the required percentage.

The indexation of the language samples of the 100 subjects by means of the CEI resulted in seven groups of language samples, the *stage corpora*, pertaining to the syntactic Stages I-VII. Table 11.3 shows the distribution of the 100 Frisian samples.

Assigning the structures to stages of syntactic development

This section explains how language structures at the levels of phrase, connectivity, pronoun and word were assigned to the syntactic stages.

The description of syntactic development poses two frequency questions in connection with the determination of the order of acquisition of syntactic structures:

(1) How many instances of a structure should a language sample contain for that structure to be considered part of the child's language system?

Criteria for emergence are bound to be arbitrary to a certain extent. Generally in child development, a newly acquired ability is 'present sometimes, absent sometimes, depending on the specifics of the task situation and perhaps other factors' (Flavell, 1985: 27). In the present study, the criterion is applied that one occurrence or token of a structure in a language

Table 11.4 Definite article *it* + *noun*: Numbers and percentages of children using the structure across Stages II–VII

Def Art *it*	N = 4 Stage II	Stage III N = 20	Stage IV N = 27	Stage V N = 21	Stage VI N = 24	Stage VII N = 4
Number	0	2	8	12	18	3
Percentage	0	10	30	57	75	75

sample is regarded as evidence of its emergence in the child's syntactic system.

(2) What percentage of subjects in a stage corpus should use a target structure for it to be entered as developing in that syntactic stage?

A 50% criterion was maintained, which means that whenever 50% of the language samples in a stage corpus contained a particular structure, this structure was entered as emerging in that particular syntactic stage.

The assignment of a structure is illustrated in the next example. As shown in Table 11.4, the definite article *it* emerges at Stage V since 57% of the children in this stage use this structure.

Bilingualism and the Frisian profile chart

Since Frisian-speaking children grow up bilingually, it is to be expected that their language samples contain Dutch elements. As Frisian and Dutch do not differ much on the levels of sentence structure, all Dutch utterances and mixed Dutch-Frisian utterances in the language samples were included in the analysis. In the same way, all phrases, whether Dutch or Frisian, were coded in the Phrase column. Conjunctions and pronouns were coded in the respective columns when the Dutch and Frisian elements were identical (e.g. the personal pronoun *ik* 'I'). Morphological structures inflected with a Frisian morpheme were coded in the Word column, irrespective of whether the head word was Frisian or Dutch (e.g. *olifantsje* 'small elephant' which consists of Dutch *olifant* 'elephant' with the Frisian diminutive marker *–sje* (instead of Dutch *–je*)). Dutch conjunctions, pronouns and morphological endings that differ from Frisian were not coded (e.g. the Dutch pronoun *hem* 'him').

Design and Description of the Frisian Profile Chart

General design

Section A of the LARSP chart has been retained, while Sections B–D are not part of F-TARSP since in clinical practice these sections were generally not used in the Dutch version. Like LARSP, F-TARSP has three columns for sentence structures: Statement, Question and Command. The other

Frisian TARSP profile chart

Name			Age	Date	SLTherapist		Total	
A	Unintelligible		Deviant	Incomplete	Ambiguous		Total A	
I	Minor	Social	Vocative No/yes Other		Stereotypes		Total Minor	
	Noun			Verb		Total	PRONOUN	Total Majors
	Adjective/Adverb						DemP (subst)	Stage
	STATEMENT		QUESTION	COMMAND	PHRASE			WORD
II	SA AX XV Other Cop		Intonation		IndefArt*in*N			Modal as Lexverb Diminutive
III	SVA SVC/O XNeg SV-Inversion XAA XAC/O Other		Tag (*Wh*)VS+	V(X)	AdjN PrN DefArt*de*N NN	CONN *en* 'and'	PronAdv *ik* 'I'	Plural Noun Compound Noun Present 1sg Present 3sg
IV	SVAC/O SVAA Other		VS(X) Wh(XY)	VXY	Modal Inf PrDN IntX DemP nn/plN Split PronAdv DAdjN AdjDN Vpart Other		*hy/er* 'he' *it* 'it'	Compound Verb Past participle
V	AVSAC/O AVSAA SVC/OC/O(X) Other		VSXY WhVSX	VXYZ+	Perfect XcX+ DefArt*it*N	*mar* (i) 'but'	*him* 'him' *wy* 'we' *my* 'me' *der* 'there' Other	Past Present 2sg Present pl
VI	6+ clause elements Coordination Subclause		VSXYZ+ WhVSXY+		PossN Postmod AdvAdjN 2 Infinitives	*want* 'for' *mar* (c) 'but' Other	*sy*(mv) 'they/them'	Infinitive+*n* Adj without –*e*
VII	Noun Phrase Tag Coordination without conj 3+ clause utterance Other				*sa'n* 'such a' N DemP nN VPrep Other	*at* 'if/when'	*je* 'one' *yts* 'some' *sy*(ev) 'she'	
			Adapted English version of F-TARSP profile chart (2008)					

Figure 11.1 The F-TARSP profile chart

columns are from left to right: Connectivity, Phrase, Pronoun and Word. The information on pronouns has been extended at the request of language therapists. The combinations of clause element and phrase that form the transitional Stages in LARSP have been omitted.

In the Question and Command columns, most structures are in italics. This indicates that these structures did not meet the frequency criteria. The reason for the low frequencies of these structures should probably be sought in the context where the language samples were taken, that is, in the presence of a previously unknown investigator. The Questions and Commands on the F-TARSP profile chart have been placed in the same stage as on the Dutch TARSP chart.

All language structures that met the criteria were placed according to the methodology presented above. This results in differences between LARSP and F-TARSP. For example the SA-structure is listed under AX in LARSP, but coded as a separate structure on the Frisian chart, since it achieved the 50%-criterion.

Frisian sentence structures have variable word order. The order of the elements in the sentence structures on the chart is the order in which the structure occurs most often; for example, the order SVA is more frequent than the order AVS, and therefore SVA is included on the chart.

Within the stages, structures were placed higher or lower according to the percentage of children using those structures. For example, SVA and SVC/O occurred in 75% of Stage-III language samples while XAA occurred in 50%, and PrN was placed at the same level as XNeg within Stage III because they were both used by 70% of the children.

Detailed description

Only the structures that deviate from the revised LARSP profile chart (1981, in Crystal *et al.* 1989) are discussed here. Structures occurring both in F-TARSP and LARSP are indicated as such in the figures pertaining to the various stages; an example is *XNeg (LII)*, which has been placed in Stage III, the LII referring to the NegX structure in Stage II on the LARSP chart.

Stage I (Figure 11.2)
- Utterances at this stage are either Minors (Socials and Stereotypes) or Majors. The Socials in F-TARSP have been split up into Vocatives (e.g. *mem* 'mum'), No/yes-responses and Other.

	Minor	Social	Vocative No/yes Other	Stereotypes		Total Minor
I	Noun				Pronoun	Total Major
			Verb	Total	DemP	
	Adjective/Adverb				(subst)	Stage

Figure 11.2 F-TARSP Stage I

	Statement	Question	Command	Phrase	Pronoun	Word
II	SA (AX LII) AX (LII) XV (SV, VO, VC LII) Other Cop (LIII)	Intonation		IndefArt in N		Modal as Lexverb Diminutive

Figure 11.3 F-TARSP Stage II

- The Majors in Stage I are nouns, verbs, adjectives/adverbs and demonstrative pronouns.
- Verbs are usually non-finite in this stage and restricted to infinitives (e.g. *ite* 'to eat').
- Demonstrative pronouns are used substantively (e.g. *dy* 'that one' or *dizze* 'this one').

Stage II (Figure 11.3)

Stage II is based on the corpora of four children only. This may indicate that children progress very rapidly from Stage II to Stage III according to our criteria.

- The most frequent structure in this stage is SA (e.g. *Skiep hjirre* 'Sheep here').
- SV does not meet the 50%-criterion in Stage II and has therefore been combined with C/OV in XV (X = S, C/O) (e.g. *Poppe koese* 'Baby sleep'; *Toer bouwe* ('Tower build' > 'Build tower')).
- The Copula emerges in Stage II.
- Only the 3rd person singular *is* 'is' is found at this stage (e.g. *Is mem* 'Is mum').
- Stage-II children only ask questions by means of a rising intonation at the end of the utterance (e.g. *Pakke?* 'To get?').
- The Stage-II Phrase column shows the indefinite article (IndefArt*in*N) (e.g. *in poes* 'a cat').
- In the Word column we see the modal used as a lexical verb (1st and 3rd person present tense) (e.g. *Wol fyts* 'Want bike').
- The diminutive is produced by all Stage-II children in the Frisian data. The diminutive is also extremely frequent in the language spoken to children. However, the children in Stage II probably do not yet know the difference between *mûs* 'mouse' and *mûs-ke* ('mouse'-dim > 'small mouse').

Stage III (Figure 11.4)
- In Stage III five types of three-clause-element structures emerge and one two-clause-element structure: XNeg. XNeg is an immature structure that increases towards 81% of the children in Stage V and declines

	Statement	Question	Command	Phrase		Pronoun	Word
III	SVA (LIII)			AdjN (LII)			
	SVC/O (SVC, SVO LIII)				Conn		
	XNeg (LII) SV-Inversion			PrN (LII)	*en* 'and'		Plural Noun
						PronAdv	Compound Noun
			V(X) (LII)	DefArt *de* N		*ik* 'I'	Present 1sg
	XAA	*Tag* (LIV)		NN (LII)			Present 3sg
	XAC/O (VCA, VOA LIII)						
	Other	(Wh)VS+					

Figure 11.4 F-TARSP Stage III

towards 50% in Stage VII (see also Table 11.5). If negation takes place in an utterance consisting of three or more elements, the negative is not specifically noted but is analysed as an adverbial adjunct.

– From Stage III onwards we find the coding SV-Inversion (e.g. *Dêr is in sjiraf* ('Over-there is a giraffe' > 'A giraffe is over there')).
– In Stage III we already see a frequent use of adverbial adjuncts, which is exemplified by the structure XAA (X = S, V, C/O, A) (e.g. *Mem ek op bedsje* ('Mum also on bed-dim' > 'Mum also on (small) bed')). The X in XAC/O may be a subject or a verb.
– Children at this stage also produce invariable tag questions, for example *hin?* and *net?* as in *do ek, hin?* 'you too, don't you?'.
– In Dutch child language the first element of a sentence is often omitted (Schlichting, 1996). This is also found in Frisian. For questions, this results in the structure (Wh)VS+ in Stage III, in which the interrogative is left out (e.g. *Ø docht er?* ('does he?' > '(Ø-What) is he doing?')).
– NN is mainly an immature expression of possession (e.g. *mem hûs* ('mum house' > 'mum's house')). Sometimes children use NN structures like *slokje wetter?* ('sip-dim water?' > '(small) sip of water?').
– The definite article *de* emerges in Stage III. While in the adult language it is used only for singular non-neuter and all plural nouns, children at this stage also use *de* before singular neuter nouns (e.g. *de hûs 'the house').
– The conjunction *en* 'and' introducing an utterance or clause element emerges in Stage III (e.g. *En op har mûle* 'And on her mouth').
– In the Pronoun column we see the personal pronoun *ik* 'I' and the pronominal adverb (e.g. *dêryn* ('there-in' > 'in there')).
– Stage III lists several morphological structures. The two regular plurals of nouns are developed (e.g. *appels* 'apples' and *bananen* 'bananas'), as are compound nouns (e.g. *bistetún* ('animal-garden' > 'zoo'); *glydsbaan* ('slide-track' > 'slide')).
– The 1st and 3rd person singular of the lexical verb also develop in Stage III (e.g. *Nim ik dizze* ('Take I this-one' > 'I take this one'); *Dy wennet yn in kastiel* ('That-one lives in a castle' > 'That one lives in a castle')).

Table 11.5 Stage-II and Stage-III declaratives with the percentages of children using this structure at least once and the mean frequency of this structure from Stages II–VI

		Stage II N = 4	Stage III N = 20	Stage IV N = 27	Stage V N = 21	Stage VI N = 24
Stage-II declaratives						
SA	Percentages	75	90	96	100	88
	Mean	8.0	10.3	6.5	3.2	3.1
AX	Percentages	75	80	100	100	100
	Mean	2.3	4.5	5.1	5.0	3.1
XV	Percentages	75	100	100	95	100
	Mean	1.7	6.7	5.6	4.5	3.3
Stage-III declaratives						
SVA	Percentages	75	75	100	100	100
	Mean	1.7	4.7	9.5	14.6	13.8
SVC/O	Percentages	25	75	93	100	100
	Mean	1.0	1.9	7.3	11.8	15.6
XNeg	Percentages	25	70	81	81	67
	Mean	1.0	3.1	3.1	2.4	2.0
XAA	Percentages	0	50	78	86	79
	Mean	–	2.6	3.1	3.3	3.3
XBC/O	Percentages	0	50	93	95	75
	Mean	–	2.1	2.4	2.0	1.9

Stage IV (Figure 11.5)
- Stage IV shows two four-element structures in the Statement column.
- The first *yes/no*-questions and *wh*-questions are listed, though only Wh(XY) meets the 50%-criterion (e.g. *Wêr is dy?* ('Where is that-one?' > 'Where is that one?')).

	Statement	Question	Command	Phrase	Conn	Pronoun	Word
IV	SVAC/O (SVOA, SVCA LIV) SVAA (AAXY LIV)			Modal Inf (LIII) PrDN (LIII) IntX (LII)		hy/er 'he'	
		VS(X) (LIII)		DemP nn/plN Split PronAdv DAdjN (LIII)		it 'it'	Compound verb Past participle
	Other	Wh(XY) (LIII)		AdjDN Vpart (LII)			
			VXY (LIII)	Other			

Figure 11.5 F-TARSP Stage IV

202 Assessing Grammar

- In the Phrase column we see the modal plus infinitive (e.g. *Kin net omfalle* ('Can not down-fall' > 'Cannot fall down')).
- Towards the end of Stage IV, Vpart is developed, that is, the inflected compound verb present or past tense (e.g. *De oaljefant yt se op* ('The elephant eats them up' > 'The elephant eats them')).
- PrDN emerges here, along with IntX.
- The demonstrative pronouns used with non-neuter and plural nouns are used here (i.e. *dy* 'that / those' and *dizze* 'this / these').
- The split pronominal adverb emerges as well (e.g. *Dizze kin der net út* ('This-one can there not out' > 'This one cannot get out')).
- The phrase DAdjN is developed in Stage IV along with AdjDN (e.g. *noch in boek* ('yet a book' > 'another book')).
- In the Pronoun column we see that the pronouns *hy/er* 'he' and *it* 'it' emerge in Stage IV. *It* can be used both as a subject and as an object (e.g. *Hy docht it sa* ('He does it so' > 'He does it like this')).
- The infinitives of compound verbs are developed (e.g. *opite* ('up-eat' > 'to eat') or *skjinmeitsje* ('clean-make' > 'to clean')). The past participle of both regular and some irregular verbs also emerges in Stage IV.

Stage V (Figure 11.6)
- The abundance of adverbial adjuncts, often consisting of one adverb only, shows clearly in the five-clause-element structures of Stage V: AVSAC/O *Ik kin pop wol even temperatuere* ('I can doll well just take-temperature' > 'I can just take the doll's temperature'), and AVSAA *No moat er wer yn de kontenerauto* ('Now must he again in the container-lorry' > 'Now he must go into the container lorry again').
- The third structure in the Statement column is SVC/OC/O(X) which contains two Complement/Objects (e.g. *Dy hie de foet stikken* ('That-one had the foot broken' > 'That one had broken his foot')). Sometimes this structure has a fifth clause element, mostly an A.
- The question WhVSX meets the 50%-criterion (e.g. *Wat docht se no?* ('What does she now?' > 'What does she do now?')).
- The perfect emerges in Stage V, with either the auxiliaries *wêze* 'to be' or *hawwe* 'to have', (e.g. *Ik bin achterút gongen* ('I was backwards gone' > 'I

	Statement	Question	Command	Phrase	Conn	Pronoun	Word
V	AVSAC/O AVSAA SVC/OC/O(X) Other	 VSXY (LIV) WhVSX (LIV)	 VXYZ+ (LIV)	Perfect (LIII) XcX+ (LIV) DefArt it N	 mar (i) 'but' (i)	 him 'him' wy 'we' my 'me' der 'there' Other	Past Present 2sg Present pl

Figure 11.6 F-TARSP Stage V

went backwards'); *Ik ha twa trekkers pakt* ('I have two tractors taken' > 'I took two tractors')).
- The definite article *it* meets the criteria in Stage V. This article only precedes singular neuter nouns (e.g. *it strân* 'the beach').
- In Stage V, the conjunction *mar* 'but' is used only to introduce an utterance, not as a coordinative (e.g. *Mar hy is der ek* ('But he is there also' > 'But he is also present')).
- The Pronoun column in Stage V includes the following pronouns: *him* 'him', *wy* 'we', *my* 'me', and *der* 'there', as in *Hy is der hast* ('He is there almost' > 'He is almost there').
- Stage V lists three morphological verb structures. The coding Past represents the simple past tense of both modal and lexical verbs. The 2nd person singular of the simple present tense ending in *–(e)st* emerges in Stage V. Present tense plural is only analysed as such when there is subject-agreement.

Stage VI (Figure 11.7)
- Declaratives with six clause elements (or more) meet the 50%-criterion at Stage VI (e.g. *Dy lizze wy straks ek oan de kant* ('That put we later also on the side' > 'We put that on the side too later on')).
- In this stage coordination emerges – for example, *Ik soe him hast deryn dwaan, mar dat lukt my net* ('I should him almost there-in do, but that manage my not' > 'I was going to put it in there, but I did not manage to').
- The Subclause also meets the criteria in Stage VI. It is mostly a complement clause or an adverbial clause (e.g. *Ik tink dat er hjir moat* ('I think that he here must' > 'I think that it must go here')).
- Possessive attributive pronouns meet the criteria in Stage VI (e.g. *syn auto* 'his car').
- The postmodifier emerges in this stage as well. This structure is often used to express possession (e.g. *de auto fan heit* ('the car from dad' > 'dad's car')).
- Another Stage-VI phrase is the adverb intensifying an adjective (see also IntX) before a noun (AdvAdjN), as in *hiele grutte skilpad* 'very big turtle'.

	Statement	Question	Command	Phrase	Conn	Pronoun	Word
VI	6+ clause elements Coordination (LV) Subclause (LV)	 VSXYZ+ WhVSXY+		Poss N Postmod (LV) AdvAdjN 2 Infinitives	want 'for' mar (c) 'but' (c) Other	sy(mv) 'they/them'	 Infinitive+n Adj without -e

Figure 11.7 F-TARSP Stage VI

- We also see phrases consisting of the auxiliary and two infinitives (2 Infinitives). For example, *Dat wol ik even sjen litte* ('That want I just see let' > 'I just want to let (you) see that').
- Stage VI includes the coordinating conjunctions *want* 'for' and *mar* 'but' (e.g. *Net deze auto, mar in gewoane auto* 'Not this car, but a regular car').
- The plural personal pronoun *sy* 'they / them' is developed in this stage. *Sy* can be used both as a subject and an object.
- The infinitive ending in *–n* meets the 50%-criterion. For example, *Hy sil te silen* ('He will to sail' > 'He is going to sail') (instead of *sile*).
- The uninflected adjective used attributively in phrases consisting of an indefinite article followed by an adjective and neuter noun emerges here (Adj without *–e*) (e.g. *in rôs stikje* 'a pink part').

Stage VII (Figure 11.8)
Stage VII is an experimental stage because it was based on the language samples of four children only.
- The noun phrase may be placed at the beginning or end of a sentence. It refers to and clarifies a pronoun in the main sentence (e.g. *Dat famke, dat past der net yn* ('That girl, that fit there not in' > 'That girl, she does not fit in there'); *Sy binne te wurch, de plysjes* 'They are too tired, the policemen').
- Two sentences may be coordinated by intonation only, without a conjunction, as in *Hjir is in motor, (Ø-en) dêr is motor* 'Here is a motorbike, (Ø-and) there is motorbike'.
- The 3+ clause utterance may consist of coordinated clauses or a combination of coordinated and subordinated clauses. For example, *Wy hiene al in kear socht, mar pake wit net wêr't se binne* ('We had already one time looked, but grandfather knows not where they are' > 'We had already looked once, but grandfather does not know where they are').
- The phrases listed in Stage VII are the demonstrative *sa'n* 'such a' followed by a noun (e.g. *sa'n hammer* 'such a hammer'), and the demonstrative pronouns before neuter nouns singular, *dit* 'this' and *that* 'dat'.
- Prepositional verbs are also listed in Stage VII (e.g. *Wachtsje op my!* 'Wait for me!').
- The conjunction *at* 'if / when' emerges in Stage VII (e.g. *At it reint, dan is er droech* ('When it rains, than is he dry' > 'When it rains, he is dry')).

	Statement	Question	Command	Phrase	Conn	Pronoun	Word
VII	Noun Phrase Tag Coordination without conj 3+ clause utterance Other			sa'n 'such a'N DemP nN V Prep Other	at 'if/when'	je 'one' yts 'some' sy(ev) 'she'	

Figure 11.8 F-TARSP Stage VII

Frisian TARSP. Based on the Methodology of Dutch TARSP   205

Namme			Leeftyd		Datum	Logopedist			Totaal
A	Onverstaanbaar		Afwijkend		Niet af	Twijfel			A totaal
I	V.U.	Soc.:	AangP Nee/ja Divers			Ster			V.U. totaal
	Zn						VOORN	G totaal	
			W		tot:		Avn		
	Bv/B							G.O.Fase	
	MEDEDELENDE ZIN		VRAAG		GEB W	WOORDGROEPEN			WOORDSTRUCTUUR
II	OndB BX XW Ov Kop		Into			inZn			HwwZ Verkl
III	OndWB OndWVC XNeg Inv XBB XBVC Ov		hin (Vr)WOnd+		W(X)	BvZn VzN deZn ZnZn	VERB en	Vobij ik	MvZn SamZn Stam Stam+(e)t
IV	OndWBVC OndWBB Ov		WOnd(X) Vr(XY)		WXY	Hwwl VzBepZn BBv/B dy/dizzeZn Vo/bij BepBvZn BvBepZn Wdeel Ov		hy/er it	SamWw Voltdw
V	BWOndBVC BWOndBB OndWVCVC(X) Ov		WOndXY VrWOndX		WXYZ+	HwwVd XenX+ itZn	mar(i)	him wy my der Ov	VerlTijd Stam+(e)st MvTT
VI	6+ Nevens Bijzin		WOndXYZ+ VrWOndXY+			BezZn Nabep BBvZn WW	want mar(n) Ov	sy(mv)	Inf+n Bvze
VII	Aan/uit NevenszVerb Sz3+ Ov					sa'nZn dit/datZn WVz Ov	at	je yts sy(ev)	
	Adapted version of F-TARSP profile chart (2008)								

Figure 11.9 The F-TARSP profile chart in Frisian

- In Stage VII the informal use of the indefinite 'one', the personal pronoun *je*, emerges (e.g. *Dat sjogge je net sa goed op it plaatsje* ('That sees one not very good at the picture' > 'One does not see that very well on the picture')). The singular personal pronoun *sy* 'she' and the indefinite pronoun *yts* 'something' are also developed at this stage.

A Frisian language version of the F-TARSP chart is shown in Figure 11.9.

Comparing Frisian F-TARSP to Dutch TARSP

Frisian grammar is close to Dutch grammar. Comparing the two profile charts confirms this statement. Of the 95 structures on the Frisian TARSP profile chart, 81 structures are also present on the Dutch TARSP profile chart. Five structures on the Frisian chart have another name or are combined structures (e.g. XAC/O in Stage III), though they correspond to the structures on the Dutch TARSP chart. The Frisian chart shows nine structures that are not part of the Dutch TARSP chart. Seven of these structures have comparable equivalents in Dutch; two are typically Frisian structures: Present 2sg (e.g. *Kinst dit ek tekenje* ('Ø-You can this also draw' > 'You can also draw this')), and Infinitive+*n* (e.g. *Wy binne hjir oan it klimmen* ('We are here climbing' > 'We are climbing here')).

Out of the total of 86 corresponding structures, 61 structures occur at the same stage on the Frisian and Dutch TARSP charts. There are 23 structures on the Frisian chart that emerge one stage earlier or later than on the Dutch TARSP chart. Two structures, PossN and DemPnN, emerge two stages later.

Validity of the Language Chart and Application in Clinical Settings

Validation is a broad concept that mainly deals with the question of the adequacy of measures. Cronbach's point of view, as formulated in *Essentials of Psychological Testing*, that all validation is essentially construct validation, has been adopted as the basis of this section (Cronbach, 1984: 126).

Validity of the CEI: Frequencies of mature and immature clause structures

In this investigation, syntactic development has been indexed with the CEI, the Clause Element Index. Generally, children are assumed to use more mature structures and fewer immature structures as their syntactic ability develops. With regard to the mean number of frequencies of the clause element used in the stage corpora, it was found that all two-element declarative structures which are generally immature – because they do not contain both S and V – show a decrease of the mean number of structures used in the stage corpora, as children are indexed to a higher CEI, including the XV structure (see Table 11.5). Table 11.5 also shows that the mean numbers of SVA and SVC/O increase substantially towards Stage VI.

Application of (Frisian) TARSP in clinical settings

The methodology of data collection and analysis of the Dutch and Frisian studies have been designed in such a way that they could initially be used to describe normal development, as was done in the present investigation, and later be applied in clinical settings to assess individual children. The data in the F-TARSP investigation were based on language samples containing 200 utterances. In clinical settings it is almost impossible to use language samples of that length, because transcribing and analysing

Table 11.6 Mean ages and standard deviations (SD) of the children at Stages II–VII

Stage	Mean ages (days)	(year;month.days)	SD (days)
II	761.25	2;00.00	88.7
III	807.50	2;02.17	100.8
IV	953.67	2;07.10	144.2
V	1222.52	3;04.06	176.3
VI	1331.42	3;07.22	108.4
VII	1409.25	3;10.09	92.2

spontaneous data are time-consuming activities for the language therapist. For the Dutch TARSP version, Schlichting (1996) calculated that a language sample of 40 Major utterances generally indicated the right stage the child was in, using the rule that 5% of the Majors in a language sample shall contain N clause elements for a language sample to be indexed as Stage N. We assume that for F-TARSP the same number of Majors holds. The number of 40 Majors is close to Darley and Moll's findings (1960) in their study of 150 five-year-olds, where 50-utterance speech samples yielded a reliability coefficient of 0.85. The mean ages of the children at each F-TARSP stage are given in Table 11.6.

A complementary way of using the chart is the profile score. Sometimes language therapists want to have more information about their clients, especially when progress in therapy needs to be measured. A simple way to document this is to compare the pre-therapy language sample to the post-therapy sample by counting all structures used. In this method Stage-I utterances are not included. The maximum number in the Frisian chart is 95.

References

Cronbach, L.J. (1984) *Essentials of Psychological Testing*. New York: Harper & Row.
Crystal, D., Fletcher, P. and Garman, M. (1989) *The Grammatical Analysis of Language Disability* (2nd edn). London: Whurr.
Darley, F.L. and Moll, K.L. (1960) Reliability of language measures and size of language samples. *Journal of Speech, Language and Hearing Research* 3, 166–173.
Dijkstra, J.E. (2008) F-TARSP: Fryske Taal Analyze Remediearring en Screening Proseduere. In *Fryske bewurking fan 'e TARSP*. Ljouwert/Leeuwarden: Fryske Akademy/Afûk.
Flavell, J.H. (1985) *Cognitive Development*. New Jersey: Prentice Hall.
Gorter, D. and Jonkman, R.J. (1994) *Taal yn Fryslân op 'e nij besjoen*. Ljouwert/Leeuwarden: Fryske Akademy.
Provinsje Fryslân. (2011) *De Fryske Taalatlas 2011. Fryske Taal yn Byld*. Ljouwert/Leeuwarden: Provinsje Fryslân.
Schlichting, L. (1996) *Discovering Syntax: An Empirical Study in Dutch Language Acquisition*. Nijmegen: Nijmegen University Press.
Schlichting, L. (1987–2009) *TARSP: Taal Analyse Remediëring en Screening Procedure. Taalontwikkelingsschaal van Nederlandse kinderen van 1-4 jaar*. Amsterdam: Pearson.
Tiersma, P.M. (1999) *Frisian Reference Grammar*. Ljouwert/Leeuwarden: Fryske Akademy.
Wells, G. (1985) *Language Development in the Pre-School Years*. Cambridge: Cambridge University Press.

12 C-LARSP: Developing a Chinese Grammatical Profile

Lixian Jin, with Bee Lim Oh and Rogayah A. Razak

Introduction

The existence of assessment tools such as LARSP has facilitated clinical language profiling, leading to better-informed intervention plans in the West. However, in the East, by and large, the development of such assessment tools is still in its infancy, although there is a great demand for providing services for speech and language therapy (SLT) needs to both child and adult clients (Cheung, 2009). This demand is particularly urgent in Chinese-speaking communities inside and outside China. As it has been estimated that 5–10% of any population may suffer communication disorders, this presents a significant proportion of the world's population who need help from SLT services in Chinese-speaking communities. Further, for both linguistic and cultural reasons, simply importing a language assessment package from ready-made Western SLT resources is not an ideal way to tackle issues faced by local SLT clients, and currently there is a lack of locally produced, and linguistically and culturally appropriate language assessment tools in China and elsewhere.

Two main difficulties for producing a locally appropriate language assessment tool in Chinese are: (1) there is no publication available based on a comprehensive and systematic investigation on child grammatical development in Chinese, although there is an increasing number of studies on different aspects of Chinese-speaking children's language development (e.g. Zhu, 1986; Erbaugh, 1992; Li, 1995; Huang & Li, 1996; Hsu, 1996; Zhou, 1997; Li & Chen, 1998; Zhou, 2002; Zhu, 2002; Tardif & Fletcher, 2008; Law et al., 2009; Zhou & Zhang, 2009) and; (2) there is no agreed system among Chinese grammarians for the use of grammatical terms and categorization of Chinese syntactic structures.

With the challenge of producing locally appropriate SLT tool to assess Chinese speaking children, the SLT team members from De Montfort University, UK (DMU) and the National University of Malaysia (UKM) carried out a project investigating child language development of Chinese-speaking children in Malaysia and developing a Chinese LARSP (C-LARSP) for the local SLT clients in Malaysia. The funding was awarded by the Prime Minister's Initiative (PMI2) grant with contributions from both DMU and UKM. The outcomes of this project not only help Chinese speakers with SLT needs in Malaysia, but also have an impact on the development of appropriate Chinese assessment tools in China and for Chinese communities in other countries.

This chapter describes some key features of Mandarin (which is used as a term to refer to Chinese as spoken in Malaysia in order to differentiate it from the term *Putonghua* used in China). It then reports the procedure of collecting and analysing data from Chinese-speaking children in Malaysia, and presents a C-LARSP chart with explanations and examples of the organization and usage applicable to assessing Chinese-speaking children. This is followed by a discussion of suggested future clinical data-collection procedures and implications for future SLT practices and research.

Key Grammatical Features of Mandarin

This section presents major grammatical features of Mandarin so that readers and users of C-LARSP are able to refer to a brief overview of Chinese grammar. However, it is important to stress that this section does not cover all the Chinese grammatical patterns because there are different Chinese grammatical categorizations even among Chinese grammarians, and there is no book within or outside China that serves as a fully comprehensive descriptive grammar (unlike Quirk *et al.,* 1985, which offered generally accepted terminology and categorization for describing English grammar as a foundation for LARSP).

For the purpose of analysing Chinese utterances, a booklet describing Chinese syntactic structures was produced (Jin, 2009) for researchers working on the data collection and analysis. There are three principles underlying this guidance booklet. (1) The syntactic analysis adapts the framework used for LARSP, such as recognizing clause, phrase and word levels. (2) It is intended for use by native Chinese or near-native Chinese speakers rather than for teaching and learning Chinese grammar as a foreign language. Thus the more commonly taught terms and classifications are used, since C-LARSP will be used by Chinese-educated professionals. However, this does not exclude the possible application of the approach by users of Chinese as a foreign language. (3) The description of Chinese syntactic structures uses information from books (e.g. Huang & Liao, 1981; Guo, 2000; Xin, 2003; Chao & Han, 2005) containing the more commonly accepted Chinese grammatical terminology taught in Chinese universities, as well as from some well-known Chinese grammar books in English (e.g.

Chao, 1968; Huang & Li, 1996; Yip & Rimmington, 2004) used in some universities outside China. The following shows some key Chinese syntactic features in two types: those similar to English syntactic structures and those perceived as particular to Chinese.

Sentence types

In Chinese, there are four types of sentences, as in English: Statement (陈述句 chenshuju), Question (疑问句 yiwenju), Command (祈使句 qishiju) and Exclamation (感叹句 gantanju). However, Chinese may be divided into two further major types of utterances: Subject-Predicate (SP) and Non-Subject-Predicate (NSP) (Guo, 2000). Nevertheless, it is important to differentiate between NSP utterances and elliptical SP utterances. In elliptical SP utterances, speakers can add the omitted element from the preceding utterances or non-linguistic context, but this is not the case in NSP (see Table 12.1).

Table 12.1 Examples of SP and NSP utterance types

Subject-Predicate (SP) 主谓句	Subject-Predicate utterances
	他　去　了　　　　　　北京。
	ta　qu　le　　　　　　beijing
	S　　P
	S　　V　aspect marker (am)　O
	he　go aspect　Beijing
	'He went to Beijing'
Non-Subject-Predicate (NSP) 非主谓句	Non-Subject-Predicate utterances
	是 他。
	shi ta
	P
	V O
	'Is him'
	Elliptical SP utterances
	要去　　　　北京。
	yaoqu　　　beijing
	P
	V　　　　　O
	'Want to go to Beijing' (subject omitted)

Single clause sentences and double/multiple clause sentences

Chinese grammarians (e.g. Lü 1947; Huang & Liao, 1981; Guo, 2000) also classify sentences into *single-clause sentences* (单句 danju) and *double/multiple-clause sentences* (复句 fuju). Many of the single-clause sentences would be regarded as complex sentences in English. Chinese grammarians (Huang & Liao, 1981; Lu, 1996; Guo, 2000) state that the main difference between a single-clause sentence and a double/multiple-clause sentence is that the clauses in the latter are relatively independent from each other, but are meaningfully related (Guo, 2000: 165). A single clause cannot act as a clause element of another single-clause sentence (Lu, 1996: 255).

Chinese double/multiple-clause sentences are often linked by conjunctions (these are termed in C-LARSP as *paired conjunctions*) such as 因为 [yinwei], 所以 [suoyi] ('because', 'therefore') and 不但 [budan], 而且 [erqie] ('not only', 'but also') or adverbs such as 就 [jiu] ('then') and 也 ('also'). There are two main types of double/multiple-clause sentences (Lu, 1996: 256): compound (联合复句, lianhefuju) and endocentric (偏正复句 pianzhengfuju), each containing sub-types (not discussed here). There is another type of double-clause sentence: the compressed sentence (紧缩句 jinsuoju), which can be either compound or endocentric. The main difference between a double-clause sentence and a multiple-clause sentence is that the latter has two or more layers of relationships (Huang & Liao, 1981: 403).

Clause elements

Clause-level elements include subject (S, 主zhu), predicate (P, 谓wei), verb (V, 述shu), object (O, 宾bin) and verb complement (Cv, 补bu). A subject can be formed by a noun, pronoun, classifier, adjective, verb, or a *de* construction, or an SV, VO or VCv construction (Guo, 2000: 103). It is normally placed at the beginning of an utterance. A predicate can be a verb, adjective, noun, time noun, or a classifier or an SV, VCv, SP construction. Thus a verb is, in fact, one kind of predicate. Chinese grammarians may put SP as the first clause level. At the following clause level(s), they further divide the P into SV, VO, VCv, VA and so on. For the purpose of fitting into the format of the LARSP chart, if the P is a verb, the SP level is normally omitted (but the example in Table 12.2 shows a level with SP and then a further level with SV). Since SP can act as one of the clause elements, when it contains a verb, an English translation of a Chinese sentence would show that this sentence is complex, but Chinese grammarians do not classify it in this way (see Table 12.2).

In Chinese, there is no independent clause-level element of subject complement as in English (e.g. SVC (*I'm happy* or *I'm a student*)). The attributive

Table 12.2 An example of P containing a verb as a clause element

这人	他不喜欢。	(P is a SV construction. It can
zheren	ta bu xihuan	
S	P	also be classified as S SV.)
	S neg V	
this person	he not like	

This is the person he doesn't like.

(定语 dingyu) is a component regarded by Chinese grammarians as a clause-level element, the same as a subject or an object, but it mainly modifies the following head word, most likely a noun (Guo, 2000: 137–46; Huang & Liao, 1981: 334–40; Xin, 2003: 117–25). It is also called an endocentric construction (偏正结构 pianzhengjiegou). A noun, adjective, pronoun, a classifier, a verb, an SV, a VCc, a VO and a *de* construction can be an attributive used to modify the head noun. This attributive tends to appear before the head word.

Clause structures

Key Chinese clause structures include those shown in Table 12.3. Like English, one or more adverbial elements can be added to any of the Chinese structures in Table 12.3. As explained earlier, there is no subject complement in Chinese syntactic categorization, thus in the example of *My Mama is a teacher*, the structure in Chinese is SVO.

There are some special Chinese clause constructions, as shown in Table 12.4. Cv refers to the verb + complement construction, which further elaborates the verb (Chao, 1968: 435; Huang & Liao, 1981: 140; Guo, 2000: 343). A verb complement can be made from an adjective, verb, adverb, classifiers or a prepositional phrase. There are at least seven kinds of Verb + Complement (Cv) constructions: resultative, degree, directional, positional, classifier, time and potential. In Chinese, Cv is one of the most complicated structures in description and analysis. The example given in Table 12.4 is a verb-complement construction for degree.

According to Yip and Rimmington (2004: 209), there are three types of expressions used to form the passive voice in Chinese: the *notional passive* which does not use any passive marker; the *formal passive*, which employs the passive marker *bei* 被 [bei]; and the *lexical passive*, which uses words 得到 [dedao] ('receive', V+Cv) to indicate a passive action. Thus the main function of the *bei* construction is to show that the subject of the utterance is actually the object of the verb action. In colloquial Chinese, other function words such as 让 *rang*, 叫 *jiao*, and 给 *gei*, 让…给 [rang…gei], 叫…给 [jiao…gei] are used to replace *bei* to form the passive function (see Table 12.5).

Table 12.3 Chinese clause structures and examples

Clause level structures	Examples
Subject-Predicate (SP) 主谓句 zhuweiju	他们 来 了。(S is a pronoun) tamen lai le S P they come am 'They have come' (P is a verb) 妈妈 高兴。(S is a noun) mama gaoxing S P Mama happy 'Mama is happy' (P is an adjective; there is no verb)
SAV 主状述句 zhuzhuangshuju	主语-------状语-------述语 zhuyu zhuangyu shuyu 哥哥 已经 走了。 gege yijing zoule S A V elder brother already go am '(My elder) brother has already left'
SVO 主述宾句 zhushubinju	兔子 笑 乌龟。 tuzi xiao wugui S V O hare laugh tortoise 'The hare laughs at the tortoise' 我妈妈 是 老师。 womama shi laoshi S V O my mama is teacher 'My Mama is a teacher'
SVOiOd 主述双宾句 zhushushuangbinju Double-object constructions	妈妈 给 了 我 一块 蛋糕。 mama gei le wo yikuai dangao S V Oi Od Mama give am I one piece cake 'Mama gave me a piece of cake'

Table 12.4 Special clause structures with examples

Special clause structures (1)	Examples
Clause (S-P) Subject + Predicate (Chao's term in English, 1968: 109) 主谓谓语句 (zhuweiweiyuju) S SV 主语--- 主语--- 述语 zhuyu zhuyu shuyu	龟　兔赛跑　大家　都　要看。 gui tu saipao dajia dou yaokan S　　　S　　A　V tortoise hare race everyone all want watch 'That the race between the tortoise and the hare hold will be wanted by everyone to watch'
Serial verb constructions 连谓句 (lianweiju) SV(O)V(O) 主语---述语--- (宾语)--- 述语--- (宾语) zhuyu shuyu binyu shuyu binyu	妈妈　回　家　做　饭。 mama hui jia zuo fan S　　V　O　V　O Mama return home make meal 'Mama goes home to cook a meal'
Pivotal constructions 兼语句 (jianyuju) SVOsV(O) 主语--- 述语--- 兼语--- 述语--- (宾语) zhuyu shuyu jianyu shuyu binyu	乌龟　叫　兔子去　森林。 wugui jiao tuzi qu senlin S　　V　Os　V　O tortoise ask hare go forest 'The tortoise asked the hare to go to the forest'
Verb + complement constructions 主述动补句： (zhushudongbuju) SVCv 主语---述语--- 程度补语--- (宾语) zhuyu shuyu chengdubuyu binyu	乌龟　跑　得　慢。 Wugui pao de man S　V　Cv tortoise run *de* slow 'The tortoise ran slowly'

Table 12.5 Chinese clause constructions led by function words

Special Chinese clause structures (2) Utterances led by *function words*	Examples
Ba constructions 把字句 (baziju)	把门　打开。 bamen da kai *Ba*O　V *Ba* door beat open 'Open the door'
Bei constructions and the passive voice 被字句(beiziju)	兔子　被乌龟　赶　上　了。 tuzi beiwugui gan shang le S　*Bei*O　　V hare *Bei* tortoise catch up am 'The hare is caught up by the tortoise'
Bi constructions 比字句(biziju)	兔子　跑　得　比　乌龟　快。 tuzi bao de bi wugui kuai S　V Cv.. *Bi*　O　..Cv hare run *de* Bi tortoise fast 'The hare runs faster than the tortoise'

Question constructions

There are three types of question structures in Chinese: *yes/no*-questions, tag questions and *wh*-questions. There are commonly six ways to form questions (see Tables 12.6 and 12.7).

Table 12.6 Main constructions for *yes/no*, choice, and tag questions in Chinese

	Yes/no, choice and tag questions	Examples
1	Statement + question particle (Qp) 陈述句 + 疑问词 chenshuju yiwenci	他们 来 了 吗? tamen lai le ma S V they come am Qp 'Have they come?'
2	Statement + *hai-shi* + statement 陈述句 + 还是 + 陈述句 chensuju haishi chenshuju	他们 回 家, 还是 回 学校? tamen hui jia haishi hui xuexiao S V O or V O they return home or return school 'Do they go back home or return to their school?'
3	Tag questions 1) S+V-*neg*-V+ (the rest of the statement) 主语+述语 (动词-不- 动词) + zhuyu shuyu dongci bu dongci 陈述句 其它成分 chenshuju qitachengfen 2) Statement + x-negative-x (x can be a verb, noun, adjective, etc) 陈述句+词-不-词 (如动词, 名词 或 形容词等) mingci huo xingrongci deng	1) 他们 来 不 来? tamen lai bu lai S V *not* V they come not come 'Do they come or not?' 2) 我们 赛跑 好 不 好(or行不行, 干不干)? women saipao hao bu hao xing bu xing gan bu gan we race good not good can not can, do not do 'Shall we have a race?'

Table 12.7 Main constructions for *Wh*-Questions in Chinese

Main wh-questions (WhQ)	Examples
1 WhQ (Who, Why) + rest of statement 疑问词 (谁，为什么)+ yiwenci (shei, sheishenme) 陈述句 其它成分 chenshuju qitachengfen	谁 赛跑？　　　为什么 赛跑？ shei saipao　　weishenme saipao WhQ V　　　　WhQ　　V who race　　　why　　race 'Who has a race? Why is there a race?'
2 S + V + WhQ (+X, which can be V, O, etc) 主语+述语+疑问词 (+句子 zhuyu shuyu yiwenci juzi 成分，如 述语，宾语，等) chengfen ru shuyu binyu deng	你们 去 哪儿？　　你们 买 什么 菜？ S　　V　WhQ　　S　　V　WhQ O you go where　　you buy what vegetable 'Where do you go? What vegetable do you buy?'
3 S + WhQ + time + rest of statement 主语 +疑问词+时间词+ zhuyu yiwenci shijianci 陈述句　其它成分 chenshuju qitachengfen	你们 什么 时候 回 家？ nimen shenme shihou hui jia S　　WhQ　　time　V　O you what time return home 'What time do you go back home?' 你们 几 点 回 家？ nimen ji dian hui jia S　WhQ time V O you which o'clock return home 'By what o'clock do you return home?'

Phrase-level elements

Phrase-level elements refer to a word or a group of words categorized below the clause level according to the head-word class. The common phrase elements in Chinese include: noun phrase (NP), verb phrase (VP), adverb phrase (AdvP) and prepositional phrase (PP). A word can be classified as a noun, verb, adjective, adverb and so on, depending on where it appears in a phrase or a clause. Chinese word-classes include: noun, verb, adjective, adverb, classifier, pronoun, preposition and conjunction. A phrase is determined by the head word in a phrase, and further analysis of phrase level shows individual word classes as phrase elements, as illustrated in Table 12.8.

A unique Chinese phrase-level construction is called the *endocentric construction* (偏正结构, pianzhengjigou), made up of premodifier(s) (pronoun, adjective, noun, classifier (cl) , *de* construction, adverb, SP construction, VO construction, etc.) and head word (noun or verb) (Xin, 2003: 117–125). The Direct Object (Od) in Table 12.8 shows an endocentric construction

Table 12.8 An example of phrase-level elements

SVOiOd	妈妈	给 了	我	一块	蛋糕。	
主述双宾句	mama	gei le	wo	yikuai	dangao	
zhushushuangbinju	C:	S V	Oi	Od		
Double object constructions		Mama give am	I	one piece	cake	
C: clause level	P:	NP VP	NP	NP		
P: phrase level		n v am	pron	cl	n	
cl: classifier						

'Mama gave me a piece of cake'

Table 12.9 *De*-N construction patterns and functions

De-N construction and functions	Examples
的 *de*-N showing possession	这 书 是 他的。(pronoun + *de*-N) zheshu shi ta de C: S V O P: NP VP NP pron*n v pron *de*-N this book is he *de*-N 'This book is his' *This pronoun would be called a determiner in English.
的 *de*-N indicating composition	金 的 是 这 个。(noun + *de*-N) jin de shi zhe ge C: S V O P: NP VP NP n *de*-N v pron classifier (m-w) gold *de*-N is this piece 'Gold one is this one'
的 *de*-N nominalizing the previous adjective	这 是 最大的。(adjective + *de*-N) zhe shi zuida de C: S V O P: NP VP NP pron v adv adj *de*-N this is most big *de*-N 'This is the biggest one'
的 *de*-N making an attributive element	漂 亮 的 孩子 (adjective + *de*-N) piaoliang de haizi P: NP adj *de*-N n beautiful *de*-N child 'A beautiful child'

218   Assessing Grammar

Table 12.9 continued

的 *de*-N used after a verb as an emphasis indicator
V + *de*-N + (noun)
	他 买的 笔*。(S is emphasized)
	ta maide bi
	C: S P
	P: NP NP
	pron V *de*-N n
	he buy *de*-N pen
	'It was him who bought the pen'.
	(Stress is on *ta* 'he')
	
	*It is possible to treat it as a phrase:
	他 买的 笔
	<u>ta maide bi</u>
	       NP
	Pron v *de*-N n
	'The pen he bought'
	but the emphasis may be changed.
	(Stress is on *bi* 'pen')
	
	兔子 是 昨天 输的。(Time is emphasized.)
	tuzi shi zuotianshude
	C: S V O
	P: NP VP NP
	   n v n v *de*-N
	  hare is yesterday lose *de*-N
	'It was yesterday that the hare lost his race'

的 *de*-N used after a verb as a confirmation indicator
V + *de*-N
	我 知道的。
	wo shidaode
	C: S P
	P: NP NP
	  pron v *de*-N
	   I know *de*-N
	'I confirm I know this'

consisting of a classifier (一块, yikuai) premodifier with a noun as head (蛋糕, dangao).

The *de* construction is a way of forming noun phrases. There are three *de* particles, using three different Chinese characters with the same pronunciation but with different functions.

- The first *de* (的, de) tends to nominalize or make an attributive contribution to the following noun (see Table 12.9). This *de* is labelled as *de*-N. An element + *de*-N can be used as a subject, object or part of a verb complement. It shows a possessive quality in combination with the preceding word, which can be a pronoun (Yip & Rimmington, 2004: 48) or a noun. A *de*-N is added to a preceding adjective so that this element characterizes the following noun. The headword noun does not need to appear. Often one can add a noun to show this is a noun phrase (see further examples in Table 12.9).

- The second *de* (得, de) tends to postmodify a verb preceding it, making the element following it a verb complement, thus it is placed between a verb and a verb complement (Cv) 跑得快 [paodekuai] ('run *de*-Cv fast'). This *de* is labelled as *de*-Cv.
- The third *de* (地, de) makes the element (which tends to be an adjective) preceding it into an adverb (*de*-ly), e.g. 高兴 [gaoxing] > 高兴地 [gaoxingde] ('happy' > 'happily').

Word-level elements

In Chinese, word-level elements are words which do not function independently in a phrase, such as the aspect marker *le* 了 in Table 12.10, which is a bound morpheme functioning as a past aspect marker for the verb 'give'.

Such word-level morphemes include aspect markers (am) for the past-aspect marker ('-ed') *le* (了), the continuous aspect marker ('-ing') *zai* (在) or *zhe* (着), the compound noun suffix *zi* (子), the number prefix or initiator *di* (第) and different *de* suffixes.

Table 12.10 An example of word-level elements

SVOiOd		妈妈	给	了	我	一块	蛋糕。
主述双宾句		mama	gai	le	wo	yikuai	dangao
zhushushuangbinju	C:	S	V		Oi	Od	
Double objects constructions		Mama	give	am	I	one piece cake	
C: clause level	P:	NP	VP		NP	NP	
P: phrase level		n	v	am	pron	cl	n
cl: classifier	W:			am			
W: word level		'Mama gave me a piece of cake'					

Data Collection and Analysis

A number of research methods have been used for collecting data related to Chinese child language development. These include individual case studies (e.g. Li & Chen, 1998); experiments (e.g. Xin, 1982); recording children's utterances or screening data collection (primary source data, e.g. Wong *et al.*, 1992); and collecting carers' recalls of children's language development (secondary source data, e.g. Zhang *et al.*, 2008). Researchers may use observation, note taking, audio and/or video recording, filling in prepared forms or questionnaires and conducting semi-structured or open interviews as ways of collecting data. Existing research into Chinese-speaking children's language development show that two kinds of data analysis methods are mainly used: qualitatively keeping a record and classifying the recorded utterances of a child's language with researchers' interpretations of the data samples; and using statistics to analyse data collected with comments to interpret the statistics. In some studies (e.g. Zhou & Zhang, 2009), both methods have been employed.

For C-LARSP, 130 Chinese-speaking children were recruited following the ethical approval procedures regulated by both DMU and UKM and with the consent given by participants' carers. The key criteria for including these children were that: (i) they were reported to have normal language development with no history of a speech, hearing or other known disorder at birth; (ii) they were aged between 1;0 and 6;11; and (iii) Mandarin was the dominant home language with a minimum of 80% language input and output reported by carers. The age breakdown can be seen in Table 12.11:

There are three types of language data collected by audio or video recording: *free conversation*, *story-telling* with a specially designed picture book and *self-generated narratives* of the children's own past experiences. For the younger children aged between 1;0-3;11, only the first two types of data were gathered. For the other children all three methods are used.

According to Crystal (1979: 22), it should be adequate to establish a profile of a child's grammatical production by collecting 'a 30-minute sample broken down into two 15-minute parts, one in which T [Therapist]

Table 12.11 Age range and number of children in the data set

Age interval	Age groups of children	No. of children in each age group with equal numbers in gender
3 months	1;0-1;2, 1;3-1;5, 1;6-1;8, 1;9-1.11, 2;0-2;2, 2;3-2;5, 2;6-2;8, 2;9-2;11	10 children x 8 age groups
6 months	3;0-3;5, 3;6-3;11,	10 children x 2 age groups
12 months	4;0-4;11, 5;0-5;11, 6;0-6;11	10 children x 3 age groups
Total	13 age groups	130 children

talks to P [Pupil] about P's immediate environment, actions etc., and one in which the conversation is about an absent situation'. In the present study, a decision was made to have a cut-off point for the number of utterances for all participants rather than by time in free conversation because the researchers needed to have a way to compare the production of children from different age ranges with a similar number of utterances. The rationale for this was that, following the experience of a pilot test, the researchers found that younger participants needed more time to produce the number of utterances required, hence it was perceived that the number of utterances was more important than the time spent in interaction. It was decided that the first 50 utterances in free conversation would be included in the grammatical analysis. The second and third methods were developed to give participants opportunities to show their language competence from a type of oral communication which might not be collected from the free conversation method. Further, the team noted that narrative skills are essential for daily communication situations and educational achievements (Cortazzi & Jin, in press). Basic information regarding the social, family and personal information of the targeted child was also collected through a questionnaire.

For the *free conversation*, it was found that most children, irrespective of gender or age within the range, were familiar with certain topics, especially food, cooking and shopping. It is believed that the cultural environment in Malaysia has provided this familiarity to children from a very young age. Thus the team later produced an assessment pack which contains some toys with fruit, vegetables, cooking and shopping items as helpful assessment stimuli for use in educational and clinical settings. This provision fits well with the argument made by Schieffelin and Ochs (1986) and Duranti (1997) that children are socialized into language, but the way this occurs varies from culture to culture. This set of conversational topics may not suit children from other cultural backgrounds.

The *picture-book story-telling* activity was developed specially for this project by adapting the widely-known story of 'The Hare and Tortoise'. Pictures were produced to match with the utterances written for a Chinese version of the story. For those children below two years of age, a researcher told the story to the child once using the utterances given in the picture book, and then asked the child to retell the story with the picture book as a stimulus. The researcher sometimes gave some neutral prompts to help children start the story-telling and to encourage them to narrate the story they have heard.

With the age groups over two years old, the researcher summarized the story first with the picture book and then let the child tell the story, using the picture book as a stimulus, with minimal prompts from the researcher. Generally, the researchers found it necessary to give more prompts with younger children than older ones. The picture book was modified for

Table 12.12 An example of utterance transcription and grammatical analysis

An example by 2;8-1-g-MY: R: researcher; C: child; No: utterance number

R	拿一个就可以了/ na yi ge jiu ke yi le 'One is enough'		
C17	拿 一 个 啊/ na yi ge a take one piece particle 'You want me to take one?' C: V　　　　0　　　Q particle P: VP　　　　NP　　Q particle P: v　　　　　cl　　Qp W :　　　　　m	Clause: Stage III VOQp Phrase: NP: cl Word: m	(point to the top)
R	/m/		
R	那个是谁? na ge shi shui? 'Who is that?'		
C18	那 个 小 姐姐/ na ge xiao jie jie that small sister 'That is the younger sister' CL :　　S　　　　　　0 PL1:　　NP　　　　　NP PL2: pron m　　adj　　n W:　　　m	Clause: Stage II SO Phrase: NP: pron-m NP: adj n	Missing verb '是' (is)

children aged 1;0-2;11 based on the researchers' feedback and initial data analysis of this age group. It was found that too much colouring and too many objects drawn in the picture distracted children and they appeared confused. So a book with simpler and 'plainer' pictures and fewer background objects was produced for this age group.

The *self-generated narrative* method used a significant or immediate past event within the children's personal and cultural experience. This tended to be about a celebration, birthday party, holiday, outing, shopping trip, visit to grandparents and so on. It is recognized that the ability to produce an appropriate narrative is closely linked with children's language development and educational achievement (McCabe & Peterson, 1991); it is useful for educational and clinical assessments (Botting, 2000) for researchers to know how children are able to produce fictional story narratives and self-generated personal narratives, as well as how the structures are developed in Chinese through age for each type of narration. There may be culture-specific language styles which emerge in children's narrative (McCabe, 1997;

Minami, 2002). However, this chapter uses the data to focus only on grammatical production rather than on the linguistic structure of narratives (Labov & Waletzky, 1967; Labov, 1977).

In total, nearly 11,000 utterances from the three types of data were transcribed and analysed following the *Guidance on analysing Chinese syntactic structures* (Jin, 2009). The main analyses include grammatical analysis, mean length of utterance (MLU), the relationship between meaning and form in an utterance (MCUS) and the analysis of narrative structures and the developmental patterns of narrative structures (McCabe & Peterson, 1991). In this chapter, only the grammatical development is reported.

The transcription includes all prompting utterances produced by researchers and children's utterances. An utterance transcription for children is produced with a *pinyin* transcription (a standard Chinese phonetic system), an orthographic form, a word-for-word translation into English and a meaning translation into English for the convenience of non-Chinese readers (see Table 12.12). The grammatical analysis is placed under each child's utterance and the contextual information and location of the LARSP stages is listed in the boxes on the right of the utterance.

Description of C-LARSP

The Chinese LARSP chart (see Figure 12.1) was created following the principles and format of the LARSP chart as described by Crystal et al. (1989). This chart reports what has been produced from the data by the participating children, and is descriptive. The ABCD sections have been adopted because these are not language specific (Ball, 1988; Samadi & Perkins, 1998) and they should be applicable to C-LARSP. The same columns have been followed in the sections of seven stages, although, in a few cases, the principle of one-element structure for Stage I and two-element structure for Stage II and so on is not strictly followed, because of the kind of data produced by the children.

Stage I features show that the children do not use any question forms; their rising intonation indicate the function of request. However, they tend to duplicate a syllable (character) in their utterances, such as *ma-ma* ('mother'), *che-che* ('car'). Chinese-speaking children in Malaysia at this age appear to have limited utterances, as expected; they are mainly vocatives, symbolic noises, nouns and verbs. However, there is evidence to show that they are beginning to produce one- and two-element syntactic constructions, such as verb command, verb, noun, and adjective, and VO, AV, pron-m (e.g. *zhe ge* ['this'] 这个), and endocentric constructions (e.g. *wo mama* ['my mummy'] 我妈妈). The two-element utterance structures are not in the English LARSP chart for this age group.

In Stage II, they continue the feature of duplicating characters and begin to produce compound nouns and verbs (x-comp). They have started

224 Assessing Grammar

Figure 12.1 A C-LARSP chart for analysing Mandarin utterances in Malaysia

to develop model auxiliary verbs and *de* constructions. The clause-level elements are similar to those in English LARSP.

The transitional stage between Stages II and III has some similarity to English LARSP, but a new element is the extended verb complement, and the adverb element is an extended noun phrase. The same pattern is repeated in the transitional stage between stages III and IV.

Stage III is an accelerated stage for many special Chinese clause structures. The *gei* ('give') construction is used to express a command. The question forms are largely produced with expressions for 'who', 'why' and 'where', and different word orders of question markers. The phrase level features show more complex combinations of phrase elements, including compound auxiliary verbs, compound verb complements, complex endocentric constructions as a noun phrase and an initiator with a classifier to modify a noun.

In Stage IV, a number of compound conjunctions (e.g. *ranhou* 然后, 'then') are produced. The tag question structures are used, alongside the question forms with more clause elements. At this stage an S SV(X) (主谓谓语句, zhuweiweiyuju) is identified, and more complex verb structures are used with up to three verb elements. Many utterances made by these children include an adverbial element at clause level. This is not shown in the clause-level elements at this stage, because an almost unlimited number of adverbial elements can be added to a sentence, and it is impossible to include all combinations. A number of complex noun formations are also recorded in the phrase-level section.

Stage V shows the paired compound conjunctions (e.g. 'because…therefore'; 'if…then…') for the creation of double-clause sentences. The compressed clause tends to use an adverb to indicate a relationship in a double-clause sentence. The compressed and double questions are developed later than the statement clause elements. The phrase-level structure appears to contain one new form which is a superlative adverb (*zui*, 最). It appears that children at this stage tend to use more of the compound forms which emerged in Stages III and IV.

Stages VI and VII contain data to show the more complex nature of Chinese utterances using conjunctions, noun phrases, and multiple clauses, as well as children's descriptive ability of narrative events and sequences. The comparative feature appears at this stage (whereas in English, comparative features appear at Stage V). The error features recorded in Stage VI are those made by these normally developing children at different stages, since there are no clinical data available for this section. This section needs further investigation by using C-LARSP for the assessment of SLT children. Stage VII also needs further research, although the narrative data are available. The four aspects listed in this stage are a useful starting point.

The word-level features have been discussed above, though this is not an exclusive list.

Discussion of C-LARSP

There are a number of issues regarding the development of this C-LARSP chart. First of all, the features shown are not a complete list for Mandarin speakers in Malaysia, or for other Mandarin-speaking communities. Secondly, there is no presentation of code-mixing information on the chart, though such mixing is a common feature in the data in children's language production (unsurprisingly, given the relationship between Mandarin and other languages, particularly English in some homes and the national Malay language in Malaysia). Table 12.13 shows an example of the influence of code-mixing in Mandarin-speaking children in Malaysia from the data collected. A proportion of their utterances is influenced by English, (i.e. they use English in their statement answers). A very small proportion of their utterances is influenced by other Chinese dialects or Malay (i.e. they used Chinese dialect pronunciation or Malay words in their statement answers). The biased use of English in their story telling may reflect the fact that the children of this age group could only name the animals in the picture, and perhaps they had previously learned the names of the animals in English. However, it appears that the proportion of code-mixing among the children reduces as their age increases.

Thirdly, it appears that some expected special Chinese sentence structures were not produced at all in these data samples. These include the *ba* construction, the *bei* construction and more complex comparative expressions. The reasons for this are unknown. One factor could be the topics of conversation. Another is the possibility that their Mandarin production was influenced by English and other languages from a young age, so that their expressions were restricted to those which conformed to the ones influencing them.

Fourthly, although this study used a systematic process to collect and analyse data, errors can occur, and data information may have been missed or misinterpreted, despite the number of checks and re-checks of data analysis carried out during the production of the profile. It is suggested that future researchers should plan the coding of data in advance and record the data using software if possible.

Fifthly, the production process of C-LARSP has enabled researchers to produce an assessment pack with a bag of toys for cooking and shopping

Table 12.13 Code-mixing in children aged 1;0–1;5

	Influences by				
	Unknown Dialect	English	Cantonese	Hokkien	Malay
Free	1.27%	17.09%	0.63%	2.53%	0.63%
Story	0	77.79%	0	0	0

items, and a picture book of 'The Hare and Tortoise', as well as some standardized forms for keeping a record of the data and analysis. They seem to be effective and useful for clinical settings, saving time and offering topics which are familiar to the children. Clearly it is important to use culturally appropriate items if this method is used for future studies and for producing assessments (Gladstone *et al.*, 2009).

Conclusion

The C-LARSP chart is an important tool for Chinese-speaking children who need to be assessed for language development by educational and SLT services. It will help to establish a standard for SLT needs in those countries where there is as yet no SLT provision, and it will enhance equality of health care in those countries where SLT services are available. However, this chart is only a starting point for linguistic and SLT researchers and practitioners. While it has been formatted on the basis of data from Malaysia, it is believed that it can serve as a foundation for profiling Chinese (Putongha) in China and in other Chinese-speaking communities.

As a Chinese saying states, *pao zhuan yin yu* 抛转引玉 ('throw a stone to attract a jade'). This means a humble stone may get some reaction which leads to a real jade stone appearing. Similar to the effect of 'throwing a stone into a pond', C-LARSP hopes to make ripples and elicit reactions from future researchers.

Acknowledgements

The authors would like to thank the PMI2 funding which supported this project financially, all the students from UKM, staff from both DMU and UKM involved in this project and Dr Linhui Li from East China Normal University, who helped to check the data for the C-LARSP chart.

References

Ball, M.J. (1988) LARSP to LLARSP: The design of a grammatical profile for Welsh. *Clinical Linguistics & Phonetics* 2 (1), 55–73.
Botting, N. (2002) Narrative as a tool for the assessment of linguistic and pragmatic impairments. *Child Language Teaching and Therapy* Vol. 18, No.1, 1–21.
Chao, Y.R. (1968) *A Grammar of Spoken Chinese*. California: University of California Press.
Chao, J.Z. and Han, J.T. (eds) (2005) *Modern Chinese Dictionary* (5th edn). Beijing: Commercial Press. [晁继周 和 韩敬体 (2005编) 现代汉语词典. 第五版. 北京: 商务印书馆; chao ji zhou he han jingti (2005 bian) xiandai hanyu cidian. diwuban. beijing: shangwuyinshuguan]
Cheung, H. (2009) Grammatical characteristics of Mandarin-speaking children with specific language impairment. In Sam-Po Law, B.S. Weekes and Anita M-Y Wong (eds) *Language Disorders in Speakers of Chinese* (pp. 19–32). Bristol: Multilingual Matters.

Cortazzi, M. and Jin, L. (in press) Approaching narrative analysis with 15 questions. In S. Delamont (ed.) *Handbook of Qualitative Research in Education*. Cheltenham: Edward Elgar.

Crystal, D. (1979) *Working with LARSP.* London: Edward Arnold.

Crystal, D., Fletcher, P. and Garman, M. (1989) *The Grammatical Analysis of Language Disability* (2nd edn). London: Cole & Whurr.

Duranti, A. (1997) *Linguistic Anthropology*. Cambridge: Cambridge University Press.

Erbaugh, M. (1992) The acquisition of Mandarin. In D. Slobin (ed.) *The Cross-Linguistic Study of Language Acquisition* (vol.3) (*pp.* 373–454). Hillsdale, NJ: Lawrence Erlbaum Associates.

Gladstone, M., Lancaster, G.A., Umar, E., Nyirenda, M., Kayira, E., Nynke R., Broek, N.R. and Smyth, R.L. (2009) Perspectives of normal child development in rural Malawi – A qualitative analysis to create a more culturally appropriate developmental assessment tool. *Child Care Health and Development* 36 (6), 346–53.

Guo, Z.H. (2000) *A Concise Chinese Grammar*. Beijing: Chinese Language Teaching Press. [郭振华 (2000) 简明汉语语法. 北京：华语教学出版社; guozhenhua (2000) jianming hanyuyufa. beijing: huayu jiaoxue shubanshe]

Hsu, J.H. (1996) *A Study of the Stages of Development and Acquisition of Mandarin Chinese by Children in Taiwan*. Taipei: Crane.

Huang, B.R. and Liao, X.D. (eds) (1981) *Modern Chinese*. Lanzhou: Ganshu People's Press. [黄伯荣 和 廖序东(1981)现代汉语. 兰州：甘肃人民教育出版社; huangborong he liaoxudong (1981) xiandai hanyu. lanzhou: gansu ranmin jiaoyu chubanshe]

Huang, C.J. and Li, Y.A. (eds) (1996) *New Horizons in Chinese Linguistics*. Dordrecht: Kluwer.

Jin, L. (2009) Chinese Syntactic Structures: A Grammar Guide to Language Profiling. Unpublished booklet.

Labov, W. (1977) *Therapeutic Discourse: Psychotherapy as Conversation*. New York: Academic Press.

Labov, W. and Waletzky, J. (1967) Narrative analysis: oral versions of personal experience. In J. Helm (ed.) *Essays on the Verbal and Visual Arts* (*pp.* 12–44). Seattle: University of Washington Press.

Law, S., Weekes, B.S. and Wong, A.M. (eds) (2009) *Language Disorders in Speakers of Chinese*. Bristol: Multilingual Matters.

Li, Y.M. (1995) *Child Language Development*. Wuhan: Huazhong Normal University Press. [李宇明 (1995) 儿童语言发展. 武汉：华中师范大学出版社; liyuming (1995) ertong yuyan fazhan. wuhan: huazhong shifan daxue chubanshe]

Li, Y.M. and Chen, Q.R. (1998). *Language Comprehension and Occurrence: The Comparative Study of Children's Comprehension and Occurrence of Question Utterances*. Wuhan: Huazhong Normal University Press. [李宇明，陳前瑞 (1998) 语言的理解与发生：儿童问句系统的理解与发生的比较研究. 武汉：华中师范大学出版社; liyuming, chenqianrui (1998) yuyande lijie yu fasheng: ertong wenju xitongde lijie yu fashengde bijiaoyanjiu. wuhan: huazhong shifan daxue chubanshe]

Lu, F.B. (1996) *Practical Chinese Grammar for Teaching Chinese as a Foreign Language*. Beijing: Beijing Language and Culture University Press. [卢福波 (1996) 对外汉语教学实用语法. 北京：北京语言文化大学出版社; lufubo (1996) duiwai hanyu jiaoxue shiyong yufa. beijing: beijing yuyan wenhua daxue chubanshe]

Lü, S.X. (1947) *Outline of Chinese Grammar*. Shanghai: Shanghai: the Commercial Press Shanghai [吕叔湘(1947)中国文法要略. 上海：上海商务印书馆; lüshuxiang (1947) zhongguo wenfa yaolüe. shanghai: shanghai shangwu yinshuguan].

McCabe, A. (1997) Developmental and cross-cultural aspects of children's narration. In M. Bamberg (ed.) *Narrative Development* (pp. 137–74). London: Lawence Erlbaum.

McCabe, A. and Peterson, C. (eds.) (1991) *Developing Narrative Structure*. Hillsdale, NJ: Lawrence Erlbaum.

Minami, M. (2002) *Culture-Specific Language Styles, the Development of Oral Narrative and Literacy*. Clevedon: Multingual Matters.
Quirk, R., Greenbaum, S., Leech, G. and Svartvik, J. (1985) *A Comprehensive Grammar of the English Language*. London: Longman.
Samadi, H. and Perkins, M.R. (1998) P-LARSP: A developmental language profile for Persian. *Clinical Linguistics & Phonetics* 12 (2), 83–103.
Schieffelin, B.B. and Ochs, E. (eds) (1986) *Language Socialization Across Cultures*. Cambridge: Cambridge University Press.
Tardif, T. and Fletcher, P. (2008) *Chinese Communicative Development Inventories*. Beijing: Peking University Medical Press.
Wong, V., Lee, P.W.H., Lieh-Mak, F., Yeung, C.Y., Leung, P.W.L., Luk, S.L. and Yiu, E. (1992) Language screening in preschool Chinese children. *International Journal of Language & Communication Disorders* 27 (3), 247–64.
Xin, A.T. (1982) Educational experiments to children aged below three years old for their language development. In Zhu, Z.X. (ed.) *Psychological Development of Children Below Three Years Old*. Beijing: Beijing Normal University Press. [辛安亭 (1982) 对三岁前幼儿语言发展教育的实验. 朱智贤主编, 三岁前儿童心理的发展. 北京: 北京师范大学出版社; xinanting (1982) dui sansuiqian youer yuyan fazhan jiaoyude shiyan. zhuzhixian zhubian, sansuiqian ertong xinlide fazhan. beijing: beijing shifan daxue chubanshe]
Xin, J. (2003) *Modern Chinese: The Study of Grammatical Rhetoric*. Taiyuan: Shenxi Booksea Press. [辛菊 (2003) 现代汉语-语法修辞研究. 太原: 山西书海出版社; xinju (2003) xiandai hanyu – yufa qiuci yanjiu. taiyuan: shanxi shuhai chubanshe]
Yip, P. and Rimmington, D. (2004) *Chinese: A Comprehensive Grammar*. London: Routledge.
Zhang, Y.W., Jin, X.M., Shen, X.M., Zhang, J.M. and Hoff, E. (2008) Correlates of early language development in Chinese children. *International Journal of Behavioral Development* Vol. 32, No. 2, 145–151
Zhou, G.G (1997) *The Study of Structural Acquisition of Chinese Sentences*. Hefei: Anhui University Press. [周国光 (1997) 汉语句法结构习得研究. 合肥: 安徽大学出版社; zhouguoguang (1997) hanyu jiufa jiegou xide yanjiu. hefei: anhui daxue chubanshe]
Zhou, J. (2002) *Pragmatic Development of Mandarin-Speaking Children*. Nanjing: Nanjing Normal University Press. [周兢 (2002) 儿童语言运用能力的发展. 南京: 南京师范大学出版社; zhoujing (2002) ertong yuyan yunyong nenglide fazhan. nanjing: Nanjing shifan daxue chubanshe]
Zhou, J. and Zhang, J.R. (eds) (2009) *Studies on Language Development of Chinese-Speaking Children*. Beijing: Educational Science Publishing House. [周兢 和张鑑如 (2009, 编) 汉语儿童语言发展研究. 北京: 教育科学出版社; zhoujing he zhangjianru (2009, bian) hanyu ertong yuyan fazhan yanjiu. beijing: jiaoyu kexue chubanshe]
Zhu, H. (2002) *Phonological Development in Specific Contexts: Studies of Chinese-Speaking Children*. Clevedon: Multilingual Matters.
Zhu, S.M. (1986) *Studies of Child Language Development*. Shanghai: East China Normal University Press. [朱曼殊 (1986) 儿童语言发展研究. 上海: 华东师范大学出版社; zhumanshu (1986) ertong yuyan fazhan yanjiu. shanghai: huadong shifan daxue chubanshe]

13 F-LARSP: A Computerized Tool for Measuring Morphosyntactic Abilities in French

Christophe Parisse, Christelle Maillart and Jodi Tommerdahl

Introduction

The version of LARSP that has been adapted for use for French-speaking children has followed the lead of Bol and Kuiken (1990) for Dutch in accurately linking stages of language development with chronological ages. Their approach used two criteria for determining whether a given structure should be included on the chart, and, if so, at which stage: the structure should be used by at least 50% of the population at a particular stage; and the median of the frequency with which a structure is used should have a value of at least 1.0. For the French adaptation (F-LARSP), a large corpus of child language in French was analysed to determine at what stage structures should be placed on the new chart and how many of these structures should be included. Further details of the adaptation can be found in Maillart *et al.* (in press). In the present chapter, we focus on the design and implementation of a computerized system for accurately carrying out F-LARSP much more quickly than is possible with current manual methods.

Description of French Morphosyntax

French basic word order

The canonical word order of French is SVO (subject – verb – object), but exceptions occur. The use of object clitics leads to SOV structure (e.g. *il le mange* 'he eats it'); the relative clause tolerates VS order (e.g. VS – *l'homme qu'aime Marie* 'the man that Marie loves' – but also OSV *que Marie aime* 'that Marie loves'); and the interrogative structure allows VSO order (e.g. *connais-tu ce garçon ?* 'do you know this boy?'). However, in oral French, the canonical SVO order tends to be preserved in interrogative forms using a rising pattern of intonation (e.g. *La fille embrasse le garçon ?* 'The girl kisses the boy?') or the *est-ce que* locution (e.g. *Est-ce que la fille embrasse le garçon ?* 'Does the girl kiss the boy?'). Null subjects are not permitted (* *neige* 'snows'), except for imperatives when an impersonal subject is required (e.g. *il neige* 'it snows' or 'it is snowing') (Kail, 1989).

Determiners are located before the noun and have different forms including the demonstrative, indefinite, interrogative, negative and possessive (e.g. *cette table* 'this table', *une table* 'a table', *quelle table ?* 'which table?', *aucune table* 'no table', *ma table* 'my table'). In contrast, adjectives are placed after the noun they modify (e.g. *une table ronde* 'a round table') with the exception of a small set (e.g. *petit* 'small'), which are placed after the determiners and before the noun.

French morphology

French is a moderately inflected language. Due to historical erosion of endings, its morphology is characterized by significant homophony in the spoken language. Verbal forms with different inflections are pronounced in a similar way (e.g. *je mange, tu manges, il mange, ils mangent* 'I/you/he/they eat'). Ninety-four percent of the verbal forms are homophonous for several inflections (e.g. *il chante/ ils chantent* 'he/they sing') (Paradis & El Fenne, 1995). In French, the gender/ number of many nouns/adjectives is made clear only by the determiner. When audible, these inflections are formed by a vocalic (e.g. *cheval / chevaux* 'horse/horses') or consonantal (e.g. *petit / petite* 'little' masculine vs. feminine) morphophonological alternation (Dubois, 1965). The vocalic alternations are so infrequent that they tend to be lexicalized. The morphophonological alternation « consonant/Ø » is more frequently used to mark the number of the verb (e.g. *part - partent; dort – dorment*). This alternation is used in many different morphological mechanisms, such as verbal, nominal and adjectival morphology, derivation and liaison (e.g. *un petit enfant* 'a little child' where the *t* of *petit* is pronounced, vs. *un petit garçon* 'a little boy', where it is not).

The article system contains definite and indefinite forms. An article precedes the noun and agrees with it in number and gender. The inflections of number or gender within pronouns and determiner classes are based on a vocalic alternation. Lexical adverbs are often formed from their adjectival form plus the addition of *-ment* (e.g. *calme-ment* 'calmly').

Past events are expressed by different tenses, depending on several factors. Finished events occurring in the past are expressed by the 'passé composé' with the auxiliaries *avoir* ('have') or *être* ('be') plus the past participle (e.g. *J'ai mangé puis je suis parti* 'I ate then I left'). Interrupted events occurring in the past are expressed by the 'imparfait' with the stem of the verb plus the endings *-ais, -ais, -ait, -ions, -iez , -aient* (e.g. *je mangeais lorqu'il est arrivé* 'I ate when he arrived'). Upcoming events are expressed by two frequent tenses: 'futur simple' for future events and 'futur périphrastique' for very close future events. The formation of simple future is the same for the three different groups: the stem of the verb plus the endings *-rai, -ras, -ra, -rons,- rez, -ront* (e.g. *je mangerai* 'I will eat'). The 'futur périphrastique' is formed from the addition of the semi-auxiliary *aller* and the infinitive form of the verb (e.g. *je vais manger* 'I'm going to eat'). Complex verb constructions, auxiliaries followed by a past participle, and modals including *aller* ('to go') followed by an infinitive are very productive and frequently used to express aspect and mode.

From E-LARSP to F-LARSP

The adaptation of the English language LARSP (E-LARSP) to F-LARSP was made in six steps:

Step 1

The two first steps were carried out in joint meetings of the three authors, who are all fluent in French and English, with two being native French speakers and the third being a native English speaker. Target structures existing in English but not French were identified and omitted from the developing F-LARSP chart. This included structures such as the plural forms of nouns, which are present in French writing but not audible in speech, the contraction *n't* from the Word column, the genitive and the contracted copula.

Step 2

New target structures specific to French were identified as potential items to be added to the chart. Examples include structures containing lexical morphology such as *n&FEM* indicating the feminine form of a noun such as *la patineuse* (the female ice skater), and *dislo-G* and *dislo-D,* which represent dislocations (repetitions of noun phrases by a pronoun) to the left and right, as in the following sentences:

<u>Moi</u> je suis contente.
<u>Elle</u> est belle <u>la jeunesse</u>.

Dislocations are frequent in oral language (Blasco-Dulbecco, 1999), even in the speech of young children (Parisse, 2008), and are likely to represent an important step in language development.

Step 3

Software identifying the potential morphosyntactic targets of the F-LARSP was developed by the first author.

Automatic coding of the F-LARSP

F-LARSP automatic processing is itself a three-phase process: (a) part-of-speech tagging, (b) extraction of grammatical forms, and (c) statistical analysis and creation of an editable chart. The final user can intervene between phase (b) and phase (c) to check the accuracy of the extraction of grammatical forms and correct the results from the automatic process. F-LARSP, including charts, statistics and software, is available at www.modyco.fr/flarsp/. The present 1.0 version is partly based on the CLAN software from the CHILDES project (MacWhinney, 2000), and on Windows-based separate applications for phase (b) and phase (c). Future versions will be available for Apple Mac OS and other systems, and will integrate all phases into a single piece of software.

Phase (a). Transcriptions of the recordings were grammatically coded for part of speech using CLAN. This software is able to produce a part-of-speech syntactic analysis (Parisse & Le Normand, 2000). It is based on two CLAN commands, MOR and POST. MOR provides all possible parts of speech for a given word out of context, as shown in example (1) below. The whole dictionary used in the MOR command was created by the first author (see childes.psy.cmu.edu/mortags/). Examples (1) and (2) below provide an example of an utterance and all the possible tags that its words can have in French. Elements analyzed by MOR are represented by a main grammatical category followed by a '|', the base of the word (infinitive for a verb, masculine singular for a noun) and, whenever it is necessary, affixes separated by '-' for regular morphology and '&' for irregular morphology (see MacWhinney, 2000). The symbol '^' codes the ambiguity between two categories.

(1) *CHI: je crois qu' ils sont passés là+bas .
             [= I think that they went (have gone) there]
(2) %mor: pro:subj|je&1S v|croire pro:rel|qu'^pro:int|qu'^prep|que^conj|qu'^adv|que^adv:int|qu' pro:subj|ils&MASC v:exist|être^v:aux|être n|passé^adj|passé^v|passer-PP adv:place|là+bas.

In (2), two words are ambiguous. One is *qu'* ('that'), which can have a variety of functions, such as referential (e.g. relative pronoun (pro:rel)) and linking (e.g. as a conjunction). The other is *passés,* which can be a noun ('the past'), an adjective ('passed') or part of a verb construction (a past participle). There are many such ambiguities in French, and a specific CLAN command, POST (created by the first author – see Parisse & Le Normand, 2000), uses the distributional properties of French to propose a best candidate out of the various options from MOR. (It can be used for other languages, and in one example it has been successfully adapted to English by Brian MacWhinney. See childes.psy.cmu.edu/mortags/ for further information about the language adaptations that are available.) An example of the result of POST is given in (3). In this example, the parser did a fully correct job, but the actual results can vary from 95% to 97% of correct tagging depending on the type of language analysed.

(3) %mor: pro:subj|je v|croire conj|qu' pro:subj|ils&MASC v:exist| être v|passer-PP adv:place|là+bas .

Phase (b). The second tool is applied directly to the output of the first phase. A set of hand-coded rewrite rules was designed and implemented with a tool compatible with the CHAT files format. Rewrite rules are applied first to the results from phase (a) and are recursively introduced until no further rule can be applied. An example of the final result is presented in (4). The results are presented as a text representation of a *n*-ary tree. A sub-tree is represented between square brackets with a similar number, for example [4 @Cop ... v|passer-PP 4], line 3 and 4 of example (4). The highest node is [1 ... 1]. Elements between square brackets in a node are sub-trees. The other elements belong to the node, such as '@Cop' and 'v|passer-PP' above.

(4) %ctr: [1 @SV [2 PROV [3 @PronP [4 pro:subj|je 4] 3] VB [3 iVB [4 v|croire 4] 3] 2] @Conj [2 conj|qu' 2] @ExpV_SVA [2 PROV [3 @PronP [4 pro:subj|ils&MASC 4] 3] VV [3 @AuxPP [4 @Cop [5 iCop [6 v:exist|être 6] 5] v|passer-PP 4] 3] SmpAdverbial [3 iSmpAdverbial [4 @Locatif [5 adv:place|là+bas 5] 4] 3] 2] . 1]

In example (4), many rewrite rules were used. It is easier to explain how they are applied by following the construction of a specific tree branch. In example (4), the copula *v:exist|être*, corresponding to the word *est* ('is'), is rewritten as 'iCop', which is one of the ways the copula can be produced in French (it is not a complex copula construction), and this in turn is analysed as a '@Cop', which is the generic name for copula constructions in the rewrite rule system. The '@' which is in front of the construction name means that this construction is to be counted in the final F-LARSP chart, whereas 'iCop' is not, because it is a transient category used only for technical purposes. In turn, the elements '@Cop' and 'v|passer-PP' are grouped together in a '@AuxPP' construction. The '@AuxPP', which will be stored in the F-LARSP chart, is in turn rewritten as a 'VV', which, preceded by a 'PROV' (subject personal pronoun) and a 'SmpAdverbial' (a simple adverbial), makes it a '@ExpV_SVA' (a subject + verb + adverbial construction that includes an expansion of the verb), which is part of the top level description of the utterance, which in our example is '@SV' (subject + verb) @Conj (conjunction) @ExpV_SVA.

The hand-coding approach of this tool has the advantage of offering good control of the identified structure, but is limited in the way that it can handle unusual constructions because handling complex constructions supposes the creation of a very large number of rules. This explains why the tool does not tend to produce incorrect F-LARSP elements, but is not successful in identifying all F-LARSP elements, and especially elements belonging to Stages IV and V. Success is much better for elements from Stage I to III. Nonetheless, after systematic work on all F-LARSP constructions, the tool produces up to 95% of the expected constructions. To facilitate rule design, all computation done on isolated words is performed using a separate set of rules.

Some specific features of French, such as dislocations, were difficult to code by machine. Features of Stage VI and VII from E-LARSP as well as some features of Stage V could not be recognized by the new program due to their variety of possible forms and were therefore not coded. Some of these limitations could be minimized with further improvements in the coding procedure, which will hopefully appear on the F-LARSP website with versions higher than 1.0.

After the process carried out in phase (b), it is possible to edit the results by hand and provide a better final F-LARSP evaluation. The manual process is carried out directly in the intermediate result file from the F-LARSP tool, which contains all necessary information for this, such as the original transcription, the linking with external sound or video if this feature was present in the original file and the results of the MOR+POST analysis. It is not necessary to correct the tree analysis, but only to suppress, add or modify information in the tree analysis line that begins with an '@', as the tree information and precise format are not necessary for further processing. The '@' information corresponds to the F-LARSP information relevant to the LARSP analysis and is used during phase (c) (see below).

Phase (c). The third tool is used on the output of the second phase, after manual editing where necessary. All tags generated by phase (b) (automatically or manually edited) that belong to a specific set are extracted and listed. Also, the number of words appropriate to the 'Word' column of the F-LARSP chart is measured. This set of elements is then organized and presented in a format that corresponds to the F-LARSP chart. The format available for the 1.0 version is Excel or OpenOffice worksheets, but PDF presentations could also be computed in the future.

Step 4

The software was evaluated using a large set of language transcriptions to identify and count potential target structures. This corpus of child language was created by Le Normand (1986; Parisse & Le Normand, 2006). Typically developing participants, all native speakers of French, were recruited from homes and nurseries in Paris and its immediately surrounding areas. This transversal corpus contains 316 recordings of 20 minutes each, from children ranging in age from 2;0 to 4;0. For the needs of this project, additional recordings (Vial, 2010; Dumez, 2010) were carried out of children aged 18 and 21 months.

The corpus was gathered using the following methods. Each child participated in a dyadic interaction with a familiar adult partner (parent or nursery teacher) either in the child's home, nursery or school. The child and adult were seated at a small table, and the same standardized set of 22 Fisher-Price toys (house, family members, dog, beds, chairs, tables, rocking horse, stroller, cars, staircase) was used with all children. Similar but slightly modified play material was used for the younger children: the material was more recent and from the brand Playmobil, and some elements were changed to avoid choking hazards. Basic information about the corpus data is shown in the first line of Table 13.1 below.

Step 5

Accuracy checks compared the software's identification of target structures to those carried out by hand. An error rate of approximately 5% was calculated, mainly consisting of the software's lack of labelling of a structure. When errors detected in Step 5 could be corrected by improving rules used in Step 3, an iterative process (going back to Steps 3, 4 and 5) was used to improve the coverage of F-LARSP features.

Step 6

Statistical analyses were performed on the children's corpus to evaluate the relevance and appropriate stage of all syntactically coded features according to the first standard used by Bol and Kuiken (i.e. the age that any given structure was used by at least 50% of the population). The results are presented in Table 13.1. The earliest age at which a structure attains a 50% level or higher is the age that the structure was placed on the F-LARSP chart. Except for a few key items, we have limited the chart to only include the structures that the software can identify automatically.

With these results clearly displaying the age-related stage at which particular structures become regular, it is a relatively simple matter to assign examples to the appropriate stage. This motivated the occasional use in our chart of categories produced by at least 30% of the children (see further Maillart, Parisse & Tommerdahl, in press). As we have developed a program that makes analysing a transcript automatic with regard to finding F-LARSP structures, the time constraint is considerably less problematic, although some clinicians may choose to carry out a hand check for very specific analyses. The automatic F-LARSP processing feature makes the pruning of

Table 13.1 Percentages of children producing LARSP target structures

		Age	1;6	1;9	2;0	2;3	2;6	2;9	3;0	3;3	3;6	3;9	4;0
		No. of children	10	13	41	31	37	36	40	34	34	33	32
		Mean utterances	87	117	73	83	94	110	113	130	117	114	109
		Mean words	114	181	118	185	236	364	397	457	464	475	453
New stage	Old stage	Section type	Category \ MLU	1.23	1.38	1.50	2.13	2.44	3.22	3.41	3.51	3.72	3.98	4.01
I		Quest	Questions	40	85	73	74	76	89	93	97	94	91	88
	I	Minor	Locative	100	85	83	97	97	100	100	100	97	97	97
	I	Minor	Vocative	100	100	95	100	100	100	98	100	97	94	94
	II	Phrase	Determiner + Noun	40	62	63	100	95	100	100	100	100	100	100
	III	Phrase	Pronoun Other	70	69	73	90	97	100	98	100	97	100	100
	III	Phrase	Pronoun Personal	50	69	73	90	97	100	98	100	97	100	100
		Word	Auxiliaries	20	54	59	81	84	97	93	100	97	97	100
		Word	Past Participle	20	62	66	81	89	97	95	94	97	94	97
		Word	Present Tense	60	69	78	100	97	97	98	100	100	97	100
II	I	Major	Others	0	0	76	90	73	58	50	38	44	33	47
	I	Major	Noun	0	0	90	97	89	75	63	56	65	39	66
	I	Major	Verb	0	0	73	77	84	78	73	79	71	52	59
	I	Minor	Others	60	85	93	94	95	92	98	97	91	91	94
	II	Exp. II	Adjunct	0	31	37	55	70	89	93	100	91	88	97
	II	Exp. II	Object	20	15	41	58	76	89	93	85	85	79	88
	II	Exp. II	Verb	0	23	49	71	86	94	88	100	94	100	97
	II	Clause	Adjunct + X	20	46	71	81	95	100	100	100	97	100	100

238 Assessing Grammar

Table 13.1 continued

		Age	1;6	1;9	2;0	2;3	2;6	2;9	3;0	3;3	3;6	3;9	4;0
II	Clause	Subject + Verb	20	46	63	90	95	100	98	100	97	100	100
II	Clause	Verb + Complement	10	38	76	71	92	97	95	100	97	100	100
II	Clause	Verb + Object	10	15	49	68	78	92	93	91	74	82	81
II	Phrase	Preposition + Noun	0	15	39	55	68	97	90	91	94	97	100
III	Phrase	Auxiliary + Past Participle	0	38	56	71	70	94	90	88	97	94	97
III	Phrase	Copula	40	54	78	77	92	92	95	91	94	100	97
III	Phrase	Modal + Infinitive	0	15	37	52	78	94	95	100	94	100	100
IV	Phrase	Verbal Negation	0	38	56	74	81	89	93	97	94	97	88
IV	Phrase	Other Negation	0	23	32	58	70	81	78	82	82	73	88
	Word	Infinitive	20	31	61	87	97	97	98	100	97	100	100
	Word	Modal	0	38	51	68	84	94	100	100	94	100	100
III	II	Complement	0	8	32	35	73	97	93	97	94	100	97
	Exp. II	Subject	10	8	24	39	62	83	78	91	88	85	94
II	Phrase	Subject Object	10	15	15	29	46	61	55	62	74	58	66
II	Phrase	Noun + Adjective	10	31	34	45	57	61	58	53	53	52	53
II	Phrase	Others	10	8	29	45	54	64	68	65	76	85	69
III	Exp. III	Adjunct	0	0	5	29	54	86	78	94	88	97	88
III	Exp. III	Complement	0	0	5	13	30	53	50	56	62	61	69
III	Exp. III	Object	0	8	10	45	73	83	88	97	94	100	94
III	Exp. III	Verb	0	8	17	32	62	92	83	97	82	97	94
III	Clause	Subject + Verb + Adjunct	20	54	49	77	89	94	95	97	94	97	97
III	Clause	Subject + Verb + Object	0	8	17	48	65	81	90	97	94	100	94

Table 13.1 continued

		Age	1;6	1;9	2;0	2;3	2;6	2;9	3;0	3;3	3;6	3;9	4;0
III	Clause	Verb + Complement + Adjunct	0	0	2	10	19	53	45	47	47	48	47
III	Phrase	Determiner + Adjective + Noun	10	8	15	48	62	83	80	79	76	88	84
III	Phrase	Preposition + Determiner + Noun	0	8	20	48	81	94	93	100	97	100	100
IV	Phrase	Conjunction + X	10	38	24	26	43	61	75	85	82	88	75
IV	Phrase	Pronoun + Pronoun	0	0	5	23	32	69	68	79	82	85	81
V	Phrase	Conjunction	20	46	37	42	68	83	90	94	91	97	94
V	Phrase	Relative Pronoun	10	23	5	19	35	56	68	68	53	70	69
IV	Clause	Subject + Verb + Complement	0	0	15	29	30	39	48	53	44	64	59
IV	Clause	Subject + Verb + Object + Adjunct	0	0	0	6	16	42	63	50	53	55	69
V	Phrase	Adjunct + Adjunct	0	0	7	6	11	42	30	44	68	55	47
Additional part (30% threshold)													
I	Phrase	Noun + Noun	30	23	39	39	38	28	15	9	24	33	19
III	Exp.III	Subject	0	0	5	10	11	42	28	12	29	33	34
III	Clause	Verb + Object + Adjunct	0	8	5	26	24	39	30	41	24	18	31
IV	Phrase	Preposition + Determiner + Adjective + Noun	0	0	0	3	14	31	35	35	35	39	31

Table 13.1 continued

		Age	1;6	1;9	2;0	2;3	2;6	2;9	3;0	3;3	3;6	3;9	4;0
IV	Clause	Verb + Verb	0	0	0	0	8	6	10	*32*	24	12	19
IV	Phrase	X+ Conjunction + X	0	0	0	0	5	19	*30*	12	*32*	18	28
V	Phrase	Others (3 elts)	0	0	2	6	14	17	15	12	24	21	*38*
IV	Clause	Subject + Verb + Object + Complement	0	0	2	6	11	19	15	21	24	*30*	*31*
IV	Phrase	Noun Phrase + Preposition + Noun Phrase	0	0	0	3	14	25	28	18	*38*	*39*	*31*

all less frequent categories from the chart less necessary because infrequent categories do not make the evaluation process more time consuming. For this reason, the inclusion of lesser-used structures may be of value in order to perform a more fine-grained analysis of older children or children with unusual production patterns. Of course, categories that are not used at all tend to clutter the evaluation process, so for F-LARSP 1.0 we have included items that never attain 50% but which have been used by a minimum of 30% of children at a certain stage. These categories are identified through the use of italics.

Table 13.1 contains the results for all F-LARSP structures that were kept in the final chart and the results for all age ranges.

Discussion

The main objectives of F-LARSP were (1) to provide speech therapists with precise developmental data, which had not previously been available, about the emergence of morphosyntactic structures in French and (2) to provide a complete and rapid assessment tool for analysing morphosyntactic abilities in oral language. Previously, the coding required for LARSP was very time consuming to carry out by hand, limiting its use in clinical situations. A computerized tool was therefore developed from CLAN transcriptions to reduce the effort involved in carrying out data analyses. This tool allowed us to process a large French-speaking corpus of 329 children aged 18 to 60 months and also to provide precise percentages of children producing structures that corresponded to a particular age level.

The completed F-LARSP chart presented in Table 13.2 contains, as a reference, the percentage of children producing the structure for the corresponding age level. A usable F-LARSP chart and complete statistics about children's production of LARSP structures will be made available at the web site www.modyco.fr/flarsp/.

One should note that the inclusion of a structure on F-LARSP says little about the number of times the average child uses that structure. A grammatical structure used by 50% or more of the children within an age group was included on the chart regardless of whether the average use was 1 or 30 occurrences. However, a structure greatly used by a few children and not used by most could not attain a place on the chart. Given this, it is possible that the information provided on this version of the chart is not ideal in its ability to identify individual differences or to suggest important clues about the character of certain language disorders. This problem may be purely theoretical, as work carried out with children with SLI shows that the order of acquisition of grammatical morphemes is similar to typically developing children, with (for example) present tense being acquired before past tense and determiners being acquired before clitic pronouns, regardless of their phonological form (Jakubowicz & Nash, 2001). However, even though the

Table 13.2 F-LARSP chart

F-LARSP adapted from original by Maillart, Parisse and Tommerdahl (in press)

Clause	Phrase	Word	Other
Stage 1 (1;6-2;0)	**DN ProO ProP** 62% 70% 69% NN 30%	**Aux PP Present** 54% 62% 69%	**Q Loc Voc** 85% 100% 100%
Stage 2 (2;0-2;6) AX SV VC VO SVA 81% 90% 76% 68% 77%	**AuxPP ModInf PrN Cop** 71% 52% 55% 78% NegV Neg 0 74% 58%	**Inf Mod** 87% 68%	**Exp: A O V** 55% 58% 71%
Stage 3 (2;6-3;0) SVO VCA VOA 81% 53% 39% Dislo-G Dislo-D 67,7% 83%	SO NA Others DAdjN cX 61% 61% 64% 83% 61% PrDN ProPro Conj RelPro 94% 69% 83% 56% PrDAN 31%		**Exp: S C** <u>83% 53%</u>
Stage 4 (3;0-3;6) SVC SVOA VV 53% 63% 32%	xCx 30%		
Stage 5 (3;6-4;0) SVOC 31%	Adjunct + adjunct 55% Others (3elts) 38% NP-Pr-NP 38%		
Coord 1 1+ Subord 1 1+			
S O C A			

sequence of acquisition is identical, acquisition may still be much later; for example, the omission of articles in children with SLI corresponds to the pattern seen in younger normally developing children (Paradis *et al.,* 2003). In the future it will therefore be beneficial to analyse language samples of children with language impairments in order to verify if, when compared with typically developing children with the same MLU (mean length of utterance), a similar distribution of categories is found.

Finally, we are aware that adjustments and improvements remain to be made, particularly regarding more complex structures which have not yet been computerized. At this stage, the software developed is unable to successfully identify elements at Stage V and higher, yet information regarding a child's ability to form complex sentences is vital. For this reason, Stage V of the chart, as well as the dislocations, are being retained in a nearly identical form to that of the original version, and will for the time being need to be carried out by hand. Similarly, Stages VI and VII have been omitted as they cannot yet be identified by the software, and in any case are arguably less informative than Stage V. Further work on developing software in this direction is planned.

As suggested above, the version of F-LARSP described in this chapter is unlikely to be the only one. Future plans for F-LARSP include using it in different settings and with a variety of groups including older children and those with different types of language difficulties, which we expect will provide invaluable feedback from a community of users. Versions using different criteria will then be developed and placed online to provide maximal access and to attempt to meet the needs of different users. These will be accompanied by detailed instructions explaining the construction and use of the chart, how it can be carried out automatically if desired, and how the information provided by F-LARSP can be used in clinical settings.

Acknowledgements

The authors thank Cécile Vial and Mélanie Dumez for their precious help with the collection and the transcription of the data from 18- and 21-month-old children.

References

Blasco-Dulbecco, M. (1999) *Les Dislocations en Français Contemporain.* Paris: Honoré Champion.
Bol, G.W. and Kuiken, F. (1990) Grammatical analysis of developmental language disorders: A study of the morphosyntax of children with specific language disorders, with hearing impairment and with Down's syndrome. *Clinical Linguistics and Phonetics* 4, 77–86.
Dubois, J. (1965) *La Grammaire Structurale du Français.* Paris: Larousse.
Dumez, M. (2010) *Analyse des conditions de passation et d'application du LARSP en vue de son adaptation francophone.* Mémoire inédit présenté en vue de l'obtention du titre de master en logopédie: Université de Liège.

Jakubowicz, C. and Nash, L. (2001) Functional categories and syntactic operations in (ab)normal language acquisition. *Brain and Language* 77, 321–339.

Kail, M. (1989) Cue validity, cue cost, and processing types in sentence comprehension in French and Spanish. In B. MacWhinney and E. Bates (eds) *The Cross-Linguistic Study of Sentence Processing (pp. 77–117).* Cambridge: Cambridge University Press.

Le Normand, M.T. (1986) A developmental exploration of language used to accompany symbolic play in young normal children (2–4-years-old). *Child: Care, Health and Development* 12, 121–134.

MacWhinney, B. (2000) The CHILDES Project: Tools for Analyzing Talk. Hillsdale, NJ: Lawrence Erlbaum.

Maillart, C., Parisse, C. and Tommerdahl J. (in press) F-LARSP: An Adaptation of the LARSP Language Profile 1.0 for French. *Clinical Linguistics and Phonetics.*

Paradis, J., Crago, M., Genesee, F and Rice, M. (2003) French-English bilingual children with SLI: How do they compare with their monolingual peers? *Journal of Speech, Language, and Hearing Research* 46, 113–127.

Paradis, C. and El Fenne, F. (1995) French verbal inflection revisited: Constraints, repairs and floating consonants. *Lingua* 95, 169–204.

Parisse, C. (2008) Left-dislocated subjects: A construction typical of young French-speaking children? In P. Guijarro-Fuentes, P. Larrañaga and J. Clibbens (eds) *First Language Acquisition of Morphology and Syntax: Perspectives Across Languages and Learners* (pp. 13–30). Amsterdam: John Benjamins.

Parisse, C. and Le Normand, M.T. (2000) Automatic disambiguation of morphosyntax in spoken language corpora. *Behavior Research Methods, Instruments, & Computers* 32, 468–481.

Parisse, C. and Le Normand, M.T. (2006) Une méthode pour évaluer la production du langage spontané chez l'enfant de 2 à 4 ans. *Glossa* 97, 10–30.

Vial, C. (2010) *Adaptation Française du LARSP. Aspects Linguistiques.* Mémoire inédit présenté en vue de l'obtention du titre de master en logopédie: Université de Liège.

14 Spanish Acquisition and the Development of PERSL

Ana Isabel Codesido-García, Carmen Julia Coloma, Elena Garayzábal-Heinze, Victoria Marrero, Elvira Mendoza and Mª Mercedes Pavez

Introduction to Spanish Grammar[1]

Spanish is an SVO language, although the elements have a relatively free distribution as shown in the following examples, which are all grammatical[2]:

(1) S+V+O: [el niño]_s [come]_v [una manzana]_o
 'The boy eats an apple'
(2) S+O+V: [el niño] [una manzana] [come]
 'The boy an apple eats'
(3) V+S+O: [come] [el niño] [una manzana]
 Eats the boy an apple'
(4) V+O+S: [come] [una manzana] [el niño]
 'Eats an apple the boy'
(5) O+V+S: [una manzana] [come] [el niño]
 'An apple eats the boy'
(6) O+S+V: [una manzana] [el niño] [come]
 'An apple the boy eats'

The first example is the most common for Spanish. While the following five examples are not used as much in the everyday language, they are acceptable structures. Due to the high level of inflection, agreement and traces of elements, Spanish does not need the presence of a subject, because it is included in the verbal inflection. The following examples, all grammatical, show the same VP with, successively a subject NP (7), a personal pronoun (8) and no subject (9):

(7) María abre la puerta / La luz está encendida / Pablo abrió la puerta y encendió la luz
 'Mary opens the door / The light is switched on / Pablo opened the door and switched the light on'

(8) Ella abre la puerta / Está encendida / El abrió la puerta y encendió la luz
'She opens the door / It is switched on / He opened the door and switched the light on'
(9) Abre la puerta / Está encendida / Abrió la puerta y encendió la luz
'She opens the door / It is switched on / He opened the door and switched the light on'

In all the Spanish examples the verb agrees in number with the subject. When the subject is omitted, the verb still continues to have traces of the subject, and it can be identified easily with respect to the number of subjects performing the action.

Spanish grammar is composed of variable and invariable elements. Variable elements are those that change for number (singular and plural), gender (masculine and feminine), conjugation (first: -ar, second: –er and third: –ir), time (present, past, future), mood (indicative, subjunctive and imperative), person (first, second and third), aspect (perfective, non-perfective), voice (active, passive) and form (simple, compound); invariable elements do not have any changes (see Table 14.1).

(i) **Determiners and adjectives** agree with the noun in gender and number:
   (10) *El* niño guapo / La niña guapa*
   'The handsome boy / The pretty girl'
   (11) *Los** buenos amigos / las buenas amigas*
   'The good friends / The good friends'
   * Singular form for the masculine determiner article
   ** Plural form for the masculine determiner article

Table 14.1 Spanish grammar: Variable and invariable elements

Variable elements	Changes in:	Invariable elements
Nouns	Gender, number	Adverbs
Pronouns (personal, possessive, demonstratives, numerals, indefinite, relatives, interrogative, exclamative)	Gender, number, person	Conjunctions
Adjectives	Gender, number	Prepositions
Determiners (articles, possessives, indefinite, demonstratives, numerals, relatives, interrogatives, exclamations)	Gender, number	Interjections
Verbs	Person, number, time, mood, voice, aspect, form	

(ii) **Nominal phrases (NP)** have the following structures:
  (12) *La niña bonita tiene una muñeca / las niñas bonitas tienen muñecas*
     'The pretty girl has a doll / the pretty girls have dolls'
  (13) *Los ladrones entraron en la tienda / el ladrón entró en la tienda*
     'The thieves came into the shop / the thief came into the shop'
     Nominal phrases as subject show the following structures:
  (14) *Ella compra un abrigo* (pronoun (Pr))
     'She buys a coat'
  (15) *La mujer compra un abrigo* (determiner (D) + noun (N))
     'The woman buys a coat'
  (16) *Esa mujer mayor compra un abrigo* (D + N + Adj)
     'That old woman buys a coat'
  (17) *Las flores que me has enviado me encantaron* (D + N + Relative Clause (RC))
     'I loved the flowers you sent to me'
  (18) *Comprar me gusta* (infinitive Vb) /*Amar es vivir*
     'I like shopping / To love is to live'
  (19) *Este rojo es muy oscuro* (D + Noun adjective)
     'This red is very dark'
  (20) *El coche de Pilar está roto* (D + N + Prepositional Phrase (PP))[3]
     'Pilar's car is broken'
  (21) *Que rías está muy bien* (Nominal Clause (NC))
     'It is very good for you to smile'
  (22) *Mi primo Fernando se casará mañana* (D + N + Apposition)
     'My cousin Fernando will get married tomorrow'

(iii) **Verbal phrase** structures include:
  (23) *Llueve* (Vb Impersonal form)
     'It's raining'
  (24) *Carmen abrió la puerta* (Vb + NP)
     'Carmen opened the door'
  (25) *Elena llegó agotada* (Vb + Adj)
     'Elena arrived exhausted'
  (26) *Mi tía me ha enseñado a cocinar paella* (IO + Vb + DO (PP))
     'My aunt has taught me to cook paella'
  (27) *Llegaremos mañana* (Vb + Adv)
     'We´ll arrive tomorrow'
  (28) *Nuestros padres nos recogerán en el aeropuerto* (Vb +PP)
     'Our parents will pick us up at the airport'
  (29) *Dijo que escribiría una carta* (Vb + Clause (C))
     'He said he would write a letter'

For the structures in (26) and (29), clauses following the verb inside the verbal phrase are finite subordinate clauses and they constitute complex sentences. There are two different types of subordinate clauses: substantive clauses and adverb clauses indicating place, time, mode, cause, purpose, concession and condition. The way to introduce both types of clauses is variable, and many conjunctions are used (see Table 14.2).

Table 14.2 Spanish grammar: Subordinate clauses

Substantive clauses	Introduced by *que*: *Déjame que te cuente una cosa* / 'Let me tell you something'	Introduced by an infinitive verb: *Déjame contarte una cosa* / 'Let me tell you something'	Introduced by a substantivated adjective clause *lo que*: *Dime lo que piensas* / 'Tell me what you are thinking'
Adverbial clauses			
Place clauses	***donde****, *en el que, en el cual, a donde, por donde, en donde* *Pueden quedarse **donde** están* / 'They can stay where they are'		
Time clauses	***cuando***, *mientras, apenas, después de, antes que, antes de, al* + infinitive *Comenzó a cocinar **cuando** estaba terminando mis deberes* / 'She began cooking while I was finishing my homework'		
Mode clauses	***como***, *según, sin* + gerund *Hazlo **como** te dije* / 'Do it as I told you'		
Cause clauses	***porque***, *ya que, como, que, pues, puesto que, dado que, en vista de que, por, de, al* +infinitive ***Como** Carlos no estaba, regresó a casa* / 'As Carlos was not there, he went back home'		
Purpose clauses	***para***, *para que, a* +infinitive, *a que* + subjunctive, *a fin de* +infinive, *a fin de que* + subjunctive, *que* +subjunctive, *por* + infinitive, *por que* + subjunctive *Te daré un mapa **para que** encuentres el camino a casa* / 'I will give you a map so that you can find the way home'		
Concession clauses	***aunque***, *a pesar de, si bien, aun cuando, con* + infinitive, *aun* + gerund, *por más* + N + *que, por* + Adj + *que, por* + Adv + *que* ***Aunque** es pobre, es honesto* / 'Though he is poor, he is honest'		
Conditional clauses	***si***, *con que, siempre que, con tal que* ***Si** bebes, no conduzcas* / 'If you drink, do not drive'		
Comparison clauses	*más . . . que, menos . . . que, tanto . . . como, tan . . . como, igual . . . que, tal . . . como* *Es **más** tarde de lo **qu**e pensaba* / 'It is later than I thought'		
Consecutive clauses	*tan . . . que, tanta . . . que, tanto . . . que, tal . . . que* *Jugó **tan** bien al futbol **que** el equipo ganó* / 'He played football so well that the team won'		

* Shown in bold are the main conjunctions for each type of adverbial subordinate clause.

(iv) **Negative sentences, passive sentences, asking questions**
Negative sentences can be constructed with adverbs *no* or *tampoco*. *No* is always placed before the verb, while *tampoco* corroborates the negation or is an extension of the negation to other elements of the structure:
(30)   *Pablo no irá al zoo*
         'Pablo will not go to the zoo'
(31)   *Pablo no irá al zoo tampoco*
         'Pablo will not go to the zoo either'

There are two ways of asking questions: one can rely on an interrogative prosody while using an affirmative syntactic structure; or one can place the verb at the beginning of the interrogative sentence. Adults use the first type of construction for information focus. Children use the SVO structure very frequently, presented here in comparison to the VO alternative:

(32)   *¿Tú vas a comprar un libro?* (SVO) / *¿Vas a comprar un libro?* (VO)
         'Are you going to buy a book?'
(33)   *¿Llueve?* (V)
         'Is it raining?'

Unlike in English, the acquisition of auxiliary verbs is not crucial for producing negative and interrogative sentences.

Passive sentences are infrequent in Spanish, especially in the speech of small children. Their use is not expected during infancy, nor even in adolescence:

(34)   *El perro lamió a la niña* > *La niña fue lamida por el perro*
         'The dog licked the girl > The girl was licked by the dog'

Main Difficulties for Children when Acquiring Spanish

In relation to grammar, difficulties can be seen in the canonical use of pronouns, determiners and noun agreement, irregular verbs, and in the construction of complex sentences.

It is very common to observe pronominal inversion or omission when children are beginning to talk or to self-identify with their names:

(35)   Question: *¿Cómo te llamas?* / 'What is your name?'
         Answer: *Te llamas Elena* / 'Your name is Elena' (instead of *Me llamo...* / 'My name is ...')
(36)   Question: *¿Quién está en casa?* / 'Who is staying at home?'
         Answer: *Está Elena* / 'Elena is staying' (instead of *Estoy yo* / 'I am staying')
(37)   Question: *¿De quién es este lápiz?* / 'Whose is this pencil?'
         Answer: **Es de mí* / **'It is of me' (instead of *Es mío* / 'It is mine')

When small children begin to use personal pronouns, they tend to create redundancy due to the fact that the information is already represented in the verbal inflection:

(38) ¿*Por qué tú te vas*?
      'Why are you going?'
(39) ¿*A dónde se va ella*?
      'Where is she going to?'
(40) ¿*Por qué yo no voy a casa de Matías*?
      'Why am I not going to Matías house?'

At the age of four and even five, Spanish children have some difficulties with the personal pronouns *conmigo* and *contigo*:

(41) **A mi padre le he regalado un marco con yo* / *'I have given my father a frame with I' (instead of conmigo")
(42) *Yo me voy con ti / 'I'm going with you' (instead of *contigo*)

Irregular verbs and subjunctive forms are perhaps the main difficulties for Spanish children. Some verb inflections may not be mastered until quite late. The improper use of some irregular verbs can be prolonged even until the age of seven or eight.

(43) *Matar: Te <u>he matado</u>* > *Te he *morido*
      'To kill: I have killed you > I have deaded you.'
(44) *Venir: <u>Ha vuelto</u> del trabajo* > *Ha *volvido del trabajo*
      'To come: He came back from work > He comed back from work'
(45) *Decir: Papá <u>dijo</u> que iríamos al zoo* > *Papá *deció/ *deciba/*dició/ *dijió que íbamos al zoo*

'To say: Daddy said we were going to the zoo > Daddy sayed we were going to the zoo' Spanish verb inflection is complex, and perfective and imperfective systems contribute to this complexity. The contrast is overtly marked, which has a direct effect on the use of some type of adverbs that require the presence of certain verbal forms and not others. At the age of four the perfective/imperfective contrast is not established, and adverbs such as those for 'yesterday' or 'tomorrow' are frequently combined with incorrect verbal forms.

The subjunctive is a complex form for children that is not well mastered until they are six or 6;6 years. Some examples of their difficulty with this form are given below. It is interesting to note that, although they cannot use the subjunctive properly, children can provide very complex structures in which both subjunctive mood and sense are involved:

(46) *Mi padre ya se *habriera dado cuenta de que su coche estaba roto* > *Mi padre ya se hubiera/habría dado cuenta de que su coche estaba roto* (5;5-year-old)
'My father would already have noticed that his car was broken.'

(47) *Si la *hubrieran hecho tres veces, ahora estaría mejor* > *Si la hubieran hecho tres veces, ahora estaría mejor* (5;8-year-old)
'If they had done it three times, now it would be better.'

PERSL, Procedimiento de Evaluación, Rehabilitación y Screening Lingüístico: The Spanish LARSP[4]

In Spain, LARSP has been known since the mid-1980s, as a Spanish translation of the procedure was made in 1984 (Crystal *et al.,* 1984). However, this was not an adaptation, for the syntactic structures matched the original English version. Spanish is a language with a rich morphology, and differences are also found in syntactic constructions and in their development. Not only do the types of structures differ, but the numbers of elements do as well. Articles and auxiliary verbs can be found early on in children's utterances (Stage II), and expanded structures are very common at each stage. There is also considerable freedom in word order; in most of the structures mentioned below, the order of constituents can be varied, as seen in the examples.

The taxonomy of the present proposal was made according to that of Boehm *et al.* (2005), while retaining the most common labels used in our academic environment. The corpus used for Stages II to VI is from the Spanish CHILDES database (MacWhinney, 1995). Morphological transcription has been made with a computer tool, AyDA (Albalá & Marrero, 2001), and disambiguated by Marrero *et al.* (2001). The last stage has been elaborated from a specific corpus of Chilean Spanish, obtained by a story-telling task, from ten children aged five to six years (five of each age). The current version of PERSL is shown in Figure 14.1 towards the end of the chapter.

Stages of PERSL

Stage I (approximately 0;9–1;6 years)[5]

Stage I allows single-word utterances to be placed into the categories of *verb, noun, verb* (command form), *question word, other* or *problem*. Even if the child might not yet have a clear notion of what nouns and verbs represent, they are placed in the nearest adult-like categories. Children use about 50 single words (holophrases) in a similar way to create sentences. The number of words used increases rapidly at very short intervals during this first stage. As a benchmark, we take the data provided by the Spanish adaptation of the

Table 14.3 Profile form for Stage I: Summary

Sentences					
Minor	*Response*	*Vocativos*	OTHER		
Major	*Commands*	*Questions*	*Statement*		
	Verbs	'where, who, which …'	Verbs	Nouns	Other

MacArthur Communicative Development Inventory (Ornat López et al., 2005), which marks the following average values of the number of words:

- 12 months: 8 words
- 13 months: 10 words
- 14 months: 18.53 words
- 15 months: 33 words

In the profile form presented below (Table 14.3), two functional possibilities are recognized:

Major sentences

Questions: the child uses question words. Usually at this stage the most commonly used pronouns are *dónde* 'where', *quién* 'who' and *qué* 'what'.

Mandates: the child uses a verb in its basic form, and accompanying behaviour clearly indicates that we must interpret it as an instruction to do something. Generally, directional verbs are used.

Minor sentences

Responses. A reply to a question
Vocatives: Calling a name (e.g. *mamá*, 'mummy')
Other: Counting '1, 2, 3, 4', saying the alphabet, and so on.

Stage II (approximately 1;6–2;0 years)[6]

Children form two-element sentences to convey a variety of functions, such as questions, commands and statements. The LARSP chart splits these into clause level and phrase level. The clause level is based on any combination of two of the five possible clause elements: *subject, verb, object, complement* and *adverbial*. The phrase level shows two-part combinations of phrasal elements. Examples include the combinations of determiner and noun (*DN*), adjective and noun (*Adj N*), and verb followed by particle (*V part*).

Based on recordings from five subjects in the age range 1;6–2;0, the most frequent structures are as follows (see summaries in Figures 14.1–14.3 and Table 14.4).

Clause level
(a) *Statements*
- Adverbial (Adv) + Verb-Copula (Cop)
  ya(es)tá 'that's it' (used by 80% of subjects); *Ahí (es)tá* 'There he/she/it is'; *Sí (es)tá,* 'Yes he's /she's / it's here'
- Negative (Neg) + VCop
  No (es)tá 'He / she / it isn't here' (100% of subjects)
  Expanded constructions[7]: *No está el niño* 'The boy isn't here/there'; *El oso no está* 'The bear isn't there'; *No está el perro* 'The dog isn't here'
- *se* + Verb (V)[8]
  Se acabó 'that's it' – *se ha acaba(d)o* 'It's finished' (60% of subjects)
  Expanded constructions: *No se puede* 'It can't/you can't'; *Se cae e(l) nene* 'The child is falling'; *S(e) ha cai(d)o la tapa* 'The lid fell off'
- V+Object (O)
  Como pan 'I eat bread'; *He hecho caca* 'I did a poo'; *Te(ng)o t(r)es* 'I have three'
- Neg + V
  No puede 'He / she / it can't'; *No oigo* 'I can't hear'; *No sé* 'I don't know'; *No t(i)ene* 'He/she/it doesn't have'; *No ten(g)o* 'I don't have'

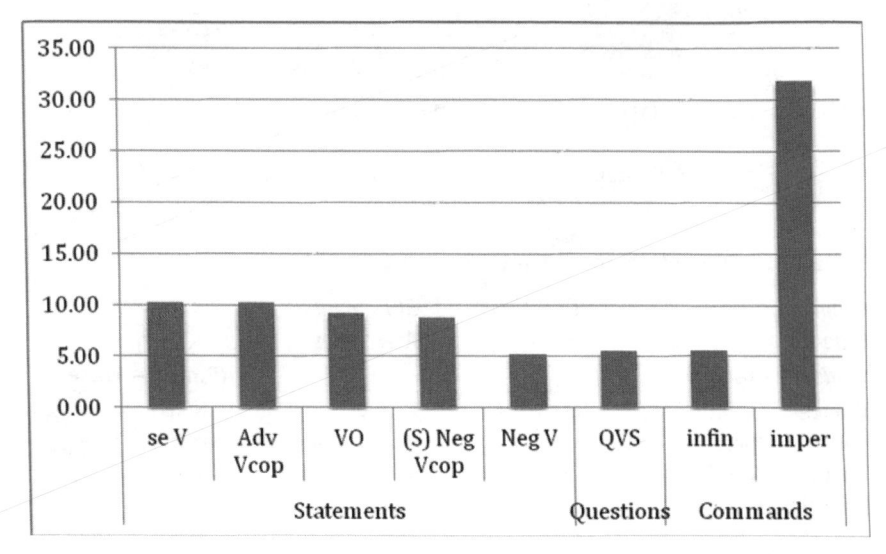

Figure 14.1 Stage II. Clause level. Frequency of structures (%). 399 clauses

254 Assessing Grammar

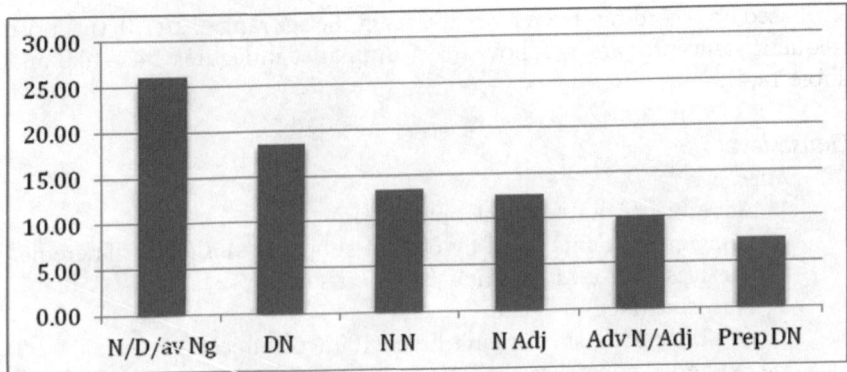

Figure 14.2 Stage II. Phrase level. Frequency of structures (%). 119 phrases

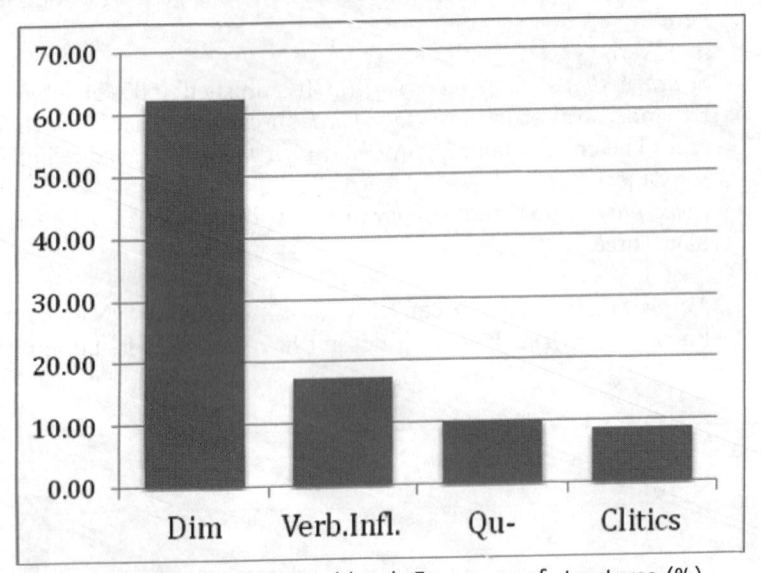

Figure 14.3 Stage II. Word level. Frequency of structures (%). 69 selected tokens

Table 14.4 Profile form for Stage II: Summary

Commands Órdenes	Questions Preguntas	Statements Aserciones	
Clause – Oración			**Phrase – Frase**
V-imper	Qu + V (+S)	se + V	X Neg
Neg + V-imper		adv + VCop	Det N
V-imper + N =		Neg + VCop /	N Adj
N + V-imper		V VO	N N
			Adv N = N Adv
			Pr (Det) N

(b) *Questions*
Qu (Question, Pronoun *wh*) + V (+ Subject, from 1;8–1;9)[9]: *Qué pasa¿* 'What's up?'; *Qué pasó¿* 'What happened?'; *(D)ó(nde) (es)tá mamá* 'Where's mummy?'; *Quién es* 'Who is it?'

(c) *Commands*
Imperative (100% of subjects): *Ten* 'Take'; *Mira* 'Look'; *Ven* 'come'
- Neg. + Imperative (= subjunctive[10])
  No tire todo 'Don't knock everything'; *No escupas* 'Don't spit'; **Quita no* 'Don't take it'; **No chupa* 'Don't suck'; **No ven* 'Don't come'
- Imperative + N = N + imperative
  Mira ese pelito 'Look at that little hair'; *Quita guaguau* 'Take away the dog'; *Ven mamá* 'Come on mummy'; *Mamá, mira* 'Mummy, look'; *Nacho, ten* 'Nacho, take it'
- A + Infinitive > *Ir a* + Infinitive[11]
  A dormir 'Off to sleep'; *A ver* 'Let's see'; *A callar* 'Be quiet'
  Expanded constructions: *Voy a dibuja(r)* 'I'm going to draw'; *Voy a esc(r)ibi(r)* 'I'm going to write'

Phrase level
- X[12] + Neg
  aquí no 'not here'; *agua no* 'not water'; *hoy no* 'not today'
- Determiner (Det) + N
  ese t(r)en 'that train'; *mi papá* 'my daddy'; *una niña* 'a girl'; *ot(r)a vez* 'once more'
- N + Adjective (Adj)
  nene grande 'big baby'; *mamá mala* 'bad/naughty mummy'; *Tello feo* 'ugly Tello'
- N + N
  mamá silla 'mummy chair'; *lápi(z) planta* 'pencil plant'; *barba papá* 'beard daddy'
- Adv + N = N + Adv
  sí grande 'yes big'; *sí mamá* 'yes mummy'; *papá aquí* 'daddy here'; *aquí mamá* 'here mummy'
  Preposition (Prep) + (Det) + N > Det + N + Prep + Det + N
  en el agua 'in the water'; *pa(ra) ti* 'for you'
  Expanded constructions: *eso lapicito de Koki* 'Koki's little pencil'; *e(l) pant(al)ón (d)e papá* 'Daddy's trousers'

Word level
A column labeled 'word' is also present on the chart listing morphological inflections in their acquired order. The structures are said to develop throughout Stages II through IV. In this study, the most relevant morphological inflections will be mentioned at the corresponding stage

- Diminutives (more frequent in American dialects of Spanish)
  pillín 'little rascal'; *cuidadito* 'be careful'; *besito* 'kiss'; *compañerito* 'pal'
- First verbal inflection contrasts (not very frequent):
(a) Sg/Pl: *vienen/viene* 'they come – he / she comes'; 1st person / 3rd person: *peino-peina* 'I comb – he/she combs'
(b) Non-personal forms
  (i) Participle: *roto roto* 'broken' ; *sentadita así* 'seated like this';
  (ii) Gerund: *bañando* 'bathing/taking a bath'; *mojando* 'wetting'
  (iii) Infinitive (see above)
- Qu-
  ¿Dónde? 'Where?'; *¿Po(r) qué?* 'Why?'; *¿Qué?* 'What?' *¿Quién?* 'Who?'
- First clitics
  cerrar-lo 'to close it'; *dá-me-lo* 'give it to me'; *quíta-te* 'get away/out'

Stage III (approximately 2;0–2;6 years)

Stage III is reserved for three-element utterances. At clause level, this might consist of combinations such as SVA or SVO. At the phrase level, along with three-part combinations such as Det Adj N or Pr Det N, there is also use of the copula, auxiliary and pronouns. Children use simple three-word sentences with a correct word order and a range of structures to convey a variety of functions, such as questions, commands and statements. Word endings develop throughout this stage and beyond.

Clause level
Statements

Figure 14.4 reflects the frequency of clause structures at Stage II, and is derived from language samples of five subjects within the relevant age range. (For other summaries at this Stage see Figures 14.5–14.7 and Table 14.5)

(1) VO
  - O = [Det+N]: *Chupa el vestidito* 'He/she sucks the little dress'; *Pintamos un caballo* 'We're drawing a horse'; *Hay t(r)es bolas* 'There are three balls'
  - V = [VAux+Past Participle]: *Me ha pegado* 'He / she hit / smacked me'; *He hecho una casa* 'I made a house'; *La ha pintado* 'he/she drew it / her'

Expanded constructions:
V = [periphrastic *ir a* + inf / *estar* + ger]: *(Es)tá viendo una vaca* 'He's / she's watching a cow'; *Va a tomar una caña* 'He's / she's going to have a glass of beer'; *Los vamos a pegar* 'We're going to glue / stick them'
  - Vocative, VO: *Daniel, quiero tostadas* 'Daniel, I want some toast'; *Coge más cosas, mamá* 'Take some more things, mummy'

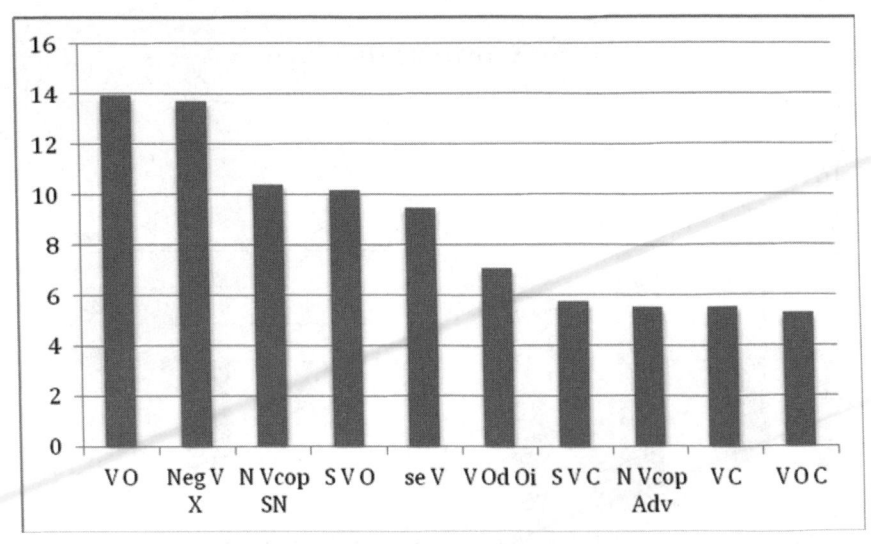

Figure 14.4 Stage III. Clause level. Statements: Frequency of structures (n = 400)

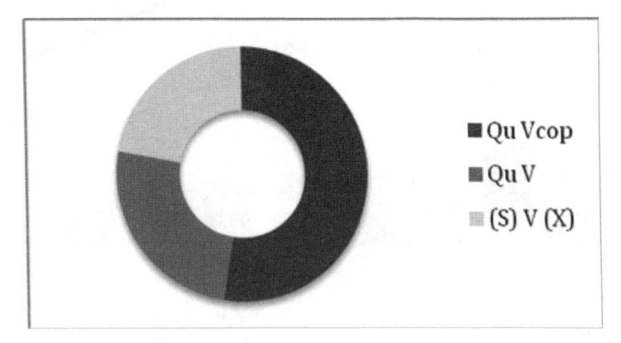

Figure 14.5 Stage III. Clause level. Questions: Frequency of structures (n = 97)

(2) Neg V X
   - Neg V S: *No sabe Koki* 'Koki doesn't know'; *No sé yo* 'I don't know'; *Yo no sé* 'I don't know'; *No v(i)ene Óscar* 'Oscar isn't coming'
   - Neg V O: *No lo miro* 'I don't see it'; *No enciendes las luces* 'Don't turn on the lights'
(3) N1 Vcop N2: *Ese es mío* 'That's mine'; *Esto son cuentos* 'These are stories'; *Yo soy mayor* 'I'm older'
   Expanded constructions[13]:
   - N2 = [Det + N]: *Esta es la moto* 'This is the scooter / motorbike'; *Esa es su casita* 'That's his / her house'; *Este es un puente* 'This is a bridge'

258 Assessing Grammar

Commands

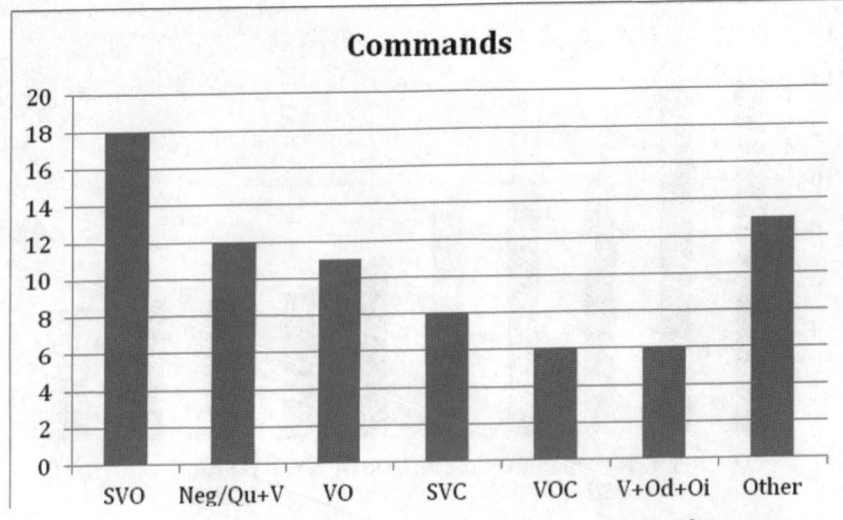

[Bar chart showing frequency of command structures: SVO ≈18, Neg/Qu+V ≈12, VO ≈11, SVC ≈8, VOC ≈6, V+Od+Oi ≈6, Other ≈13]

Figure 14.6 Stage III. Clause level. Commands. Frequency of structures. 75 commands

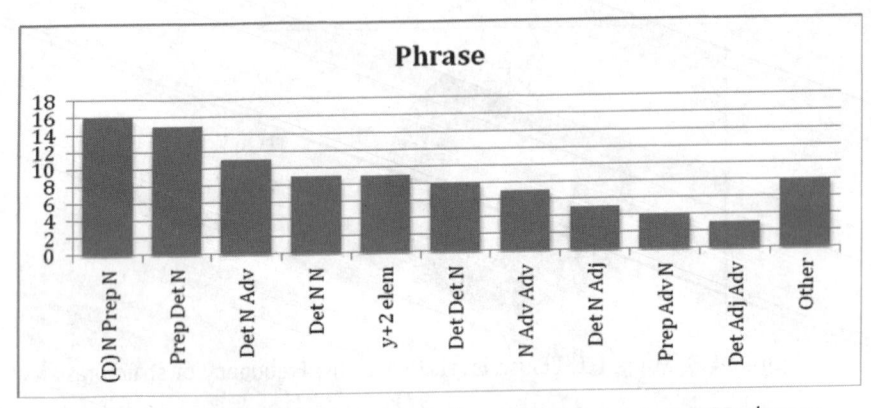

Phrase

[Bar chart showing frequency of phrase structures: (D) N Prep N ≈16, Prep Det N ≈15, Det N Adv ≈11, Det N N ≈9, y+2 elem ≈9, Det Det N ≈9, N Adv Adv ≈8, Det N Adj ≈6, Prep Adv N ≈5, Det Adj Adv ≈4, Other ≈9]

Figure 14.7 Stage III. Phrase level. Frequency of structures. 95 phrases

Table 14.5 Profile form for Stage III: Summary

Commands *Órdenes*	Questions *Preguntas*	Statements *Aserciones*	
Clause – Oración			**Phrase – Frase**
S Vimper O=Vimper O S	*Qu* Vcop N	V O	(D) N Pr N
Neg/*Qu*- Vsubj	*Qu* V X	Neg V S/O	Pr Det N
Vimper O= O Vimper	¿(S) V (O)?	N VCop N	Det N Adv
		S V O	Det N N
		Se V X	Det Det N
		Other	Other

- N2 = [Det + N + X]: *Estaba una niña mala* 'She was a naughty girl'; *Ese* es la casita de los barriletes* 'This is the little house for the kites'
(4) S V O: *Yo veo a niñas* 'I see girls'; *Tiene pecas Cecilia* 'Cecilia has freckles'; *Tú tienes ba(r)ba* 'You have a beard'
Expanded constructions
Yo quiero un coche más 'I want another car'; *La abuelita me la comp(r)ó* 'My granny bought it for me'; *El pequeño tiene su cola* 'The small one has a / his tail'; *Mamá, tú pones eso* 'Mummy, you put this on'
(5) se V X
    - *Se cayó solito* 'He fell on his own'; *Sí se pega* 'Yes it sticks'; *Esa se cayó* 'That fell over'
    - V = [complex form]: *Se ha caído* 'It fell'; *Se han acabado* 'They've run out'; *Se van a perder* 'They're going to get lost'
Expanded constructions
Se ha perdido pelota 'The ball is lost'; *Se han escapado las orejas* 'The ears got away'; *Se caen al suelo* 'They fall on the floor'; *Esto se va a caer* 'This is going to fall over'
(6) Other
    - V Od Oi: *Le da besitos* 'He / she gives him / her kisses'; *Me compra un caballo* 'Buy me a horse'; *toma la mano a Ca(r)litos* 'Take Carlito's hand'
    - S V A: *Uno va aquí* 'One goes/you go here'; *Bárba(ra) cae (al)suelo* 'Barbara fell over' ; *Este vive aquí* 'He lives here'
    - N Vcop Adv: *Entonces (es)taba una niña* 'So, there was a girl'; *(Con)ejo aquí está* 'Here's the rabbit' ; *Ya está uno* 'That's one'
    - V A: *Sale de aquí* 'He / she leaves here'; *A piscina voy* 'I'm off to the pool'; *Pasa por el puente* 'Go over the bridge'
    - V O A: *Lo dejo aquí* 'I'm leaving it here'; *Así los pegamos* 'We stick them like this'; *Ya he hecho un pipí* 'I already did a pce'

Questions
- Qu- VCop N: 50 tokens (*qué* = 39; *quién* = 6; *dónde* = 5); *¿Qué es eso?* 'What's that?' (100% of subjects); *¿Este quién es?* 'Who's this?'; *¿Dónde está la vaca?* 'Where's the cow?'
- Qu- V X: 26 tokens (more variety of *wh*-pronouns): *¿Cómo se llama?* 'What's it called?' (50% of subjects); *¿Dónde va Nacho?* 'Where's Nacho going?'; *¿Quién la compró?* 'Who bought it?'
- ¿(S)V(X)?: 21 tokens. Ten different structures: *¿Ese se deja?* 'Is that one being left here?'; *¿Me lo das?* 'Will you give it to me?'; *¿En Soto hay moras?* 'Are there any blackberries in Soto?'

Commands
- SVO=VOS: *Abre la pue(r)tita tú* 'You open the door'; *Papá quita el p(i)e* 'Daddy take your foot off'

- Neg/Qu- Vsubj: *No te vayas* 'Don't go'; *Mamá, que juegues* 'Play, mummy'
  VO: *Toma una pelota* 'Take a ball'; *Haz un castillo* 'Make a castle'

Phrase level
- (Det) N Pr N: *cucharadita de azúcar* 'spoonful of sugar'; *a mí (cos)quillas* 'I'm ticklish'; *las otras en Morelia* 'the others in Morelia'
  Expansions: *Entonces niña a cama* 'Then the girl goes to bed'; *este tachito de Koki* 'Koki's little bucket'; *los niños de aquí* 'the children from here'; *de la casa* 'from the house'
- Pr Det N: *en e(l) culo* 'on your / my / his / her bottom'; *con *la limón*[14] 'with the lemon'; *Ese pa(ra) ti* 'That one's for you'
  Expansions: *Ese para la señora* 'That's for the lady'; *ahora la de Pulgarcito* 'now Tom Thumb's story'; *en la ducha sí* 'in the shower, yes'
- Det N Adv: *ot(r)a cosa más* 'one more thing'; *un niño no* 'not a boy'; *mañana las canicas* 'tomorrow, the marbles'; *¿estas tres también?* 'these three as well?'
- Det N N: *tú un coche* 'you, a car'; *su tía Marta* 'his / her aunt Marta'; *el bebé pollito* 'the baby chick'
  a. Det Det N: *ese ot(r)o babito* 'that other little baby'; *el gato ese* 'that cat'; *todo el mundo* 'everybody'

At Stage III, we also find combinations of two elements, typical of stage II, joined by a coordinative particle *y*: **uno oso y *uno (con)ejo*[15] 'a bear and a rabbit'; *y eso no y este sí* 'and not that one, this one'; *el teja(d)o y la pistola* 'the roof and the gun'.

Word level
Several types of verbal inflection need to be recognized.

(i) Periphrases
  - *r a* + infinitive: the most frequent; it is almost always used to convey future value (in agreement with the adult tendency): at this stage we found three tokens in the future tense, as opposed to 43 periphrastic constructions, in 100% of subjects: *Voy a ver* 'I'll see'; *Vamos a cantar* 'We're going to sing'; *Va a dormir aquí* 'He's / she's going to sleep here'; *Sí voy a dar* 'Yes I'm going to give'.
  - *estar* + gerund (durative value): *E(s)tá durmiendo* 'He's / she's sleeping'; *Está volando e(l) globo* 'The balloon is flying'; *Estoy haciendo* 'I'm doing / making'
(ii) Auxiliary verbs
  Children at this stage expand the verbal paradigm with the 'composed' (*compuestos*) tenses, mostly the past perfect: *Se ha perdido* 'He / she has disappeared'; *Ya he mordido* 'I've already bitten it'; *Las has perdido* 'You've

lost them'. In American Spanish the use of this tense is different and less frequent than in Castillian Spanish (Kany, 1969); our sample is mostly composed of Castillian subjects, with the exception of K (Mexican).

(iii) Subjunctive

Negative and temporal constructions force the emergence of the subjunctive in such constructions as *no te vayas* 'don't go', *no se vayan* 'don't go' (plural) , and *c(u)ando vaya a la guardería* 'when I go to the crèche' (in alternation with incorrect uses of the indicative in this context).

(iv) Overregularizations

The progressive richness of verbal morphology has the consequence of an increasing number of overgeneralizations in irregular forms at Stages III and IV: **venió* < *vino* 'I comed < I came'; **rompido* < *roto* 'breaked < broken'; **poní* < *puse* 'I putted / I put'; **pusí* < *puse* 'I putted < I put'; **sabo* < *sé* 'I knowed < I know'; **hagado* < *hecho* 'maked < made'.

(v) Clitics and pronouns

The system is increasingly complex (*-me, -te, -se, -lo, -los, -la, -las, -le, -les, -se*) and requires pronominal agreement (*yo-me-mí; tú-te-ti*). Children at this stage sometimes achieve these grammatical requirements (*Tú te llamas* 'You're called'; *Yo me quedo* 'I'll stay') but at other times they fail: *No gusta *a mí* < *No me gusta* 'Me no like < I don't like'; *Dame conejo *yo* < *Dame conejo a mí* 'Give the rabbit to me'; *Una para *tú* < *Una para ti* 'One for you'; **Mí no (em)puja* < *Yo no empujo* 'I don't push'.

At this Stage the first conversational markers appear in children's speech samples, becoming very frequent in some subjects (this feature is said to be dependent on personal communicative styles): *Venga* 'Come on'; *¿Vale?* 'OK?'; *¿Eh?* 'What?'; *¿A que sí / no?* 'Don't you think?' and so on. They will be used continuously from now on.

Stage IV (approximately 2;6–3 years)

Children consolidate simple sentence structure with combinations that are increasingly rich and wide-ranging. Even if complex sentences are typical of the next stage, in our sample 20% of long statements (four elements or more) are complex or quasi-complex sentences. The long phrasal combinations are less frequent than in previous stages. As before, frequency statistics are based on five children within the relevant age range (see summaries in Figs 14.8–14.11 and Table 14.6).

Clause level

A sample of 728 clauses was collected: 77% statements, 13% questions and 10% commands. A total of 10% of the clauses longer than three elements were negative statements. 18% were copular verbs (*ser, estar,* 'to

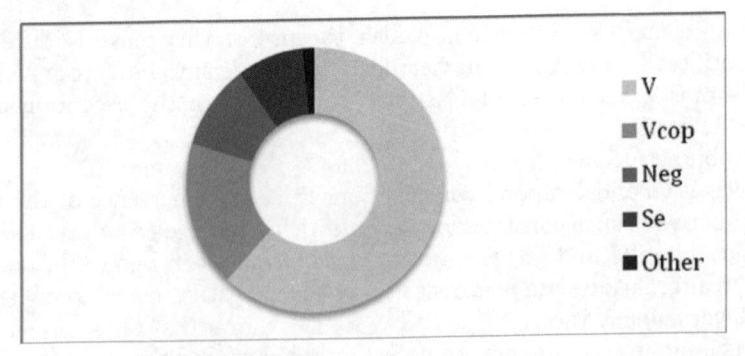

Figure 14.8 Stage IV. Clause level. Frequency of structures by type. 728 clauses

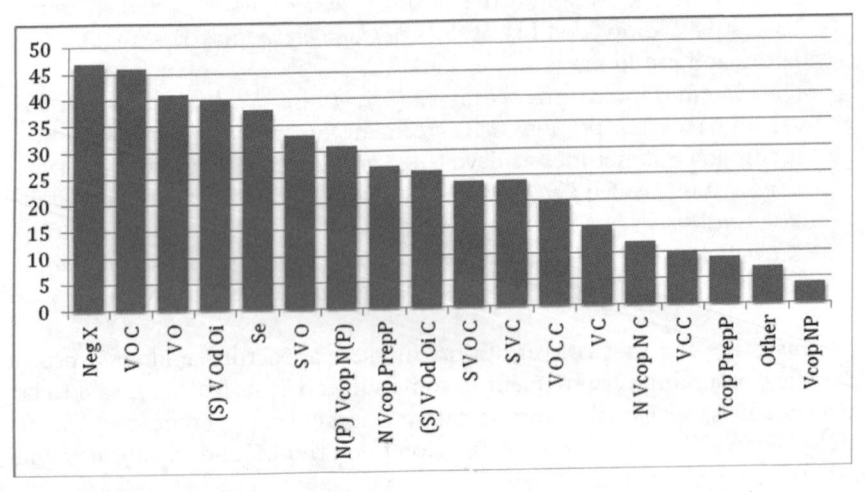

Figure 14.9 Stage IV. Clause level. Frequency of structures. 728 clauses

be'), and 62% were other verbs. A total of 8% of the constructions use the particle *se*, mostly with an impersonal or reflexive value (see Figure 14.8).

Statements

In the Stage IV sample, negative clauses are the most frequent structure. This is probably a question of style within the interactions. The relevant fact is that the internal construction of these negative clauses is complex, and follows the same preferences that can be seen in their affirmative correlates:

- V O A: *Voy a buscar el ort(r)o tenedor luego* 'I'll look for the other fork later'; *Me ha dado unas gotas para la oreja* 'He / she has given some drops

for my ear'; *(L)o p(u)ede hace(r) dep(r)isa* 'He / she can do it quickly'; *Ya han *ponido[16] la luz* 'They've already putted on the light'
- V O[17]: *Estoy mirando a mamá* 'I'm looking at mummy'; *Hay dos elefante *e hijo* 'There are two elephants *e son'; *lo saco todo esto* 'I'm taking all this out'; *Vamo(s) a pone(r) ese de cinta* 'Let's put the ribbon one on'
- (S) V Od Oi[18]: *Me he pintado las uñas* 'I've painted my nails'; **Ese[19] la encontró el papá* 'Daddy found that'; *Me lo *regalaban[20] abuela* 'Granny gave that to me as a present'; *(Es)tá gua(r)dando el regalito pa(ra) mí* 'He / she is keeping the present for me'
- Se X: *Por eso se enoja* 'That's why he/she gets angry'; *Se ha roto un poco* 'It's a bit broken'; *Se cae a mi bolsillo* 'It falls into my bag; *Eso no se pinta* 'You don't paint that'
- S V O: *Yo lo puedo llenar* 'I can fill it'; *Lucio hace muchas cosas locas* 'Lucio does a lot of crazy things'; *Le sale *e(s)te[21] rayita* 'He / she got a scratch'; *La han puesto los señores* 'The men have put it on'
- N Vcop N = NP Vcop NP: *Este es un avión* 'This is a plane'; *Esa casa es grande* 'That house is big'; *Está muy buena el agua* 'Water is very good'; *(L)a mía es (n)a(r)anja* 'Mine is orange'
- N Vcop PrepP: *Esto es para mí* 'This is for me'; *Estos rebozos son de la Inocencia* 'Those shawls belong to Inocencia'; **O[22] perro (es)tá e(n) la calle* '*0 dog is in the street'
- (S) V Od Oi A: *Me lo dio Isabel para *tú[23]* 'Isabel gave it to me for you'; *Te voy a tirar un día agua* 'One day, I'm going to throw water on you'; *Tú se lo quitaste ayer* 'You took it away from him / her yesterday'; *Yo le saqué antes punta al verde* 'I sharpened the green one before'; *A(ho)ra te enseño una canción* 'I'm going to teach you a song now'
- S V O A: *Tú haces una casa así* 'You make a house like this'; *Yo la dejo ahí* 'I leave it there'; *Ot(r)o día Rafa a@ rompió uno* 'The other day Rafa broke one'; *Parados los quiero yo* 'I like them standing still'
- S V A: *Este va junto de estos chiquititos* 'This goes with those little ones'; *Ellos a dormir ahí* 'They're going to sleep here'; *Yo voy a la (es)cuelita* 'I go to school'
- V O C A: *Ya tenemos otro tenedor allá* 'we already have another fork over there'; *Así me pongo muy nerviosa* 'This makes me very nervous'; *Gua(r)da(r)lo aquí en mi casa* 'To keep it in my house'

The first complex sentences

Complex sentences are the main characteristic of the next stage (cf. above); however, we do find at this point a certain number of adverbial subordinates, for the most part with a casual value (*porque*, 'because': *Es más grande po(r)que voy a la escuela* 'It's bigger because I go to school'), but also conditional (*si*, 'if': *Si no quieres más esto, vas a la calle* 'If you don't want this any more, you're out') or final (*para*, 'to': *Eso es pa(ra) lavar el plato* 'This is for washing the plate'). However, what should be underlined is the presence at this stage of some fixed structures that can bootstrap the emergence of complex sentences in the near future. It is the case of *es que* 'the reason is', *verdad que* 'is it true that?', *sabes que* 'did you know that?', or simply *que* 'that' + O:

- *Es que estoy cogiendo agua* 'I'm getting water at the moment'; *Es que no sale* 'It just won't come out'; *Es que se ha acabado* 'It's just that it's finished'
- *Sabes que después me pican las peñas?* 'Do you know that the stones hurt me afterwards'; *Verdad que tengo muchos?* 'I have a lot, haven't I?'; *A que tú quieres uno rojo?* 'I bet you want a red one'
- *Que está muy malo* 'It's really bad'; *Que pongas el disco de Parchís* 'Put on the Parchís CD'

Questions

The data here comprised 82 utterances, 83% of which were *Qu-* clauses and 17% (S) V (O)? clauses.

Qu- questions

- 22% Vcop (*Qu-* + *ser* 'to be', *estar* 'to be'); 31% Vperiph (*Qu-* + *estar* 'to be' + gerund /*ir a* + infinitive); 47% other V.
- 33% *dónde* 'where'; 26% *por qué* 'why'; 18% *qué* 'what'; 9% *cómo* 'how'; 8% *cuál* 'which'; Other 7%

At this stage, we highlight the presence of complex verbal forms in questions as periphrases: *Cómo estaban bailando estos patos* 'How those ducks were dancing'; *Quién me va a quitar el jersey?* 'Who is going to take off my jumper?'; *Por qué estabas gritando, papá?* 'Daddy, why were you shouting?'. *Qu-* pronouns are much more varied than before.

Commands

There is a very distinct construction that appears at Stage IV in our Spanish corpus. It occurred in 100% of the subjects and two to three of all commands, although in the previous stage it only occurred rarely. Formally it is a command, functioning as a discourse marker (calling the attention of the listener). It always has the same structure: *mira,* 'look' / *oye,* 'listen' / *toma,* 'take it' + O[24]:

- *Mira, se está cortando la nariz* 'Look, he / she is cutting his / her nose' ; *Mamá, mira cómo sale* 'Mummy, look how it's coming out'; *Toma, se ha roto* 'Take it, it's broken', *Mira, este es el papá* 'Look, this is the daddy'; *Oye, me siento aquí* 'Listen, I'm going to sit here'; *Está guardada en el coche, mira* 'It's in the car, look'

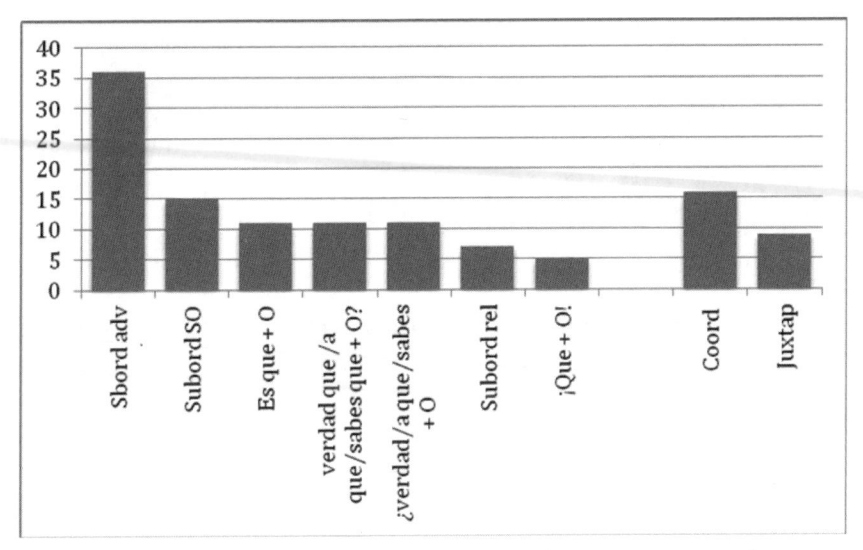

Figure 14.10 Stage IV. Clause level. First complex sentences.121 clauses

Table 14.6 Profile form for Stage IV: Summary

Commands	Questions	Statements	
Órdenes	Preguntas	Afirmaciones	
Clause – Oración			**Phrase – Frase**
Mira/oye/toma/espera+O	Varied qu- pron	Neg V S/O	Expansion + Adv
other	Complex verb	(S) V O C	Expansion + PrepP
		(S) V O	Qu- phrases
		(S) V Od Oi	Coord
		N(P) VCop N(P)	Other
		Se V X	
		Other	

Phrase level

Previous structures can be expanded at this stage with the addition of adverbs (*una comidita muy rica* 'yummy food'), prepositional phrases (*con las manos en las peñas* 'with my hands on the stones'), *qu-* pronouns (*con qué otra cosa?* 'with what other thing?', *qué regalos más bonitos* 'what lovely presents'),[25] or coordination (*los pantalones y las botas* 'pants and boots', *mi papi, mi mami* 'my daddy, my mammy', *un mono y una flor* 'A monkey and a flower'). However, as mentioned above, phrases longer than four elements are rather uncommon in our sample (55 examples, of which 11 are nouns followed by a subordinate clause: *en mi piscina que se llama bañera* 'in my swimming pool which is called a bathtub'; *el mes que viene* 'next month'; *un huevito para coser* 'an egg to cook'.

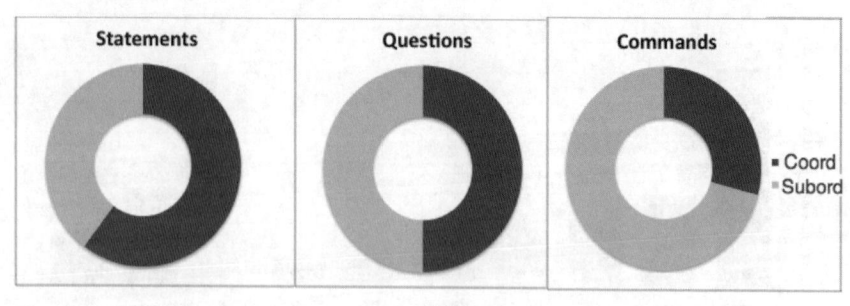

Figure 14.11 Stage V. Clause level. Frequency of complex/compound sentences by communicative function. 180 clauses

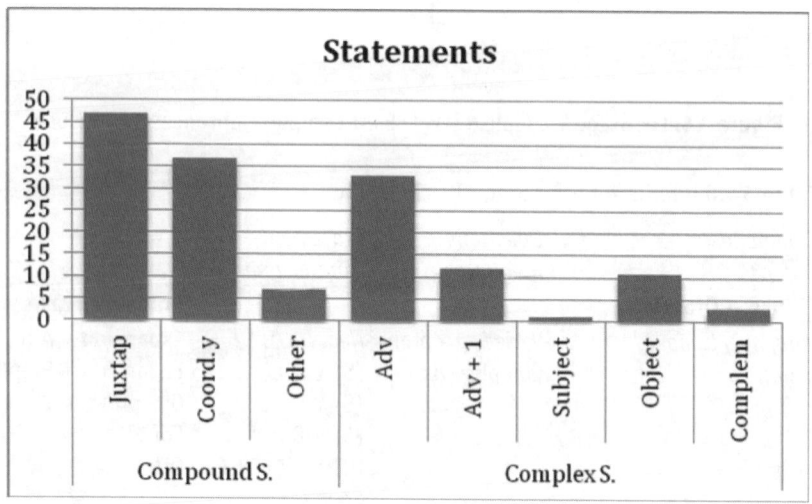

Figure 14.12 Stage V. Clause level. Statements. Frequency of structures. 151 sentences

Word level
- Double negative: *No me voy a casar con nadie* 'I'm not going to marry anyone'; *No hago nada* 'I'm not doing anything'; *No canté nada* 'I didn't sing anything'
- First comparatives in phrases (not yet in clauses): *Este es rojo como la cuchara* 'This is red like the spoon'; *Más dulce es este* 'This one is sweeter', *Qué palos más malos* 'What bad sticks'
- Complex verb forms: *tener/hay que* 'you have to' + inf (*Tienes que tomar* 'You have to take', *Hay que comerse eso* 'You've got to eat that'); *poder* 'to be able' + inf (*Se pueden esperar* 'They can wait'; *Ay, que no puedo mover!* 'Oh no, I can't move!' , *Se puede abrazar* 'You can hug')

Stage V (approximately 3–3;6 years)

This is the stage of recursion. Coinciding with their first attendance at school, children can join simple clauses to form compound and complex sentences linked by diverse conjunctions or adverbs. At this time, of course, the previous structures established in Stage IV are still present (periphrastic verbal forms such as *tener que* 'to have to' + inf; *hay que* 'you need to' + inf; commands headed by *mira* 'look', *oye* 'listen', *espera* 'wait' ... as a way of introducing a sentence), but they are not included in the following computations, which are based on language samples from nine subjects.

Clause level

The data comprised 180 complex or compound sentences, of which 84% were statements, 13% commands and 3% questions. The proportion of complex *versus* compound sentences in each group can be seen in Figure 14.11, and a summary is presented in Figure 14.13 and Table 14.7.

Statements

Compound sentences (91 utterances)

– The most frequent situation is simple juxtaposition where clauses are joined together without any grammatical connector: *esta es muy fea, la nuestra es más bonita* 'this is very ugly, our one is nicer'; *yo no lo tengo que hacer, yo tengo que hacer puntitos* 'I don't have to do it, I've got to make little dots'; *se va a caer el otro, se va a caer* 'the other one is going to fall, it's going to fall'.

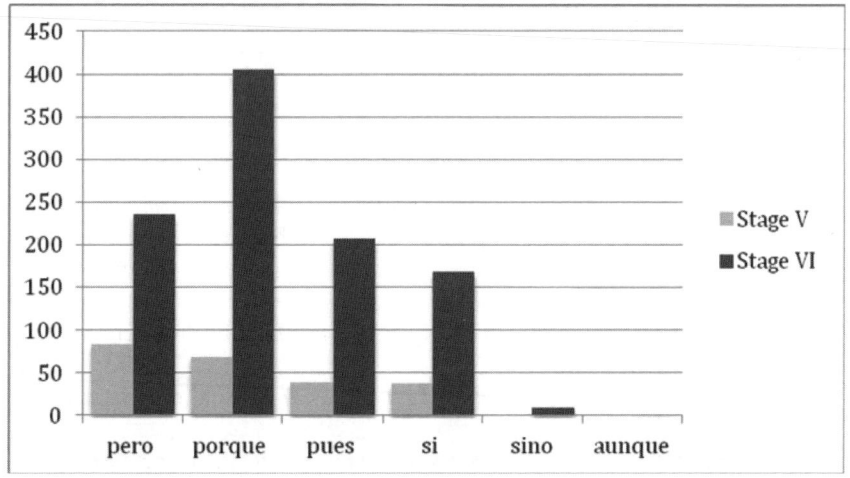

Figure 14.13 Use of conjunctions, Stage VI *vs.* Stage V

Table 14.7 Profile form for Stage V: Summary

Conn	Clause level					Phrase level
	Commands	Questions	Statements			
y	Subord. *que*	Coord	Coord-Juxtap	1	1+	Relative
Coord	Coord	Subord	Subord			Adv
Subord	Other		Adv	1	1+	+1
Other			0			
			Other			

- In coordinated sentences, the conjunction *y*, 'and', is by far the most common: *y te curo yo, y soy la médica yo* 'and I cure you, and I'm a doctor'; *cogió el jabón y le estaba echando al niño* 'he/she grabbed the soap and was putting it on the child'; *y pisa el suelo y hace tonterías* 'and he/she walks around and does silly things'.
- Nevertheless, a few other conjunctions can be found in the sample: *pero*, 'but' (*ya tengo reloj, pero e(s)pera que te llame* 'I've already got a watch, but wait until I call you'); *pues*, 'since' (*qué guapo va a quedar, pos[=pues]está quedando guapísimo* 'how lovely he's going to look, he's looking gorgeous').

Complex sentences (61 utterances)
Adverbial clauses (76% of subordinated clauses)

(a) 56% =*Adv* = main clause + subord. The types of adverbial clause are listed below by frequency order:
  - Temporal, *cuando*, 'when': *Cuando le *trayó[26]la manzana la mordió* 'When he / she *bringed the apple, he / she bit it'; *Cuando te llame lo coges tú, ¿vale?* 'When I call you, you'll pick up, right?'
  - Final *para que* 'to, in order to': *Ahora apago la luz pa(ra) que duermas* 'I'm turning off the light so you can sleep'; *Haciendo bocadillos así pa(ra) que coman* 'Making sandwiches like that so that they eat', or simply *que*: *Haciendo patatas fritas *que coman* 'Making chips so that they eat'
  - Cause: *porque*, 'because': *Pero sólo era uno porque sus hermanos estaban trabajando en el pueblo* 'It was only one because his/her brothers were working in the village'; *Es una bruja de mentira porque me dio un globo* 'She's not a real witch because she gave me a balloon'; *que* with causal value: *Me la voy a llevar, que está rota* 'I'm going to keep it because it's broken'
  - Place, *dónde*, 'where': *Le dije yo dónde e(s)taba* 'I told him / her where I/it was'.
  - Condition, *si*, 'if': *La hacemos si sale mi película de María* 'We'll do it if my film of María comes out'

(b) 20% = main clause + two or more subord (*Adv+1*): *Porque aunque haya un poco de bulto, como está el colchón* 'Because even if it's a little bulky, since the mattress is there'; *Toma, que él te pre(s)ta ése que e(s) tuyo* 'Take it, he is lending it to you so it's yours'; *Pero mis amigos no sé si cabrán, porque van mis tíos y tú* 'But I don't know whether my friends will fit, because my aunt and uncle and you are going as well'
- Object clauses (18% of subordinate clauses): *Me dijo que iba a pe(s)car* 'He / she told me that he / she was going to go fishing'; *Ya pensaba que se cayó el Mora* 'I already thought that the Mora fell down'; *Entonces, yo creía que íbamos a la escuela* 'Then, I thought we were going to school'
- Other: subject clauses and complement clauses are scarce in our sample (subject: *Es mejor que no le pongas esto* 'It's better not to put that on him / her'; complement: *Tiene m(i)edo a que quede esto un poco así* 'He / she is afraid that it's going to stay a little like that')

Questions

We only have eight examples of questions using complex or compound sentences: coordinated (*Y qué dijo la niña y qué *dijo[27] los ositos?* 'And what did the girl say and what did the little bears say?'); subordinated (*Te acuerdas de que en Madrid salió María?* 'Do you remember that María went out in Madrid?').

Commands

As seen before (Stage IV), commands present a particular structure in which subordination is preferred to coordination. Nonetheless, the same pattern is always followed: main clause (Vimper) + *que* 'that' + subordinate clause: *Dámelo que te tapo* 'Give it to me and I'll cover you'; *Ciérralos que me da miedo* 'Close them because I'm scared'; *Dibuja la mariposa de lunares que yo dibujo mi gato y mi perro* 'Draw the spotted butterfly and I'll draw my cat and dog'.

Phrase level (20 utterances)

- Relative clause, 14 examples: *Había un tobogán que resbalaba* 'There was a toboggan which slid'; *Y aquí hay otro pollito que va caminando* 'And here is another little chicken walking around'; *Los pajaritos que van por el aire* 'The little birds that fly'
- Adverbial clause (five examples): *Y esto pa(ra) qué es?* 'And what's this for?'; *El martes cuando vinimos del cole* 'On Tuesday when we came from school'; *A ti no, porque e(res) mala* 'Not for you, because you're naughty'
- Combinations (more than one clause): *Y después que acabe los tres cerditos porque yo la sé* 'Afterwards, I know what happens to the three little pigs'

Stage VI (approximately 3;6–4;6 years)

Throughout Stage VI, children continue to develop the use of sentence structures, and improve their awareness of irregularities and of other complex devices of language. They eliminate most errors from their speech. As a way of showing these new achievements, Tables 14.8–14.10, and Figures 14.13–14.15 compare some relevant grammatical markers in the previous stage and in the sixth stage.

Table 14.8 Conjunction use at Stage VI

Conjunctions	Stage V	Stage VI
Absolute number of items (tokens)	228	1027
Absolute number of different items (types)	4	6
Sample size (in words-tokens)	40,154	32,483
% (tokens)	0.57	3.16

Table 14.9 Adverb use at Stage VI

Adverbs	Stage V	Stage VI
Absolute number of items (tokens)	1326	3576
Absolute number of different items (types)	63	81
Sample size (in words-tokens)	40,154	32,483
% (tokens)	3.30	11.00

Table 14.10 Adverb use Stages V and VI

		Stage VI	Stage V
mañana	tomorrow	18	2
hoy	today	17	0
ayer	yesterday	11	2
nunca	never	24	0
siempre	always	7	0
bueno	well	16	6
mal	bad	27	5
claro	of course	46	4
todavía	yet	18	2
tan	as / so	20	4

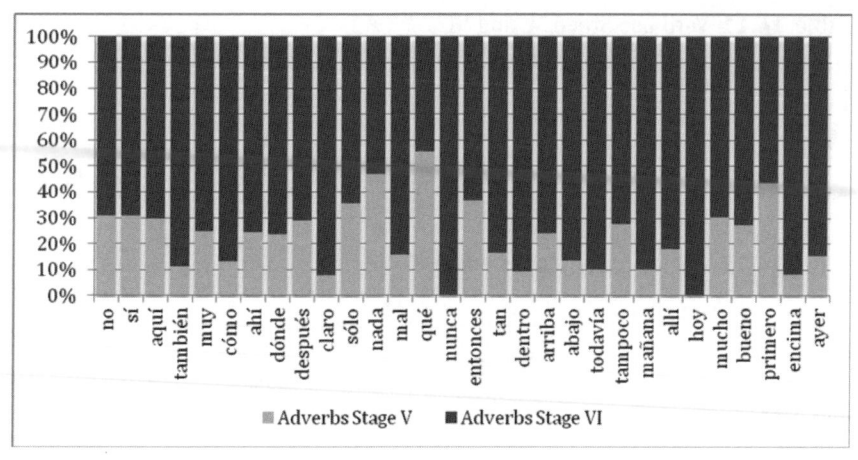

Figure 14.14 Use of adverbs, Stage VI *vs.* Stage V

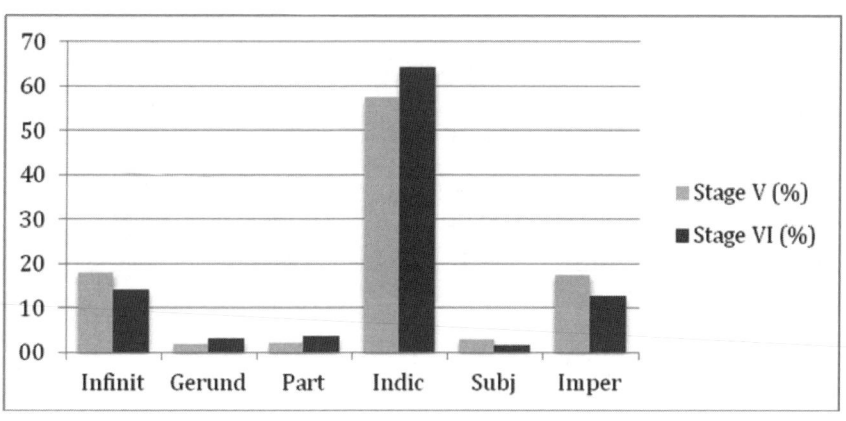

Figure 14.15 Proportion of use of verbal forms. Stage VI / V

In terms of frequency order, the main positions are similar in both groups: *no-sí*, 'no-yes'; *aquí-ahí*, 'here-there'; *muy-mucho-nada*; 'very / many-nothing'; *cómo* 'how'; *dónde*, 'where'; *entonces* 'then'. However, it is interesting to consider cases such as those shown in Table 14.10, where there is a high frequency in Stage VI but low in Stage V:

We do not find any use of passive voice in our sample. Errors to be marked at this stage can be seen in Table 14.13.

Table 14.11 Verb use Stages V and VI

Verbs	Stage V	Stage VI
Absolute number of items (tokens)	2111	7057
Sample size (in words-tokens)	40,154	32,483
% (tokens)	5.25	21.72

Table 14.12 Use of *haber* Stages V and VI

Use of aux. *haber* 'to have'

	Stage VI	Stage V
Ind pres	210	54
Ind past	31	2
Ind fut	3	
Infin	1	
Cond	1	
Subj	1	1
	247	57

Table 14.13 Errors to be marked at Stage VI

Connectors	Phrase		Clause	Word
	NP	VP		
y	Det	Omission	Omission	Overreg
coord	Omission	Substitution	Substitution	Other
subord	Substitution	Vcop	Agreement	
	Prep	Vaux		
	Omission			
	Substitution			
Other		Ambiguous		

Stage VII (over 4;6 years)[28]

Analysis of narratives

At this stage, children have already mastered the basic morphosyntactic structures in different types of sentences. This development is manifested in their use of complex syntax, especially in subordinate clauses. Consequently, we analysed narratives from children in this age range to find evidence for the increased use of complex syntactic structures. The language samples were obtained in the telling of three stories by 10 children aged five or six years (five of each age). A total number of 275 sentences was identified. Subsequently, we analysed the simple and complex sentences, the latter defined as those that contain subordinate clauses. In the latter, we determined the type of subordinate (nominal, adjectival and adverbial) clauses. The results of the use of simple and complex sentences are shown in Figure 14.16.

The predominant use of simple sentences is noteworthy, although more than one third of the sentences are complex. In this regard, it is important to note that in 104 complex sentences, 119 subordinate clauses were identified. In these cases, coordination can be seen among the subordinates. For instance: < *se trataba de* 'it was about' > *que el sapito era muy saltarín y que el sapito no dejaba dormir a los otros amiguitos de la laguna* 'The little frog was very restless and he kept his other little friends in the pool awake'. The subordinate can also be embedded: *Y después le construyeron un gimnasio para que pueda saltar* < *lo que él quiera* > 'Afterwards, they built a gym for him so he could hop – what he wants-'.

The percentage of ungrammatical sentences is higher in complex sentences (23%: **Después le prometió a sus amigos que nunca iba a hacer ruido más,* instead of *despúes leS prometió a sus amigos que nunca más iba a hacer ruido,* 'Afterwards, he promised his friends that he was never going to make any more noise') than in simple sentences (8.7%). Complex syntactic structures involving subordination are not totally dominant, as evidenced by the grammatical mistakes found in some of the responses.

Subordinate clauses

The subordinate substantive clearly dominates the other types of sentences. The characteristics of the various subordinates used by the children in their stories are listed in Table 14.14 and are ordered from the highest to lowest percentage of use.

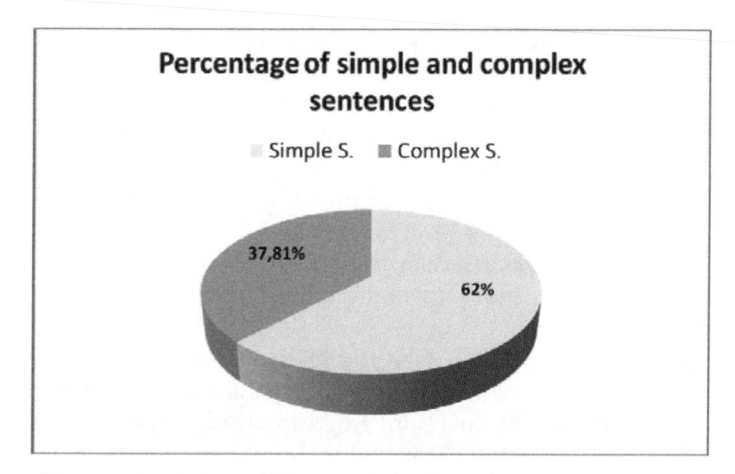

Figure 14.16 Stage VII. Use of simple and complex sentences

Table 14.14 Substantive subordinate clauses

SUBSTANTIVE SUBORDINATE CLAUSES	%
With subordinating conjunction que	50.6
With infinitive	41.0
Direct style	8.2

Substantive subordinate clauses
(i) Subordinates with subordinate conjunction *que*
 These are the most commonly used, presenting structures of varying complexity.
 – With subordinate conjunction *que*, 'that': *Y vio que los conejitos eran muy amables* 'And he / she saw that the little rabbits were very friendly'
 – With *que* connected by coordination (usually expressed by the conjunction *y,* 'and'). They are also frequently used with verb clauses: *Y después prometió que no iba a comer más y que no iba a quitar la comida de ellos* 'And afterwards he/she promised not to eat any more, and that he/she wasn't going take away their food'; *Y prometió que nunca más le va a robar la comida a sus amigos y nunca más va a comer mucho* 'And he/she promised never to steal food from his/her friends, and never to eat too much any more'.
 – It should be noted that some of the subordinates can contain another subordinate embedded clause: (*Se trataba de* 'It was about') *que el sapito era muy saltarín y que el sapito no dejaba < dormir a los otros amiguitos de la laguna >* 'The little frog was very restless and he kept his little friends in the pool awake'.
(ii) Subordinates with an infinitive:
 – As direct object: *Y ellos decidieron curarle la patita* 'And they decided' to cure his / her foot'; *Prometió nunca robarle las cosas a los conejos* 'He / she promised never to steal things from the rabbits'
 – In prepositional phrases: *Por robar la estufa se quemó la cola* 'He / she burnt his/her tail while trying to steal the stove'; *Sus amigos la invitaron a jugar* 'Her friends invited her to come and play'; *Entonces le pusieron muchas cosas para comer* 'Then they prepared lots of things to eat'
(iii) In direct style: children can use subordinates in a fairly simple direct style which move towards indirect style structures with the conjunction *que,* 'that':
 – *Dijo ¡socorro, socorro!* 'he/she said: 'Help! Help!''
 – *Y muy agradecido el sapito saltarín dijo que entonces dijo muchas gracias* 'And then the grateful hoppy frog said, thank you very much': there is an attempt to use the subordinate conjunction *que*, corrected to use direct style.

— *y el lobo dijo ¡socorro!, ¡ay! que se quemaba la cola* 'And the wolf said, help!, Ouch, his tail was burning': a structure with direct style is used simultaneously with a subordinate using *que*.

Adverbial subordinate clauses

When using adverbial structures, the most common are those with the subordinate conjunctions *porque* and *para que* (see Table 14.15). Both have already been acquired, but at this stage they are used with greater complexity.

(i) Adverbial causal clauses with conjunction *porque*, 'because': This early-acquired structure offers, at the seventh stage, different levels of complexity and could appear even in very complex structures.
- (Examiner: ¿*Pedían socorro los conejitos*? 'Did the little rabbits ask for help?')*Porque les robaron la estufa* 'Because they stole their stove'; *Pero no cabía porque estaba muy gorda* 'He/she didn't fit because he/she was very fat'. Both structures are quite simple subordinates, being affirmative and negative respectively.
- *La ardillita no podía salir de su casa porque estaba muy gorda, gorda* 'The little squirrel couldn't leave her house because she was really quite fat'; *Y después ella no podía salir porque estaba muy pero muy gorda* 'And after she couldn't go out because she was fat, I mean very fat'. In these subordinate clauses can be noted the use of resources to intensify (repetition of the adjective 'fat' and repetition using the conjunction *pero, muy pero muy*).
- (*Se trataba de*) *que también le hicieron una trampa al sapito saltarín < porque no dejaba dormir a sus amigos >* 'They also set a trap for the little hoppy frog < because he wouldn't let his friends sleep >'. The subordinate with *porque* is embedded in another subject (substantive with *que*) and, in turn, contains a subordinate with an infinitive (*dormir a sus amigos*, 'sleep to his friends').

(ii) Adverbial final clauses, with the preposition *para* + *que*, 'to, in order to', 'for ... to'. In these cases the verb is in the subjunctive mood: *Y le*

Table 14.15 Adverbial subordinate clauses

ADVERBIAL SUBORDINATE CLAUSES	%
Causal with *porque*, 'because'	26.6
Final with *para que*, 'in order to', 'for ... to'	26.6
Temporal with *cuando*, 'when'	16.6
Comparative with *tanto que*, 'so ... that', 'as much ... as'	13.3
Causal with *como*, ,'since', 'as'	10.0
Gerund subordinate	6.6

hicieron un gimnasio para que saltara de día 'And they made a gym for him so that he could hop during the day'; *Después lo invitaron a la casa pa que se calentara ahí* 'Afterwards, they invited him home so that he could warm himself'; *Y después se fue corriendo muy rápido para que los conejitos no lo alcanzaran* 'And afterwards, he ran off really quickly so that the little rabbits couldn't catch him'.

(iii) Adverbial temporal clauses, with the conjunction *cuando*, 'when'. Different levels of complexity can also be observed in this type of structures. Sometimes we find two subordinate clauses coordinated (without conjunction or with *y*, 'and'), in the same level of the syntactic hierarchy: *Y cuando se mejoró le hicieron un gimnasio* 'And when he / she got better they made a gym for him/her'; *La ardillita cuando está gordita cuando podía ver por la ventana no podía salir por la ventana ni por la puerta* 'When the little squirrel is fat, when she could see through the window, she couldn't get out either through the window or the door'; *Y después cuando le acercaron la estufa y se derritió el hielo prometió que nunca más le iba a robar las cosas a nadie y nunca más que le iba a robar algo* 'And afterwards, when they had brought him / her near the stove and the ice had melted, he/she promised that he / she would never again steal anybody's things and he / she was never going to steal anything again'.

(iv) Adverbial comparative clauses with *tanto que* or *tan . . . .que,* 'so . . . that', 'as much . . . as'. These structures are used as intensifiers: *Comió tanto que no podía salir* 'She ate so much that she couldn't get out'; *Hacía tanto frío que se convirtió en hielo* 'It was so cold that he/she froze'; *El lobo se sentó tan cerca de la estufa que se le incendió la cola* 'The wolf sat so close to the stove that his tail caught fire'.

(v) Adverbial causal clauses with subordinating conjunction *como,* 'since', 'as': *Y como tenía mucho frío robó la estufa de los conejitos* 'And since he was so cold, he stole the little rabbits' stove'; *Como estaba tan cerca de la estufa se quemó su cola* 'As he was so close to the stove he burnt his tail'.

(vi) Adverbial clauses with gerunds: *Y quedó llorando de día y de noche* 'And he / she spent all day and night crying'; *Había una vez un sapito saltarín que pasaba de día y de noche saltando* 'There once was a little hoppy frog who spent all day and night hopping'.

Phrase structure: Adjective clauses

These subordinates are less frequent in children's stories and are always structured with the relative pronoun *que*: *Había un lobo que les robó la estufa* 'There was a wolf who stole their stove'; *Una ardilla comía to(d)a la comi(d)a que había* 'A squirrel who ate all the food there was'. Occasionally, this type of subject is substantivized: *Y después le construyeron un gimnasio pa que pueda saltar lo que él quiera* 'And afterwards they built a gym for him so that he could hop to his heart's content'.

Table 14.16 Details of sample

Stage	Subjects	Age	Corpus (CHILDES Spanish database)	Recordings	Total no. words	Mean MLU
II	E(milio)	1;06-1;07	Vila	16	9236	1.76
	J(uan)	1;07-1;09	Linaza			
	K(oki)	1;07-1;11	Montes			
	M(aría)	1;08-1;11	Ornat			
	A(lfonso)	2;00	Marrero&Albalá			
III	E(milio)	2;01-2;06	Vila	17	8102	2.54
	J(uan)	2;03-2;04	Linaza			
	K(oki)	2;01-2;06	Montes			
	M(aría)	2;01-2;06	Ornat			
	A(lfonso)	2;03-2;06	Marrero&Albalá			
IV	E(milio)	2;11	Vila	10	8418	3.25
	J(uan)	2;08	Linaza			
	K(oki)	2;07-2;11	Montes			
	M(aría)	2;07-2;08	Ornat			
	A(lfonso)	2;10	Marrero&Albalá			
	I(daira)	3;00	Marrero&Albalá			
V	J(uan)	3;05-3;06	Linaza	10	10719	3.96
	M(aría)	3;01	Ornat			
	I(daira)	3;03	Marrero&Albalá			
	C(hild)300a=06	3;00	Díez-Itza			
	C(hild)300b=07	3;00	Díez-Itza			
	C(hild)302=01	3;02	Díez-Itza			
	C(hild)303=08	3;03	Díez-Itza			
	C(hild)304=10	3;04	Díez-Itza			
	C(hild)304b=09	3;04	Díez-Itza			
VI	J(uan)	3;09	Linaza	15	25703	6.24
	M(aría)	3;07-3;11	Ornat			
	A(lfonso)	3;08	Marrero&Albalá			
	I(daira)	3;07-4;00	Marrero&Albalá			
	C(hild)307=05	3;07	Díez-Itza			
	C(hild)307b=14	3;07	Díez-Itza			
	C(hild)307c=16	3;07	Díez-Itza			
	C(hild)307d=12	3;07	Díez-Itza			
	C(hild)309b=13	3;09	Díez-Itza			
	C(hild)309c=17	3;09	Díez-Itza			
	C(hild)309d=19	3;09	Díez-Itza			
	C(hild)311=18	3;11	Díez-Itza			
VII	5 children	5;00-5;11	Pavez y Coloma	10	–	–
	5 children	6.00-6;11	(not in CHILDES)			

Assessing Grammar

Nombre   Edad   Fecha de muestra
Tipo

A No analizada	Problemática
1. Ininteligible 2. Sonidos simbólicos 3. Alterada	1. Incompleta 2. Ambigua 3. Estereotipos

B. Respuestas

	Totales	Rep	Normal				Anómala		Probl
Tipo de estímulo				Mayor		Menor			
			Elípticas	Reduc	Completas		Estruct	∅	
Preguntas			1 2 3+						
Otros									

C. Espontáneas

D. Reacciones   General   Estructural   ∅   Otros   Problemas

Etapa I

Minor *Menores*	Responses *Respuestas*	Vocatives *Vocativos*	Other *Otros*	Problems *Problemas*
Major *Mayores*	Commands *Órdenes*	Questions *Preguntas*	Statement *Aserciones*	
	Verbs *Verbos*	Qué 'what', quién 'who' dónde,'where'...	Verbs *Verbos*	Nouns *Nombres*	Other *Otros*

Etapa II

Conect

Clause – Oración

Commands *Órdenes*	Questions *Preguntas*	Statement *Aserciones*	**Phrase - Frase**
V-imper. Neg + V-imper. V-imper+N = N+V-imper	Qu + V (+S)	se + V adv + VCop Neg + VCop / V VO	X Neg DN N Adj NN Adv N = N Adv Pr(D)N

Etapa III

Commands *Órdenes*	Questions *Preguntas*	Statements *Aserciones*	**Phrase - Frase**
S Vimper O = Vimper O S Neg/Qu- Vsubj Vimper Od = Od Vimper	Qu Vcop N Qu V X ¿(S) V (O)?	Neg V S/O N VCop N S V O Se V X Other	(D) N Prep N Prep Det N Det N Adv Det N N Det Det N Other

Etapa IV

Commands *Órdenes*	Questions *Preguntas*	Statements *Afirmaciones*	**Phrase - Frase**
Mira/oye/toma/espera +O Other	Varied qu- Complex verb	V(c) + O(d) Neg V S O (S) V O C (S) V O (S) V Od Oi N(P) VCop N(P) Se V X Other	Expansión + Adv Expansin + PrepP Qu- phrases Coord. Other

Etapa V

y coord.
subord
other

Commands *Órdenes*	Questions *Preguntas*	Statements *Afirmaciones*	**Phrase - Frase**
Subord. que Coord. Other	Coord. Subord.	Coord-Juxtap 1 1+ Subord Adv 1 1+ 0 Other	Relative Adv +1

Etapa VI

coord
pero
subord
porque
pues
sino
si
other

	Clause – Oración		**Phrase - Frase**	**Word - Palabra**
SV Complex - Verb perif. - Complex tenses	Clause Complement claro, también - temporal nunca-siempre , hoy-ayer-mañana, todavía - locative aquí-ahí-allí, dentro, encima, arriba-abajo	Errors Element ∅ Concord	SN D P D∅ P∅ D P	SV Aux > ∅ Cop	N V irreg reg

Etapa VI

Discurso   Comprensión sintáctica   Estilo

N.º total de oraciones: Media de oraciones por turno: Longitud media de las oraciones:

Conclusions

We have outlined a *preliminary* adaptation of LARSP to Spanish. Our main goal has been to provide some clear indications about syntactic development profiles that could be useful to Spanish-speaking speech-language pathologists. However, we are well aware of the shortcomings of our proposal; the sample size the chart is based on is far from the one used by Klee and Gavin (2010) for English or by Maillart et al. (2010) for French. Table 14.16 summarizes the main characteristics of our sample.

The translation of the results to LARSP charts is also under revision, and for Stage VII this is still absent; the error chart and information about word level must also be systematized. The current version of PERSL is shown below in Figure 14.1, and it should be noted that it contains some revisions of the partial stage diagrams given in the body of the chapter. Still, we hope that this contribution is a first step towards the production of a Spanish LARSP, or in general, towards an increasing use of assessment and screening procedures in syntactic development in Spanish-speaking environments. We do not have many tools for this purpose. There are several proposals which use data obtained through standardized tests, such as Aguado (1989), and there are important studies using natural speech samples to determine profiles of syntactic development in Spanish, such as Fernández and Aguado (2007). Although their sample is limited to the ages of 3;0, 3;6, and four years, the number of subjects (50) was far greater than ours. The authors consider the use of verb forms, as well as subordinate clauses, mean length of utterance, mean length of the longest utterances, and syntactic complexity. As we do not have many precedents of this type, any addition must be a non-negligible contribution in this field.

Notes

(1) Ana Isabel Codesido-García and Elena Garayzábal-Heinze are responsible for the first two sections of this chapter.
(2) The grammatical terminology adopted in this work comes from the functionalist theoretical framework as described in Rojo and Jiménez-Juliá (1989).
(3) As prepositional phrases are followed by a nominal structure, they follow the same possibilities as mentioned above.
(4) This and the following sections were contributed by Elvira Mendoza, Victoria Marrero, Carmen Julia Coloma and Mª Mercedes Pávez.
(5) This subsection was authored by Elvira Mendoza
(6) The following four subsections were authored by Victoria Marrero.
(7) These kind of expansions will be usual in the next stage, but some children can produce them now.
(8) The syntactic role of *se* in Spanish is a complex matter. In our sample, it is mostly used in a reflexive way, and corresponds to a Direct Object, as well as *me* or *te*. However, we chose to maintain it as a specific category which was not included in the general VO because it is especially frequent in child language and very easy for speech therapists to detect.

(9) The brackets indicate that the element is optional and may appear or not; in this case, Subject appears in our sample when children are at least 1;08–1;09 years old.
(10) The sign * indicates incorrect use. In Spanish the construction imperative negative requires the substitution of the imperative mode by the subjunctive mode (*ven* – VERB-IMPERATIVE-2.P.SG. 'come'> *no vengas* – NEG + VERB 'come'-PRES-SUBJ-2ª P.SG; 'don't come'). At the end of Stage I children can combine negatives and imperatives, but many of them still use the imperative mode preceded by negation: *no ven* – NEG + VERB 'come'-IMPER-2ª P.SG; 'don't come'.
(11) The sign > indicates that one structure evolves, at the end of this stage into another, more complex one. In this case, the initial *a* + inf is expanded in *ir a* + inf.
(12) X = N / Adv / Pron . . .
(13) As noted previously, these expansions will be typical in the next stage, but some children can produce them now.
(14) Wrong gender agreement between article and noun.
(15) Uno instead of un.
(16) Overregularization: *ponido* < *puesto*
(17) Clearly, this structure is computed as having four elements because (a) the verbal form is periphrastic or complex; (b) the object is a Noun Phrase (Det+N). It can be observed in the examples.
(18) Od = Direct Objec; Oi = Indirect Object
(19) Wrong gender agreement
(20) Wrong number agreement
(21) Wrong gender agreement
(22) Determiner omission
(23) Instead of *ti*.
(24) A total of 65% of utterances use *mira*; 20% use *oye*; 9% use *toma*; 7% use *espera*. As in many other Spanish constructions (cf. the introduction to this chapter) word order can be varied, as shown in the examples.
(25) Cf. below, word level, comparative structure.
(26) Overregularization; *trayó* < *trajo*
(27) Wrong number agreement
(28) This subsection was authored by Mª Mercedes Pávez; Carmen Julia Coloma and Elvira Mendoza.

References

Aguado, G. (1989) *Test de Evaluación del Desarrollo de la Morfosintaxis en el Niño (TSA)*. Madrid: CEPE.

Albalá, M.J. and Marrero, V. (2001) Las características lingüísticas de *AyDA* (un analizador morfológico para el español). *III Encuentro Internacional sobre la Adquisición de las lenguas del Estado, Universidad de Málaga*.

Boehm, J., Daley, G., Harvey, S., Hawkins, A. and Tsap, B. (2005) *LARSP Users Manual*. La Trobe University. Retrieved 22 January 2012: http://www.latrobe.edu.au/communication-clinic/attachments/pdf/larsp-manual.pdf

Crystal, D., Fletcher, P. and Garman, M. (1984) *Análisis Gramatical de los Trastornos del Lenguaje: un Procedimiento de Evaluación y Reeducación* (edición española revisada por Mª Teresa Espinal Farré). Barcelona: Ed. Médica y Técnica.

Fernández, M. and Aguado, G. (2007) Medidas del desarrollo típico de la morfosintaxis para la evaluación del lenguaje espontáneo de niños hispanohablantes. *Revista de Logopedia, Foniatría y Audiología* 27, 140–152.

Kany, Ch. E. (1969) *Sintaxis Hispanoamericana*. Madrid: Gredos.

Klee, T. and Gavin, W.J. (2010) Reference Data for the LARSP Profile Chart for 2-and 3-year-old Children". *31st Annual Symposium on Research in Child Language Disorders, Madison, Wisconsin*.

López Ornat, S., Gallego, C., Gallo, P., Karousou, A., Mariscal, S. and Martínez, M. (2005) *MacArthur: Inventario de Desarrollo Comunicativo. Manual y Cuadernillos*. Madrid: TEA Ediciones.

MacWhinney, B. (1995) *The CHILDES Project: Tools for Analyzing Talk* (2nd edn). Hillsdale, NJ: Lawrence Erlbaum.

Maillart, C., Parisse, C. and Tommerdahl, J. (2010) F-LARSP, French Language Assessment, Remediation and Screening Procedure. *13th Meeting of the International Clinical Linguistics and Phonetics Association. Oslo.*

Marrero, V., Albalá, M.J. and Moreno-Torres, I. (2001) La morfología infantil en español. Datos para su estudio. *III Encuentro Internacional sobre la Adquisición de las lenguas del Estado, Universidad de Málaga.*

Rojo, G. and Jimenez-Juliá, T. (1989) *Fundamentos del Análisis Sintáctico Funcional*. Santiago de Compostela: Universidade de Santiago.

15 LARSP for Turkish (TR-LARSP)

Seyhun Topbaş, Özlem Cangökçe-Yaşar and Martin J. Ball

Introduction

Database of child speech

This chapter aims to adapt LARSP to Turkish by analysing the language samples of typically developing children. There are no large-scale normative data on developmental stages of grammatical development in Turkish, although there are some ongoing studies. Nevertheless, certain predictions can be made about language development implicit in some detailed studies (a comprehensive review can be found in Aksu-Koç (2010)). Thus, the main reasons to adapt LARSP to Turkish are: (a) to observe language acquisition from the earliest ages; and (b) to ameliorate the lack of detailed inventory tools describing grammatical development for Turkish children. The participants in this research project were 70 typically developing Turkish-speaking children. This adaptation of LARSP to Turkish was based on data from 20 of these children at different stages of language development from 0;9 to 3;6 years of age (Stage I: 0;9–1;6, 4 children; Stage II: 1;7–2;0, 4 children; Stage III: 2;1–2;6, 5 children; Stage IV: 2;7–3;0, 5 children; Stage V: 3;1–3;6, 2 children).

The language samples were collected both longitudinally and cross-sectionally. The spontaneous speech samples of each child were transcribed and divided into utterances for analysis beginning from Stage I. The speech samples were elicited by semi-structured techniques, using picture compositions during mother-child and therapist interaction in the children's homes. The data were recorded digitally and then analysed qualitatively. In this chapter, the first five stages of the adapted TR-LARSP profile will be discussed.[1]

Brief outline of Turkish grammar

Turkish, belonging to the Turkic family, is an agglutinative language allowing predominantly suffixation. Derivational and inflectional suffixes, as well as clitics, are added to the root of the words with rich combinations to create new meanings. Some prefixes and infixes can also be seen in foreign borrowings. The order of morphemes is fixed in that derivational morphemes precede the inflectional ones in stem words.

The neutral word order is subject-object-verb (SOV), but is flexible for pragmatic purposes of signalling topic-focus (Erguvanlı-Taylan, 1984). Basic grammatical relations depend on the use of inflectional marking on verbs and nouns. In general, sentence-initial position is the topic position, whereas pre-verbal position is the focus position. Noun Phrases (NPs) are made transparent via case-marking, permitting word-order variation. The pronouns *ben* ('I') and *siz* ('you') are typically omitted since *-ım, -sunuz* indicate the person and number of the subject being marked as predicates. Object nouns may also be omitted depending on the context of utterance. If the sentence has more than one object, and if one of them is a direct object, the order whereby the direct object is closer to the verb is the more common. Gender is not expressed in nouns or pronouns; it does not affect agreement (Yavaş, 2010). Basic simple sentences are sentences with verbal predicates and those with non-verbal predicates (nominal or adjectival predicates and with existential predicates).

Definiteness is partly marked by word order and partly by morphology. Underhill (1972) illustrates how word order changes can signal differences in definiteness on subject and object NPs. For example, in the sentence 'oğlan topu köpeğe attı' ([the] boy ball+def to+dog+def threw = the boy threw the ball to the dog), the position of the subject implies definiteness (the direct and indirect objects are marked morphologically for definite). If the word order is changed to 'köpeğe **bir oğlan top** attı' then both 'ball' and 'boy' are now indefinite; and in the case of 'boy' it is solely the word order that shows this.

Furthermore, word order differentiates those sentences with clefts from those with pseudo-clefts, which are made with a headless relative clause and a nominal predicate. Turkish, being a verb-final language, follows the implicational relations for the order of elements in many structures. Thus, instead of prepositions, many postpositions are allowed, and the few prepositional phrases come before the verb. Branching goes in the opposite direction from English (i.e. to the left of the head noun). Relative clauses are formed by the movement of the head noun to the end of the sentence, and then the appropriate form of participle is selected to replace the tense suffix with a participle suffix. Examples and relevant structures for adapting LARSP can be found in the following sections.

Design of TR-LARSP

The A–D sections of the original LARSP profile have been retained in TR-LARSP, as these sections are not language specific. However, the morphological richness of Turkish posed problems that led to the authors making some adjustments in order to fit the requirements of the language into the profile chart. The main profile of stages was kept similar, but Stage I was divided into two sub-stages, and a separate word-level chart was designed for morphological development covering all stages. The preliminary versions of profile charts for TR-LARSP are shown in Figures 15.1 and 15.2, located towards the end of the chapter.

Types of Utterance: Child and/or Adult

Section A, B, C, D

Unanalysed strings and problematic

The database consists of utterances from children who do not have any kind of language or articulation problems. As a result of this, all the unanalysed utterances are ones that can be seen in normal language development in Turkish. This part of the chart is unchanged from LARSP, as every language has a similar pattern at this developmental period. Turkish children at this stage use symbolic noise (instead of the object or animal name), so we can code these types of noises on to the chart easily. Deviant structures are the utterances that fit into neither adult grammatical structures nor the predicted grammatical development of normal children. However, we did not find any deviant structures in our data. This may partly be due to the fact that word order in Turkish is flexible, especially for pragmatic purposes. The meaning that was intended to be transferred to the communicative partner by the child, for example with the use of sentence stress, is accomplished, and so the structures found are grammatically normal for this developmental period. Following future analysis of more children's data, changes to this section may be made. The section for problematic utterances retains the same description as given for LARSP in Crystal *et al.* (1989).

Responses, spontaneous speech, and reactions

These parts of the initial sections of the TR-LARSP syntax chart are the same as those on the original LARSP chart, and allow for the recording, where wished, of utterance type (e.g. in terms of ellipsis) both for responses and for spontaneous speech. They also allow for the linguistic reactions of the therapist to be recorded, if this is felt to be important, such that one can trace whether the utterance types produced by the therapist have any influence on subsequent utterances of the client.

Grammatical Categories and Levels of Analysis

Clause-level categories

Questions: *Wh-*questions are formed with the particles *ne* 'what', *neden / niye / niçin* 'why', *hangi* 'which', *kim* 'who' and *nerede* 'where' in pre-verbal or sentence-initial positions. *Yes/no*-questions are signalled by an interrogative particle *–mI*.[2] The location of *–mI* is at the end of the constituent questioned. If the constituent is a whole sentence, *-mI* goes to the end of the sentence. If the constituent is not a whole sentence, then *–mI* is found at the end of that constituent. If the predicate is non-verbal, *-mI* follows the predicate but precedes the personal ending (a summary of Turkish grammar can be found in Yavaş, 2010). Examples of these structures can be observed in the following sections.

Subordinate clauses: Noun clauses, relative clauses and adverbial clauses

In English, subordinate clauses are linked to matrix clauses by complementizers such as *that, which, who* and *where*. In Turkish, subordinate clauses are linked to the main clause by attaching bound morphemes to the stem of the embedded verb. Some of the subordinating morphemes that are used to embed one clause within another are *-DIK, -(y)EcEk, -mE, -(y)Iş, -mEk*. and *-mIş*.

Noun clauses occur in the same environments as NPs. They can be replaced by NPs or by a pronoun. Likewise, the subject can be null. Noun clauses, like NPs, have nominative case if they occur at subject position. Noun clauses can also occur in direct and oblique object positions like NPs. In this case, they are assigned accusative or dative case in the object position by the main verb, just like NP objects. Thus, an object noun clause can be case-marked depending on the type of case that the main verb assigns. Noun clauses, like NPs, can function as complements of postpositions and can also function as predicates. The difference between NPs and noun clauses, however, is that NPs have head nouns, while noun clauses have a subject-predicate (NP-VF) structure. The subordinating noun clause suffixes are *-DIk, -EcEk, -(y)Iş, mEk,* and *-mE*. Noun clauses that are obtained by the morphemes *-DIk* and *-EcEk* usually correspond to English *that*-clauses, while those that are obtained by *–mE and -mEk* are similar to English infinitival clauses or gerunds.

Subordinate clauses can also be used as NP modifiers. These clauses are known as relative or adjectival clauses. Relative clauses serve to provide additional information about the noun they modify, but are not required for the completion of the meaning of the noun. Relative clauses are on a par with adjectives in their relationship with the head noun, and are sometimes called adjectival clauses, in parallel to adverbial clauses which are adjuncts to VPs or sentences.

The relativizer is formed with a participial verb form: *-En* marks subject relatives, *-DIK, -EcEk, -mIş,* and aorist suffixes mark non-subject relatives where the element relativized may be the direct or oblique object. In non-subject relatives, the subject of the relative clause carries the genitive and the verb carries the possessive for agreement. In subject relatives there is no genitive, hence no agreement.

Adverbial clauses modify VPs or sentences and are heterogeneous both morphologically and syntactically. Some of the suffixes used as adverbials are *–ErEk, -IncA,* and *-dIğIndA.*

Phrase-level categories

Noun phrases (NP): Turkish is a head-final language, whereas English is head-initial. Since the heads of the NP, VP, and PP are at the end of their phrases, the last word of an NP is a noun and of a VP is a verb. An NP in Turkish can be illustrated as follows (all the units in parenthesis in an NP are optional), as described in Turan (2006):

NP → (referential determiner) (relative clause) (quantificational determiner) (adjective) (indefinite article) (noun) Noun

Postpositional phrases (PP): While English has prepositions, Turkish has postpositions. The functions of some English prepositions are fulfilled in Turkish by case suffixes. There are also independent postpositions which have NP complements. Sometimes a PP can have an additional adverb:

PP → (adv) NP P.

Adjective phrases (AdjP): Adjectives can appear at different positions in a sentence: as a modifier of a noun (attributive adjective) or in predicates (predicative adjective). Adjective phrases have an adjective as a head in final position, and this may also consist of a degree adverb that modifies the adjective. Some AdjPs requires PP complements and some NP complements:

AdjP → (NP/PP) (Degree adv) Adj

Adverb phrases (AdvP) and adverbials: Adverbs modify different syntactic categories and can function as adverbials. Other than being a distinct class, they can be derived from adjectives or nouns. AdvP has an adverb as its head. Syntactic functions of AdvP are: modifier of verbs, adjectives, adverbs, clauses, nouns, postpositions and complement of verbs:

AdvP → (Adv) Adv

Verb phrases (VP): Objects are complements of verbs and are obligatory elements in VPs if the verb is transitive or ditransitive (i.e. having both direct and indirect objects). On the other hand, intransitive verbs do not have any complements; that is, they are used without objects:

VP → (AdvP) (NP) (NP) Verb

Copular verbs (Vcop): In Turkish, copular verbs are *–Imek, -DIr, olmak*, and zero copula, and they cannot stand alone. Zero copula is not pronounced, but is realized in the predicate. In copular VPs, NPs, PPs, AdjPs, and clauses are subject complements.

Word-level categories

A word can belong to the following classes: nominal (nouns, pronouns, adjectives, adverbs), verb, postposition, conjunction or discourse connective and interjection (Göksel & Kerslake, 2005). During suffixation, morphophonological alternations may occur due to vowel and consonant harmony in that virtually all grammatical suffixes harmonize with the last vowel of the lexical stem. Thus, a suffix may have different forms, and the alterable sounds in suffixation are usually indicated by capital letters. For example the plural suffix *-lAr* has two forms, *-lar* and *-ler*. However, the perfective – *DI* has eight forms, as *-dı, -di, -du, -dü, -tı, -ti, -tu,* and *-tü*, where both the consonant and vowel are subject to alternation. Each morpheme is syllabic and stress is typically word final.

Derivational suffixes function to form new words and can be attached to nominals and verbs. When attached to nominals they create both verbs and other nominals (nouns, adjectives, and adverbs). As an example, the *–lIk* morpheme is added to the stem *göz* 'eye' to form another noun *gözlük* 'eyeglass / spectacles'; when the *–cE* suffix is added, it becomes a verb *gözle-* 'observe'.

Inflectional morphemes mainly express grammatical functions. When attached to nominals, they mark number/plurality, possession, and case (nominative, accusative *–(y)I*, dative, *-(y)E*, ablative *–DEn*, and locative – *DE*) in that order. The nominative case and singular are unmarked base forms that have no phonological realization. When the inflectional suffixes are attached to verbs, they mark voice (causative, passive, reflexive and reciprocal), negation, tense/aspect/modality, mood, copular and person. There are also subordinating suffixes and nominal inflectional suffixes attached to verbs that may have a single or multiple function (Turan, 2006).

Developmental Analysis

Stage I (0;9–1;6)

As shown in Figure 15.1, Stage I is divided into two sub-stages as *Stage Ia* and *Stage Ib*. Stage Ia relates to Stage I of LARSP with which there were both similarities and differences, and covers the period from 0;9 to 1;3 as the stage of one-element utterances. Since Turkish children use two elements (words with inflections) as early as 1;3, which is well documented in the

288 Assessing Grammar

Name		Age		Sample Date		Type		
A	**Unanalysed**				**Problematic**			
	1 Unintelligible	2 Symbolic Noise	3 Deviant		1 Imcomplete	2 Ambiguous	3 Stereotypes	

B	Responses			Normal Response					Abnormal		
			Repetitions	Major			Reduced	Full	Minor	Structural	∅	Problems
	Stimulus type	Totals		Elliptical								
				1	2	3+						
	Questions											
	Others											

C	Spontaneous							
D	Reactions		General	Structural	∅	Other	Problems	

		Minor	Responses		Vocatives		Other		Problems	
Stage I (0;9 – 1;6)		**Major 1a**	Comm	Quest	Statement					
			'V'	'Q'	'V'	'N'	other		problems	
		Major 1b	V XV VX	Qwh V+mI	(S)V	V	Vneg	N	Pron	Adj DemAdj
Stage II (1;7 – 2;0)		Conn.		Clause				Phrase		
			impX Ximp	XQ QX V+Q(mI) V+Q(mI)	∅OV SV OiV Other	AV OA -Ip	AdjN XIns		NN Other	
Stage III (2;1 – 2;6)			bakXY XYbak XYV	VQ(mI)X XQY QXY	SOV OAV AOV ∅OVV SOC	ASV SVV AOdAV SOOiV Other	IntAdj PronN DemAdj DemAdjN		PronAdj PronNPr NNAdj Other	
Stage IV (2;7 – 3;0)		c (ve, da) s (-mak için)	+S	QXY+ SOV+Q(mI)	Subord A 1 SOdAV Neg(hiç) Neg(değil) AO(O=XY+N)V S(S=Pron+N)cV Other		XcX XcXY XYc		Aux PronAuxN Other	
Stage V (3;1 – 3;6)		c s		XY+(mI) XY+ değil+ Q(mI)	Coord 1 Subord 1 1+					
Stage VI (3;7 +)										
Stage VII										
		Total no. Sentence		Mean No. Sentences Per Turn			Mean Sentence Length			

© Seyhun Topbaş & Özlem Cangökçe-Yaşar 2011

Figure 15.1 TR-LARSP Profile: Syntactic development

literature (Aksu-Koç, 2010) as well as in our data, Stage Ib was assigned to the period covering 1;4 to 1;6. Thus, the main difference occurring between the Turkish and English charts at this stage was the use of two-element structures.

Ketrez and Aksu-Koç (2009) determined three phases of inflectional development: premorphology as Phase I, proto-morphology as Phase II, and morphology proper as Phase III. Phase I is the earliest phase, with an MLU range 1.20 to 1.34, where children produce monosyllabic and disyllabic words with correct intonation and stress pattern. This pattern of development was also evidenced in several other studies (Aksu-Koç, 1997; Çapan, 1988; Topbaş et al., 1997; Özcan & Topbaş, 2000). Children at this stage seemed to use some inflectional paradigms based on modelling adult utterances. Although these inflectional markings do not fit any spontaneous productivity criteria, they do show evidence of sensitivity to the language. Aksu-Koç proposed that Turkish children go through a pre-categorical period like that observed in the case of English-speaking children as claimed by Radford (1990). In our analysis, this Phase I (as proposed by Aksu-Koç) is referred to as Stage Ia of TR-LARSP (see Table 15.1).

From 1;5 onwards the overall number of inflectional paradigms and the number of members of the inflections increase. Some structures which may be defined as two-element emerge and are therefore subsumed under Stage Ib (see Table 15.2). The ages of 1;5–1;6 are critical ages that can be accepted as a threshold of newly emerging three-member inflectional suffixes. It was difficult to determine the age borders, as there seemed an overlap between Stage I and Stage II. Thus, Stage Ib can be accepted as a transitional stage to Stage II.

Table 15.1 Stage 1A (0;9–1;3)

Minor	Responses	Vocatives	Other	Problems			
Major	Comm	Ques	Statement				Word
Stage 1a Major	'V'	'Q'	'V'	'N'	other	problems	

Table 15.2 Stage 1B (1;4–1;6)[3]

Major	Comm	Ques	Statement					Word
Stage 1b Major	V	Q wh	(S)V	V	Vneg N	Pron	Adj	Neg -mA
	XV	V+mI					Dem Adj	CASE-ACC, PERSON-1S, 2S, GEN
	VX							PAST -DI

Table 15.3 Stage 1B (1;4–1;6) Examples

Comm	Quest	Statement			PHRASE	
V	Q wh	V	Vneg –mA	N	Pron	Adj
Bak!	Ne?	Gel	Git-me	Araba	Ben	Güzel
'Look-IMP'	'What-Q'	'Come-IMP'	go-NEG-3S	'Car'	'I-1S'	'Beautiful'
			'Don't go'			
XV bak/bak XV	V+mI	(S)V	Ø Vneg			Det./dem.adj
Anne bak!	Ol-du mu?	Gel-di-m	(I) gel-me-m			Bu
mom look-IMP	be-PAST-Q	come-PAST-1S	come-NEG-1S			'This'
'Look mummy!'	'Is it done?'	'I came'	'I won't come'			Bu-nu
						'This-ACC'
Anni ka:k						
Mom wake up-IMP						
'Wake up mommy!'						
Bak, açtım						
Look, I open-PAST-1S						
'Look, I opened it.'						
VX/XV						
aç bu-nu						
'Open this-ACC'						
Sen aç						
You open-IMP						
'You this!'						

Any uninflected verbs are categorized under V in the Statement and Command columns. These verbs are bare forms, having the form of simple present 3rd person singular. They also mark the imperative form of commands as in *gel-* ('come'), *git-* ('go'), *kalk-* ('stand up'), *bak-* ('look') and *aç-* ('open').

The phrase level (Table 15.3) included pronoun and adjective use. The use of adjective is elicited from the context and labelled as Adj. *Bu* ('this') is coded as a referential determiner. In questions, the emergence of /-mI/ question marker is listed. In context, children use this question form to get approval for an event.

Through the end of this stage the past tense *–DI* and progressive *–yor* inflection and the negative *–mA* suffix emerge attached to verbs, as can be seen in Table 15.4. The *-mA* is always after the verb stem and precedes the inflectional markers but follows the voice suffixes. Words like *küçücük* ('very very small') and *babacığım* ('my dear daddy') are listed under the Other category. The Problem category is used for inexplicable utterances and ones that have multiple meanings.

Stage II (1;7–2;0)

At this stage, sentences that contain two elements are used more productively; however, three-element structures were also observed. This period is also marked by the productive use of verbal and nominal morphology with multi-member suffixes (Table 15.5). The inflectional development

Table 15.4 Stage 1B Suffixation

İpek 1;5 (17 months)	Utterance	Two-member suffix	Three-member suffix
One element	Oku Read-IMP 'Read this (to me).'		
	Gel Come-IMP 'Come!'	gel- di come-PAST 'He came.'	gel- me- m come-NEG-1S 'I won't come.'
Two element	Baba git Father go-IMP 'Dady go (please).'	git -ti go-PAST 'He went.'	
	Gözünü kapat Eye-POSS-ACC close '(Please) close your eyes'	göz-ün Eye-POSS	göz- ün -ü Eye-POSS-ACC
	Annesini öpüyo Mom-POSS-ACC kiss-PROG-3S' 'She is kissing he mother'	anne-si mom-POSS öp-üyo kiss-PROG-3S	anne-si-ni mom-POSS-ACC

Table 15.5 Stage II (1;7–2;0)

CLAUSE					PHRASE	WORD
Comm	Quest	Statement				
VXY	XQ	SV		AV	Adj N	PAST; EVID, FUT
XVY	QX	SOV/OVS		OA	XIns	PASSIVE
XYV	V+Q(mI)	(O)OV		VV	NN	ADVERBIAL
	OV+Q(mI)	OindV				

Table 15.6 Stage II: Commands

	V	X	Y	Extra Info	Gloss
VXY	Bak 'Look'	bu 'this'	salıncak 'swing'	V+X+Y (verb+ demAdj+noun)	'Look this is a swing'
	X	Y	V		
XY V	Bebeğim 'My doll'	burda 'here'	bak 'look'	X+Y+V (noun+ adv+verb)	My doll is here look!'

292 Assessing Grammar

at this stage is similar to Phase II proto-morphology where the MLU range is 1.58 to 3.42, as Ketrez and Aksu-Koç (2009) proposed.

The clause level categories of Stage II

Commands: The commands of the previous stage expand with elaborations as shown in Table 15.6. We see structures like XVY = *Sen ye bunu* with emphasis meaning 'You'll eat this, not me'.

Questions: There are four types of question form in Stage II. The question /-mI/ is acquired almost without error due to the flexibility of word order, requiring only that the stress is placed appropriately before the suffix /-mI/. Negation is also expressed in these question forms. The *wh-* question particles emerge at this stage as well. These forms are: XQ/QX, V+Q(-mI), OV+Q(-mI), and V+NEG+Q. Verbs are extended by appropriate suffixes, as shown in Table 15.7.

Statements: At the clause level, Stage II statements differ from LARSP. The most notable differences are in word order, since canonical word order in Turkish is SOV. Sentence-initial position is used for subject/topic, preverbal position for direct objects when they are unmarked (i.e. indefinite and nonreferential) and postverbal position for backgrounded, old informa-

Table 15.7 Stage II: Questions

Child			Extra Info	Word
Can 1;7	XQ$_{wh}$ / Q$_{wh}$X	Bu ne? this Q 'What is this?'		XQ(Adj+Q)
	V+Q$^{(-mI)}$	Bit-ti mi? finish-PAST Q-mI		PAST –dI
	OV+Q$^{(-mI)}$	Bebek gerek-ir mi? baby necessary-AOR Q-*mI* 'Does baby necessary?'		AOR –Ir 3S
Atakan 1;8	V+NEG+ Q$^{(-mI)}$+X	Çalış-mı-yor mu bu? Work -mA-PRG Q(-mI) this? 'Isn't this working?'		NEG –mA PROG –yor 3S
	V+PASS+ NEG+Q$^{(-mI)}$	Boz-ul-muş di mi? PASS(-Il)-EVD NEG(değil) Q(-mI) 'It is, isn't it?'		3S, PASS –Il PAST EVID –mIş NEG değil (not)
İpek 1;9	V+PASS+ NEG^{-mA}+ Q$^{(-mI)}$+X	Kapa- n- mı- yo mu bu? Close-PASS(-Il)-mA-PRG Q(-mI) this? 'Isn't this closed?'		PASS –In PROG –yor 3S
	A+V Q$^{(-mI)}$	Şimdi kapat-ım mi? Now close-FUT -1S Q-mI 'Shall I close it now?'		OPT- ayım 1S

tion (Erguvanlı-Taylan, 1984; Kornfilt, 1997). In children's speech four elements are recognized: subject, verb, object/indirect object and adverbial. Although they were simpler in use when compared to adult language, they can be recognized as the basic productions of more complex structures. Since pronominal subjects may be omitted, inflections were listed both syntactically and morphologically on the TR-LARSP chart. Almost all the children in our data correctly assigned grammatical roles to sentence constituents.

Although XV was common at this level, due to the flexible word order of Turkish pragmatically the order of constituents can be shifted. Children were able to use these elements with appropriate different combinations. The forms of statements were found to be SV, OV, $O_{ind}V$, AV and OA. The use of null subject with two-element clause structure is added as a developmental change. Examples are shown in Tables 15.8 and 15.9.

Owing to the agglutinative structure of Turkish, verbs carry suffixes that generate the root of the sentences. In Stage II several examples of these forms of structural constructions were observed.

Phrase-level categories of Stage II

At the phrase level there are three forms: AdjN, X_{ins}, and NN (see Table 15.10).

Word-level categories

At this stage, verbs are marked for voice, modality, negation, tense/aspect/mood and person, as can be seen from Tables 15.5–15.9. Case morphology is reflected in the emergence of specific constraints, and the generalization of productive schemas is closely tied to an increase in the lexicon. The marking of number on nominals is found later than case marking, but no difficulty is observed in its production. The question particle *–mI* and *wh*-questions are used in different word orders depending on the stress and context. Nominal inflections were number, possessive and case, marked in that order. The use of accusative and dative case was earlier and more frequent than the other cases.

At this stage the present/ progressive *-Iyor* for talking about ongoing events and the optative *-(y)A* for invitations to joint attention are used more frequently. The future *-(y)AcAk* is used to express intention for action, the inferential *-mIş* to comment on states that constitute new information and also used are the habitual/possible *–Ir and* the causative-reflexive *–Iş*. The agreement paradigms emerge together with the associated tense/aspect/mood markers. The possessive is more frequent than the genitive in the children's speech. This may be due to the possessor, which is typically one of the interlocutors who is present and can be presupposed, but the possessed object needs to be specified. A few substitution errors were also observed but were very rare.

Table 15.8 Stage II: Statements. SV/SOV/OVS

	Subject	Object	Verb	Extra Info	Word	
Ece 1;7	Ece		oku-du read-PAST			Ece read.
	(S) (she)	okul-a School-DAT	gidi-yo go- PROG-3S	(S): Null subject	-DAT -A	She is going to school
	Ben I	tenis tennis	oynu-yo-m play-PROG-1S			I am playing tennis
	(Ben) (I)	tayak comb	a:-dı-m take-PAST-1S	(S): Null Subject		I took a comb
	Gemi ship		gid-iyo go-PROG-3S			The ship is going
İpek 1;9	Ben I	bu-nu this-ACC	aç-a-mı-yo-m 'open-POT-NEG- PROG-1S'	O:Dem.Adj	Mood POT	I can't open this
			kapa-n-mı-yo (bu 'this') 'close-PASS- NEG-PROG-3S'	O:Dem.Adj Inverted sentence	PASS -In	This cannot be closed
	(Ben) (I)	kadıak-tan slide-ABL	kay-ca-m slip-FUT-1S	(S): Null Subject	-ABL-DAn Near FUT	I am going to slide
	(Ben) (I)	oyunca-n-ı toy-POSS- 2S-ACC	ver-mi-ce-m give-NEG-FUT- 3S	(S): Null Subject Indirect object	FUT	I won't give your toy
	Object	Verb	Subject			
	Sabun-u soap-ACC	al-a-ma-m take-POT- NEG-1S	ben I	Inverted sentence		I can't get the soap

The locative *-DA*, the ablative *–DAn,* the instrumental-comitative *-(y)lA* [(y)la/le], and the plural *–lAr* are added. The genitive *-(n)In* case is expanded by noun phrases. The person/number suffixes are marked for subject-verb agreement.

Stage III (2;1–2;6)

At this stage sentences usually contain three elements. In our data there are certain uses of four-element sentences. But, taking into consideration the general usage and frequency of four-element usage, we decided to exclude this from the chart. By age 2;6 children easily command verb and noun inflections in simple sentences, although this is not like adult productivity in complex sentences (see Table 15.11).

Table 15.9 Stage II: Statements (2)

		Object	Oind	Verb		Word	Extra Info	Gloss
Can 1;8	OV/OOV	ayakkabı 'shoe'		giy 'wear-IMP'				'Wear the shoe'
			makine-de 'dishwasher-LOC'	yıka-n-ıyo 'wash-PASS-PROG'				'It is washed in the machine'
		A	O	V				
Atakan 1;6		ordan 'there-ABL'	bi tane araba 'a/one car'	çıkcak 'get out-FUT'		-FUT	NP=Det. Number+N	'A car will come out from there'
		O	A	V			Extra Information	
İpek 1;8		(O) him/her	ora-ya 'there-DAT'	koy-du 'put-PAST-3S'			Adverbial-Dem pro (O:him/her): Null subject	'He put it there'
		S	V	V				
İpek 1;9		(S) Ben ('I')	gid-Ip 'go+Ip'	alim 'take +OPT 1S'	(S): Null subject -Ip: Subord	-Ip		'I will go and take it'

Table 15.10 Phrase-level categories of Stage II

	Adj	N	N	X_{ins}	Extra Info	Word	Gloss
AdjN	küçük 'small'	araba 'car'			NP=Adj+N		'small car'
NN		baba-nın 'father-GEN'	çorap-lar-ı 'sock-PL-POSS'		NP=Det+N	GEN, PL-*lAr*, POSS	'father's socks'
NXins				araba-yla 'car-INS'	PP= Nclitic		'with car'

The clause-level categories of Stage III

In Stage III clause level, the categories are mainly expansions of the previous stage. Unlike in English LARSP, suffixes play an important role in sentence configuration (see Tables 15.12 and 15.13). The question forms are expanded by one element. The /-*mI*/ question marker is still the most common suffix to make a question. The question forms are VQ(mI)X, XQY and QXY.

At the statement level, OAV, AOV, OVV, SOC, ASV, SVV and AO$_d$AV sentence forms are used. The possible combinations at clause level are listed in Table 15.14.

Table 15.11 Stage III

CLAUSE			PHRASE		WORD	
Comm	Quest	Statement				
+S	VQ(mI)X	SOC	ASV	Int Adj	Pron Adj	
	XQY	OAV	SVV	Pron N	Pron N Pr	
XYV+	QXY	AOV	AOdAV	Dem Adj	NN Adj	
		ØOVV	SOOindV	Dem Adj N		

Table 15.12 Clause-level categories of Stage III: Commands

Conn					
	Comm				
	+S				
	XYV+	Hadi,	bebeğ-im-i	ver!	'Come on, give me my
		'Come on	doll-GEN-ACC	give-3SIMP'	doll'

Table 15.13 Clause-level categories of Stage III: Questions

Questions				Gloss
VQ(mI)X	Yakış-tı	mı	gözlük?	'Do the glasses suit?'
	'suit-PAST	Q	glasses'	
XQY	Bun-lar	ne böyle?		'What are all these?'
	'Pro-PL	Qwh these'		
QXY	Ne	gelmiş	buraya?	'What came here?'
	'Qwh	come-EVD	here'	

Phrase-level categories of Stage III

Ekmekçi and Can (2000) reported evidence from the period between 1;7 and 2;4 which shows that children pay attention to restrictions on the syntactic positions of constituents within sentences and phrases, displaying awareness of the head-final property of Turkish. In noun phrases, modifiers precede the head noun (e.g. Adj + N *küçük araba* 'small car', and Relative Clause + N *ağlayan bebek* 'crying baby' (2;3)). Similarly, complements are positioned before the verb both in verb phrases (e.g. *yüz-ünü kapatmış* (1;11)) and in adjunct phrases (e.g. N + ABL *elin-den yedi* (1;11)) (Aksu-Koç, 2010). Our data supported these findings. Thus the relevant structures are placed in TR-LARSP. The examples are shown in Table 15.15.

Pronoun use in Turkish is a marked option because the subject is indicated by agreement-marking on the verb. Initially children avoid the subject

Table 15.14 Clause-level categories of Stage III: Statements

Statem	S	O	C	V	Extra information	Word	Gloss
SOC	Anne 'Mom'	o dolap 'that cupboard'	çok güzel 'very beautiful'		VP=S+A+V		'Mummy that cupboard is very beautiful'
OOindV		gözlüğümü 'glass-POSS-ACC'		takıp da 'put-Ip' da (conn)	Derivational suffix) -lık (ğ)		'I will put my glasses on to see'
(S)OVV	(ben) 'I'	seni 'you-ACC'		öp-mek 'kiss-V' gör-e-yim 'see-OPT-1S' isti-yor-um 'want-PROG-1S'	(s): Null subject	-mEk	'I want to kiss you'
				çarp-ış-mış-lar 'crash-REF-EVD-PL3'	-Iş = reflexive	-Iş	'They have crashed'
	O	A	V				
OAV	(S)	bu-na 'here-DAT'	dışarda 'outside-LOC'	bin-iyor-um 'ride-PROG-1S'	(S): Null subject		'I ride this outside'
	A	O	V				
AOV	(S)	Boynu-na 'neck-POSS'	atkı 'scarf'	tak-mış 'put-PASTEVI-3S'	(S): Null subject		'She put a scarf around her neck'
		baba-nın 'father'+GEN kitab-ı 'book'-POSS	burda 'here'	var 'exist'	(O)= noun + noun		'Here is father's book' The father's book is here

Table 15.15 Phrase-level categories of Stage III

	N	N	Dem	DAdv	Adj	N	Extra Info	Gloss
IntAdj				çok 'very'	güzel 'beautiful'		AdjP = degree adv+ adj	'Very beautiful'
Det, AdjN			bu 'this'		büyük 'big'	uçak 'plane'	NP=Det+Adj+ noun	'This is a big plane'
ProN	benim 'I-GEN1S'	bisiklet-im 'bike-POSS1S'						'My bike'
ProNPr	bizim 'we-GEN1PL'	arabamız 'car-POSS1PL'				gibi 'like'	PP=Gen Pro+N+ PPparticle	'Like our car'
Pron Adj	benim-ki 'IGEN1S-ki'				büyük 'big'		Possessive Pro+-ki +Adj	'Mine is big'
NN Adj	Ayşe-nin 'Ayşe-GEN'	saçları 'hair-POSS3PL'			kısa 'short'		NP=N+N+Adj	'Ayşe's hair is short'

when it can be recovered from the context, displaying an awareness of the pragmatic use of the null-subject option. They use null subjects in subject position, then they use full NPs and overt pronouns are less frequent (Topbaş & Özcan, 1997).

Stage IV (2;7–3;0)

During this fourth stage, children begin using complex syntactic structures that involve coordinate, adverbial, complement and relative clauses. These constructions emerge in the context of discourse with adults. Through the use of non-finite verb forms, subordinate clauses lose their canonical sentential forms and call for processing strategies that are different from those that apply to simple sentences (Aksu-Koç, 2010). Children, therefore, have difficulty in producing these constructions, particularly if the discourse genre is demanding. Thus, existing strategies are revised to accommodate the new structures.

At this stage, sentences characteristically contain four or more elements. Connectivity is found, combining two independent clauses with conjunctions. It appears that children begin using connectors productively around 2;6, with the particle *işte* 'there' and another emphatic particle, *-dA*. However, coordination is not only a way of combining clauses but is also a way of combining phrasal categories such as NP and NP, AdvP and AdvP, VP and VP, N and N in an NP and PP and PP. Such structures were rare at this stage.

The temporal connectives *sonra* 'then', *ondan sonra* 'after that' and the cause–effect connectives *için* 'for' and *onun için* 'that's why' are the most frequent ones observed in utterances. Coordinating conjunction *ve* 'and'

Table 15.16 Clause-level categories of Stage IV: Connectivity

STAGE IV	Conn	
	c *ve, da, ama*	Hiç bu gitmiyo ama
	onun için, sonra, ondan sonra	('but this never goes')
	s *V+Ip* 'having + V + ed'	Kuş koymak için
	V+mAk için	('to put birds in')
	V+IncA 'when / cause'	El sokmak için
		('to put hands in')

Table 15.17 Clause-level categories of Stage IV: Commands and questions

Comm	Quest
+S	QXY+
Git burdan dedim!	Ne var içinde?
V A V	Q X Y
'I said leave!'	'What is in it?'
	SOV+Q(mI)
	(*Sen bize gelcek misin?*)
	('Are you coming to us?')

is rarely used to connect only two elements. The conjunction *ama* 'but' appears around 3;0, as seen in Table 15.16.

A major difference between Turkish and English in connectivity is that, in English, the two clauses preserve their canonical form, and subordination is realized by the use of conjunctions in adverbial clauses. However, in Turkish, coordination can also be formed by subordination with adverbial clauses. This type of subordinate clause usage is marked as subordinate by the use of 's' in the TR-LARSP chart and has been shown under both connectivity and clauses columns, as is illustrated subsequently.

Children begin using the negative particles properly: *hiç* 'never' and *değil* 'not' for negative meanings. They can use the negative suffix /-mA/ with *hiç* to form a grammatical sentence as well in Question forms (see Table 15.17).

The clause-level categories of Stage IV

Unlike English, complex sentences with a subordinate clause undergo a number of syntactic operations such that surface form does not reflect underlying meaning in a transparent fashion as it does in simple structures (Aksu-Koç, 2010). Hence, complex sentences pose problems (see Tables 15.18 and 15.19).

In the third example in Table 15.18, the subordinate clause contains one adverbial. Because of this we marked it as *Subord A 1*. Converbs[4]

Table 15.18 Clause-level categories of Stage IV: Statements

		Extra information:
Neg (Hiç)	Hiç bu gitmiyo ama 'This isn't ever going'	git-mi-yo(r) V $_{neg}$ PROG
Neg(değil)	Diş macunu değil 'This isn't toothpaste'	
(Selin 3;0)	**Subord A 1** Sarı yanınca hazır oluyorsun. 'You have get ready when the yellow lights are on'	yan-ınca V CONV – light-CONV
SOdAV	Burcu beni pat dövdü S O$_d$ A V 'Burcu hit me suddenly pat' *(pat* is a symbolic voice of hitting someone suddenly)	
(Arzu 2;9)	Ağzı-mız kirlen-diği zaman yıka-rız A V 'When our mouth gets dirty, we wash it'	A=N+[V+dIk-I]+N
AO(O=XY+N)V	Ucunda *uzun bir iğne* var A O V 'There is a long needle on the top of it'	
S(S=Pron+N)cV	*Bizim Can* da uyudu S s V 'Our Can slept too'	S= ProP+N

most typically observed at this stage are V+*IncE* 'when/cause' expressing sequence / contingency and V+*Ip* 'having V+ed' expressing a sequential relation with the action denoted by the main verb as a background or precondition. Although V+*Ip* had emerged at the preceding stage, it is more frequently used at this stage. In previous studies (Aksu-Koç, 1994; Topbaş & Özcan, 1995) these structures were found to be absent in three-year-old children's narratives. However, in our data there were several instances of usage during conversational discourse within a picture-description play situation, as in the following example from Utku (3;0):

Sonra bi tane kırmızı yan-ıyo, hemen dur-uyo-sun   O = Det + Adj
Coord   O   V   A   V
Later one red burn-PROG immediately stop-PROG-2S
'Later, a red light turns on, you stop immediately'

Table 15.19 Clause-level categories of Stage IV: Complex sentences

Relative Clause	çarpış-an 'crush-SREL (crushing)'	otomobil 'automobile'		'Crushing car'
ProN	Benim ki de 'I-GEN-ki conn'	oldu Ol-PAST Be-PAST Aux 'happen'		'Mine is done too'
ProN	senin-ki-ler 'your-GEN-ki-PL' 'yours'	yasak 'forbidden'	değil 'not' Neg	'Yours are not forbidden'
SV	ben	salla-(y)-a-ma-m ki 'swing-POT-NEG-1S'		'I couldn't swing'
AVS (inverted sentence)	ağaçtan ağaç-ABL 'from tree'	düşecek düş-FUT 'will fall'	çocuk 'kid'	'The kid will fall from the tree'
OPostposition	bizim 'our' O: Pronp+N	lambamız lamba-POSS-1PL 'lamp'	gibi 'like'	'Like our lamp'
Oneg	ateşim ateş-POSS 'my fever'	yok Neg		'I don't have fever'

<u>Sarı yan-ınca hemen hazır ol-uyo-sun</u>
  A   c   V
Yellow burn-IncA right away ready be-PROG-2S
'When the light turns yellow, immediately you get ready'

V = compound verb
A = Adj + N(V + Inca)

<u>Yeşil yan-ınca geç-iyo-sun</u>
  A   V
Green burn-IncA pass-PROG-2S
'When the light turns green, you pass'

    Towards the end of this stage, some of the adverbial clauses formed by nominalized forms of the verb (V+ *[-mE/-mEk/-DIK]* + a postposition (*e.g. için* 'for', *zaman* 'time', *sonra* 'after')) begin to emerge in response to questions within conversation. These structures are recorded both in clause and phrase level, as well as in connectivity.
    The infinitival noun complements with *-mAk* with the desire verb *iste-* 'want' also appear. In *-mAk* complements the subject of the embedded clause is coreferential with that of the main clause, yielding syntactically

simpler constructions. Although -*mA* and -*DIK* both appear with genitive subjects, -*mA* is earlier. Subject complements with -*mA* nonverbal predicate appear around 2;8, and later object complements with -*mA* (which may or may not be the same as subject constructions) are observed. The -*DIK* and -*EcEk* noun complements appear around 3;0 but pose problems, particularly with the irregular verb *ol-* 'be', which is an auxiliary verb required in the embedding of sentences with nonverbal predicates.

As explained in the preceding sections, Turkish relative clauses are not transparent, and are not canonical in form, which results in difficulties for comprehension and production by young children. Furthermore, relative clauses are constructed in a non-uniform way across different types of relativization. Therefore, the child has to figure out the grammatical role the relativized noun plays in the subordinate clause from the relativizer used (subject if -*En* or -*DAki*, nonsubject if -*DIK*) and the grammatical role it plays in the matrix sentence (SS and SO if the subject, and OS and OO if the object) from the case-marking in the matrix clause.

Phrase-level categories of Stage IV

Table 15.20 illustrates the newly appearing categories at phrase level for Stage IV. These include phrasal coordination of both simple and complex items, the use of auxiliary verbs and pronouns with auxiliaries.

Stage V (3;1–3;6)

Stage V is generally formed from the more complex structures of Stage IV. The most frequent connectors are *çünkü* 'because' and *ve* 'and'. Other connectors are *ya da* 'or' and *ama* 'but'.

While the construction of inflectional paradigms does not pose a learning problem, given their extreme regularity, using them in appropriate sentence frames in appropriate contexts rests on a more protracted process of learning. What has been observed shows that, very early in development, morphological processes are applied in a rule-governed way.

In Turkish, complex sentences with a subordinate clause undergo a number of syntactic operations such that surface form does not reflect underlying meaning in a transparent fashion, as it does in simple structures. Hence complex sentences pose problems and need the scaffolding adults provide in discourse. Later acquisitions involve coordinate, adverbial, complement and relative clause constructions that emerge in the context of discourse with adults as the child becomes socially and communicatively more competent (see Table 15.21).

The aorist inflection -*Ir*, which presents much morphophonological variation, is not fully mastered until the age of seven.

Table 15.20 Phrase-level categories of Stage IV

PHRASE		
XcX		
O da kapı		
'That is a door too'		
XcXY		
Pamuk ve yedi cüceler		
'Snow and the seven dwarves'		
XYc		
kuş koymak için		
'To put birds in'		
El sokmak için		
'To put your hands in'		
Aux		O*lmak* ('be') is an auxiliary verb.
Hazır oluyorsun	N 'be'	In this example, *hazır* ('ready') is
'You are getting ready'	hazır ol-mak	compounding with *olmak*.
Pron Aux N		
Bizim başımıza geldi bunlar		
'These have happened to us'		

Table 15.21 Categories of Stage V

STAGE V	Conn	CLAUSE		PHRASE	
		Comm Quest	State		
	c	**XY+(mI)**	Coord	1	
		(*Bana iki kilo süt verir misin?*)			
		('Can you give me 2 kg of milk?')			
	s	**XY+değil+Q(mI)**	Subord	1	+1
		(*Merdiven gibi çıktım değil mi?*)			
		('I climb like stairs, don't I?')			
		Other			

Conclusion

In this study, a pilot analysis of data sampled from 20 Turkish-speaking children aged between 0;9 and 3;6 was used to adapt a Turkish version of LARSP. It was found that TR-LARSP comprehensively represented the children's language acquisition. This preliminary analysis is a first step towards the development of an assessment and remediation tool for language impairments. It is hoped that when the stages of TR-LARSP are fully finalized, age norms can be developed for contrastive analysis both within and across languages, and will be a useful tool for the field of

VERBAL INFLECTIONS

STAGE	TENSE				ASPECT		MOOD					COP	COMB	V(+)=V	V(+)=N
	P		AOR	FUT	PF	IMPF	IMP	OBLG	POT	COND	EVID	-IDI			
	-DI	-mIş	-r	-AcAk	-DI -mIş	-Iyor-(DI) -IDI -Ir-(DI) -mAkDA- (DIR)	-In -Ø	-mAlı	-AbIl	-sA	-mIş				
STAGE I	+	+		+		+(-Iyor)	+(Ø)								
STAGE II			+						+						
STAGE III											+		AcAk+mIş		-Ip
STAGE IV															
STAGE V											+				

VERBAL INFLECTIONS

STAGE	CAUS						PASS			REF	REC	NEG	QUEST	PL
	-DIr	-t	-It	-Ir	-Ar	-Art	-n	-In	-Il	-(I)n	-(I)ş	-mA		
STAGE I									+ (middle)			+	+	+
STAGE II		+		+										
STAGE III									+			+		
STAGE IV							+							
STAGE V														

NOMINAL INFLECTIONS

STAGE	CASE					PLURAL	POSS						QUEST	INSTR			DERIVATIONAL SUFFIXES		CONJ	NEG
	ACC	DAT	ABL	GEN	LOC	-lAr	1S	2S	3S	1P	2P	3P	-mI	Wh	-(y)lA/ile	-ki(n)	N(+)=N	N(+)=V	dA	(değil)
STAGE I	+	+	+			+	+	+					+						+(Pron+dA) (DEM+dA)	+
STAGE II				+					+					+	+					
STAGE III										+	+					ı				
STAGE IV																	-IncA		N+II	
STAGE V																				

Figure 15.2 TR-LARSP-m Profile: Morphological development

speech and language pathology and clinical linguistics to facilitate better assessment and treatment processes in Turkey.

Notes

(1) Readers will note that stages VI and VII on the TR-LARSP chart are currently blank. It is hoped to complete these in due course after further research.
(2) The use of capital letters in this and other affixes illustrates vowel consonant harmony in Turkish. For example, I for /i, cu, u, y/ (high vowels), and E, for /e, a/; Capital D represents /d/ or /t/ the vowel that is actually realized depends on the vowels of the stem.
(3) The tables illustrating structures at different stages generally contain more information than we retain in the TR-LARSP charts shown as Figures 15.1 and 15.2. This is done for illustrative purposes.
(4) Converbs are 'derived from verbs and carry out functions of adverbial linking or conjoining between clauses' (Slobin, 1995: 349).

References

Aksu-Koç, A. (1994) Development of linguistic forms: Turkish. In R. Berman and D. Slobin (eds) *Relating Events in Narrative: A Crosslinguistic Developmental Study* (pp. 329–388). Hillsdale, NJ: Erlbaum.

Aksu-Koç, A. (1997) Verb inflection in Turkish: a preliminary analysis of the early stage. In U. W. Dressler (ed.) *Studies in Pre- and Proto-Morphology (pp. 127–39)*. Vienna: Verlag Der Österreichischen Akademie der Wissenschaften.

Aksu-Koc, A. (2010) The course of normal language development in Turkish. In S. Topbas and M. Yavaş (eds) *Communication Development and Disorders* (pp. 65–103). Bristol: Multilingual Matters.

Çapan, S. (1988) Acquisition of verbal inflections by Turkish children: A case study. *Studies on Turkish Linguistics* (pp. 275–288). Ankara: Middle East Technical University.

Crystal, D., Fletcher, P. and Garman, M. (1989) *The Grammatical Analysis of Language Disability* (2nd edn). London: Cole & Whurr.

Ekmekci, Ö. and Can, C. (2000) Head parameter setting in the acquisition of Turkish as a first language. In A. Göksel and C. Kerslake (eds) *Studies on Turkish and Turkic Languages* (pp. 275–86). Wiesbaden: Harrassowitz Verlag.

Erguvanlı-Taylan, E. (1984) *The Function of Word Order in Turkish Grammar*. Berkeley: University of California.

Göksel, A. and Kerslake, C. (2005) *Turkish: A Comprehensive Grammar*. London: Routledge

Ketrez, F.N. and Aksu-Koç, A. (2009) Early nominal morphology in Turkish: Emergence of case and number. In U. Stephany and M. Voeykova (eds) *Development of Noun Inflection in First Language Acquisition: A Cross-Linguistic Perspective*. Berlin: Mouton de Gruyter.

Kornfilt, J. (1997) *Turkish Grammar*. London: Routledge.

Özcan, F.H. and Topbaş, S. (2000) The structural and semantic analysis of verbs in the acquisition of Turkish. *Current Research in Language and Communication Science* 1, 57–67.

Radford, A. (1990) *Syntactic Theory and the Acquisition of English Syntax*. Oxford: Blackwell.

Slobin, D. (1995) Converbs in Turkish child language: The grammaticalization of event coherence. In M. Haspelmath and E. König (eds) *Converbs in Cross-Linguistic Perspective* (pp. 349–71). Berlin: Mouton de Gruyter.

Topbaş, S. and Özcan H. (1995) Anlatılarda bağlaç kullanımı: Normal ve özel eğitim gereksinimli öğrenciler arasında bir karşılaştırma. *IX. Dilbilim Kurultayı Bildiriler Kitabı*. Bolu: Abant İzzet Baysal University.

Topbaş, S. and Özcan, F.H. (1997) Pronominals and their pragmatic functions in the acquisition of Turkish. In K. İmer and E. Uzun (eds) *Proceedings of the VIIIth International Conference on Turkish Linguistics* (pp. 139–48). Ankara: Dil Tarih-Coğrafya Fakültesi.

Topbaş, S., Maviş, I., and Başal, M. (1997) Acquisition of bound morphemes: Nominal case morphology in Turkish. In K. Imer and N.E. Uzun (eds) *Proceedings of the VIIIth International Conference on Turkish Linguistics* (pp. 127–37). Ankara: Dil Tarih-Coğrafya Fakültesi.

Turan, Ü.D. (2006) Chapters 9–12. In Z. Balpınar (ed.) *Turkish Phonology, Morphology and Syntax*. Eskişehir: Anadolu University Publishing.

Underhill, R. (1972) Turkish participles. *Linguistic Inquiry* 3, 87–99.

Yavaş, M. (2010) Some structural characteristics of Turkish. In S. Topbas and M. Yavaş (eds) *Communication Development and Disorders* (pp. 48–65). Bristol: Multilingual Matters.

Subject Index

The alphabetical arrangement of the index is letter-by-letter. Grammatical terms and abbreviatons in LARSP charts are not indexed

accuracy 37, 41, 233, 236
acronyms 8, 110, 165
adjective constructions
  Bengali 140, 143–6
  Chinese 211–18, 223
  Dutch 95, 97–8, 107
  French 231, 233, 238–9
  Frisian 191, 199, 203–4
  German 81–2, 84–5, 88
  Hebrew 44–5, 53–4, 58, 60, 64–6, 71
  Irish 158, 162, 163–5
  Persian 170–71, 182, 186
  Spanish 246–8, 252, 255, 275–6
  Turkish 285–97, 301
  Welsh 111–13, 120, 127–8, 130
adverb constructions
  Bengali 140, 142–6, 151
  Chinese 211–12, 219, 225
  Dutch 97, 102, 106
  French 231, 234
  Frisian 190, 192, 199–203
  German 84
  Hebrew 48, 53–4, 60–61, 63–5, 67–8, 70–71
  Irish 157, 160
  Persian 169, 178–9, 181–2
  Spanish 246, 248–50, 252–5, 268–71, 273, 275–6
  Turkish 285–6, 290–302, 305
  Welsh 121
African languages 3
agreement
  Frisian 203
  German 79, 81–4, 88
  Hebrew 44–5, 48, 51–4, 62–6, 75
  Persian 176, 185
  Spanish 245, 249, 261, 272, 280
  Turkish 283, 285, 293–4, 296
  Welsh 113
alternating verbs 15–17, 26
American Speech-Language-Hearing Association (ASHA) 41
aphasia 6
argument
  internal vs external 15
  structure 15–20, 84, 89, 112
aspect
  Bengali 140
  Chinese 210, 219
  Frisian 232
  Hebrew 45, 53, 65
  Irish 157–61, 169
  Persian 173
  Spanish 246
  Turkish 287, 293
  Welsh 117–23, 130
auxiliary verbs (Aux) 7–8, 21–2, 31–2, 47
  Bengali 140
  Chinese 225
  Dutch 97, 100, 103
  French 231–4, 237–8, 242
  Frisian 190, 202–3
  German 80–82, 84–5, 88
  Hebrew 55–6
  Irish 157–61
  Persian 172–3, 175, 177, 180–81, 185–6

Spanish   249, 251, 256, 260–61, 272
Turkish   301–3
Welsh   119–25, 138

Bengali LARSP   2, 139–48
bilingualism
  Frisian   189, 196
  Irish   150, 156
  Persian   167
  Welsh   110–12, 115, 131–3
borrowing   131–3, 282

Cantonese   3
case histories   10
caseloads   7, 38–9
case studies   8, 86–9, 96, 99, 102–7, 195
causative-inchoative   18–19
CHILDES   5, 43, 168, 233, 251, 277
child language studies   4–5, 10, 12, 71, 78–9, 93, 98–101, 112–15, 193, 208, 220–23
Chinese
  grammar outline   210–17
  LARSP (C-LARSP)   2, 208–29
Clause Element Index   194, 206
clause structure   4–5, 7, 15–26, 31–2
  Bengali   141–6
  Chinese   209–19, 223–5, 230
  Dutch   95–8
  French   237–40, 242
  Frisian   189–91, 193, 198–206
  German   77–81, 84–6, 88, 93–8, 106
  Hebrew   46–54, 56, 59–72
  Irish   153–61
  Persian   176–84
  Spanish   247–8, 252–69, 272–6
  Turkish   283–303
  Welsh   115–19, 121, 123–4, 130, 132, 137
clinical linguistics   6–7
clitics

French   230, 241
Frisian   192
Hebrew   45
Irish   154–7
Spanish   256, 261
Turkish   282, 295
code-mixing/switching
  Chinese   226
  Irish   154
  Welsh   115, 131–3, 137
commands   34
  Bengali   141–2
  Chinese   210, 223–5
  Dutch   95–6
  French   233
  Frisian   194, 196–7
  German   80
  Hebrew   54, 57–60
  Irish   153–4, 156, 159–61
  Persian   173–6, 178–81
  Spanish   251–66, 268–9
  Turkish   290–92, 296, 299
  Welsh   117, 120, 123–4, 137
Communicative Development Inventory   150
comparatives
  Chinese   225–6
  Hebrew   68
  Irish   164
  Persian   182, 187
  Spanish   248, 266, 275–6
  Welsh   128
complementation   7, 23–4
  Chinese   211–15, 225
  Dutch   95, 97 107
  French   238–40
  Frisian   190, 202
  German   80–81, 85, 88
  Hebrew   48, 51, 53, 59, 61, 65, 67–70, 72
  Irish   158, 160
  Persian   170–71, 176, 182–3, 185–6
  Spanish   252, 269
  Turkish   285–7, 296, 301–2
  Welsh   117, 120, 124, 130

complex sentences 7, 13, 22–6, 39, 67, 137, 142, 211, 243, 249, 261–8, 273, 294, 300–303
comprehensiveness 1, 10, 25, 41, 77–8, 115, 153, 162–4, 208–9, 303
computerized profiling 30–42, 90, 230–43
connectivity 23–4
　Bengali 146
　Chinese 225
　Dutch 97–8, 106
　Frisian 193–4, 202–4
　German 79, 81, 84–8
　Hebrew 48, 51–2, 56, 59, 64–5, 67–70, 72
　Irish 161
　Persian 173, 181–3
　Spanish 247–8, 260, 263–78
　Turkish 285–7, 298–303
　Welsh 117, 120–1, 123, 137
construction, defined 48
control, clinical 11
converbs 305
COPROF 77–91
copula (Cop)
　Bengali 140
　Dutch 97, 100, 103, 106–7
　French 232, 234, 238, 242
　Frisian 199
　German 84, 88
　Hebrew 47, 48, 50–53, 58–9, 61, 64, 66
　Irish 152, 158–60, 162
　Persian 168, 171–2, 176, 179, 185
　Spanish 253–65, 272
　Turkish 287
　Welsh 120, 121, 124–5, 130, 138
CORPUS module 30–31

Danish LARSP 2
definiteness 45–6, 51–2
　Bengali 140
　Dutch 98
　French 231
　Frisian 191, 196, 199–205
　Hebrew 58, 61–3, 65, 71, 72
　Irish 152, 160
　Persian 169–70, 184, 186
　Spanish 246
　Turkish 283, 286, 293
　Welsh 112–13, 125, 127, 129, 133
deixis 57–9, 125
description, importance of 10
determiners
　Bengali 140, 142, 144
　Chinese 217
　Dutch 95, 97
　French 231, 237, 239, 241
　Frisian 191
　German 79, 81–2, 88
　Hebrew 44
　Persian 177, 183–4
　Spanish 246–7, 249, 252, 255, 260, 280
　Turkish 286, 290
　Welsh 112, 121–3, 127, 130
development, importance of 10
diagnosis 7–8
diminutives 95, 106–7, 162, 191, 196, 199, 256
discourse 10
dislocations in French 232
Dutch LARSP 2, 92–109, 189
　compared to Frisian 205–6

ellipsis 50
　Bengali 142
　Chinese 210
　German 82, 88
　Hebrew 67–9, 210
　Irish 158–9
　Persian 168
　Turkish 284
　Welsh 119, 137
endocentric constructions in Chinese 212, 216
end-weighting 20

Subject Index

errors 14, 18, 32
  Chinese 225–6
  German 88
  Hebrew 50–52, 61, 63, 65–6, 69, 72
  Irish 161, 164
  Persian 184
  Spanish 270–72, 279
  Turkish 292, 293
  Welsh 114, 116, 119, 123–8, 130
ESGRAF 90
existential constructions
  Hebrew 46–8, 52, 55, 61
  Persian 184
  Turkish 283
expansion 4, 20–21
  French 234
  Hebrew 53, 58–60, 63, 65–6, 70
  Irish 158–9
  Persian 178–80
  Spanish 251, 253–63, 266, 279, 280
  Turkish 292, 294–5
  Welsh 123

Farsi *see* Persian
faultlines 12
finiteness 21–2, 71–2, 79–81, 84–6, 140, 189–92, 199, 247, 298
F-LARSP 230–44
French
  grammar outline 230–32
  LARSP 2, 230–44
Frisian LARSP 2, 189–207
  compared to Dutch 205–6

Gaelic *see* Irish
genitive *see* possessive
German LARSP 2, 77–91
Giriama LARSP 2
gradual nature of development 12, 14
GRAMAT 92–109
grammar, centrality 5–7, 14, 78
Greek LARSP 3

hardware 30
harmony in Turkish 287, 304
Hebrew
  grammar outline 44–8
  LARSP (HARSP) 1, 2, 43–76
Hungarian LARSP 2–3

ILARSP 149–66
imperatives *see* commands
indefinite *see* definiteness
individual differences 17, 56
inflections *see* morphology
insight, clinical 10–11
interaction 7–10, 32, 34, 48, 168, 221, 236, 262, 282
interrogatives *see* questions
intransitives *see* transitivity
Irish LARSP 2, 149–66, 173, 185
  grammar outline 151–2
Italian 3

Japanese LARSP 2, 3

key features
  Bengali 142–8
  Chinese 209
  Korean 3

language acquisition *see* child language studies
language vs speech 8
LARSP background
  approaches compared 2
  as state of mind 10
  choice of acronym 8
  developmental issues 2
  functions 7, 10
  history 4–11
  second edition 10
  structure of the chart 8–9
  thirty years on 12–28
LARSP chart illustrations 16
  Bengali 147
  Chinese 224

Computerized Profiling 36
Dutch 95, 96, 103–5, 109
French 242
Frisian 197–205
German 83, 87
Hebrew 74–6
Irish 154
Persian 174
Spanish 278
Turkish 288
Welsh 118, 126, 129
larsping 1
LLARSP 110–38
  –C vs –M vs –T 116

MacArthur-Bates Communicative Development Inventory 13, 252
major sentences 22, 49, 51–2, 79, 82, 84–5, 117, 137, 142, 151, 156, 173, 193–5, 207, 210, 237, 252
Malay LARSP 3
Mandarin *see* Chinese
mean length of utterance (MLU) 12, 24, 34, 38, 81–2, 88–9, 95, 99, 102–6, 141–3, 150, 223, 237, 243, 277, 289, 290
minor sentences 4, 32, 49–50, 99, 102–5, 117, 137, 156, 193, 237, 252
modal verbs 22, 32
  French 238
  Frisian 199, 201–2
  German 81, 82, 84
  Hebrew 53, 60, 65
  Persian 172–3, 175, 180, 185
  Welsh 122
morphology 2, 7, 21–2, 31–2
  Bengali 140
  Chinese 219
  French 231–3
  Frisian 190–91, 200
  German 78–9, 84

Hebrew 44–8, 51–4, 59–60, 63–4, 66–9, 71
Irish 151, 153, 162–4
Persian 171–80, 184–7
Spanish 250, 254–6, 260–61, 266
Turkish 282–3, 287, 292–4, 301–2
Welsh 116, 124–33, 137
morphophonology *see* phonology
mutation
  Irish 2, 151–2, 159, 163–4
  Welsh 2, 112–16, 120, 122–4, 128–31

narrative analysis in Spanish 272–8
negation (Neg) 19–20, 32, 39
  Bengali 140, 143, 145–7
  Chinese 212, 215
  French 231, 238, 242
  Frisian 190, 193–200
  German 80–82, 86, 88–9
  Hebrew 46–7, 54–5, 60–62, 66, 71
  Irish 151–62
  Persian 168–9, 172, 175–6, 180, 185
  Spanish 249, 253–63, 266, 275, 280
  Turkish 287–4, 296–301
  Welsh 117, 119–20, 123–5, 127, 138
non-finite *see* finiteness
Norwegian LARSP 2
noun phrases (NP) 7, 15, 19–21, 23
  Bengali 140, 142–5
  Chinese 216–19, 225
  Dutch 97
  French 232, 240, 242
  Frisian 191, 203–4
  German 79, 81, 84, 88
  Hebrew 45, 52–3, 60–71
  Irish 150, 159, 161, 163
  Persian 169, 170, 177, 178, 180, 183, 186–7
  Spanish 245, 247, 263, 272, 280

Turkish 283, 285–7, 294–6, 298–9
Welsh 119, 123–5, 127, 138

oral skills 78
Other, as a category 7
overregularizations in Spanish 261

Panjabi LARSP 3
particles
  Bengali 140
  Chinese 218–19, 225
  Dutch 193–4
  Hebrew 46–7, 52, 55
  German 81, 84
  Irish 151, 152, 157, 162, 164
  Spanish 252, 260, 262
  Turkish 284–5, 292–3, 298–9
  Welsh 120, 123–4, 130
passives
  Chinese 212, 214
  Hebrew 45, 69, 71
  Persian 183, 186
  Spanish 246, 249, 271
  Turkish 287, 291
  Welsh 123
Persian
  grammar outline 169–73
  LARSP 2, 167–88
PERSL 245–81
phonology 8, 29–30, 44–5, 52, 72, 116, 128, 131, 133, 139, 150–2, 231, 241, 287, 302
phrase structure 7, 20, 31–2
  Bengali 141–6
  Chinese 216–19, 225
  Dutch 97–8
  French 237–40
  Frisian 199–203
  German 84
  Hebrew 53, 63, 65–6, 68, 70–71
  Irish 159–60
  Persian 170, 176–80
  Spanish 252–60, 266, 269, 276–7

Turkish 290, 293, 296, 298, 302–3
Welsh 120–23
P-LARSP 167–88
Portuguese 3
possessive constructions
  Bengali 142
  Chinese 219
  Dutch 97–8, 106–7
  Frisian 191, 200, 203
  German 79, 84
  Hebrew 44, 46–8, 52, 55, 60–61, 63, 65
  Irish 152, 163
  Persian 170–71, 177–8, 184–5
  Spanish 246
  Turkish 285, 287, 293, 298
  Welsh 111, 113, 122, 130
postpositions 140, 142, 283, 285–7, 301
pragmatics 10, 49, 54, 57, 283–4, 292, 298
prepositions 7, 15, 26
  Chinese 212, 216
  Dutch 97–8
  French 238–40
  Frisian 192, 204
  German 79, 81–2, 84
  Hebrew 46, 48, 52–4, 57, 60, 62–3, 65–6, 68–70, 72
  Irish 151, 157, 160, 163
  Persian 169, 170, 179, 184, 186
  Spanish 246–7, 255, 266, 274–5, 279
  Turkish 283, 286
  Welsh 120–22, 125, 127, 129, 130
PRISM 18, 29, 132
pro-drop 140, 142, 167, 169, 177
professionalism 11
profiles 8, 29–30
  vs tests 7
pronouns 14, 23, 25, 30–31
  Bengali 140
  Chinese 211, 213–15, 217
  Dutch 95, 97–8, 106–7

French 231–4, 237, 239, 241
Frisian 191–2, 195–8, 200–205
German 79, 84, 86, 88
Hebrew 48, 50, 52–4, 57, 59, 61–64, 66, 68, 70–72
Irish 157, 160, 162
Persian 169–71, 177–8, 180, 184–5
Spanish 245–7, 249–50, 252, 255–6, 259, 261, 264–6, 276
Turkish 283, 285, 287–90, 296–7, 302
Welsh 113–14, 122, 127, 130
PROP 29
PROPH 29

questions 7, 9–10, 14, 19, 34, 39
Bengali 140–6
Chinese 210, 215–16, 223–5
Dutch 97–8, 106
French 230–31, 237
Frisian 190, 193–4, 196–7, 200–205
German 78, 80, 82, 84, 86, 89
Hebrew 47, 50, 54, 55–9, 62, 64, 68, 72
Irish 151–62
Persian 169, 172, 173, 175–6, 179, 180
Spanish 246, 249–52, 254–9, 261–6, 268–9
Turkish 284–5, 289, 292–3, 295–6, 299
Welsh 117, 120–21, 123, 124–7, 130, 137
Quirk grammar 11, 20, 21, 29, 169, 209
Quirk Report 4, 7

relative constructions 23–5
French 230, 233, 239
Hebrew 48, 63, 67–8, 70
Spanish 246–7, 268–9, 276
Turkish 283, 285–6, 298, 301–2
Welsh 123
remediation *see* therapy
responses 7, 9–10, 19
Bengali 142
Frisian 198
German 78, 82, 88
Hebrew 49–50, 64, 72
Irish 162
Spanish 252, 273
Turkish 284, 289
Welsh 125, 127, 137
Reynell Developmental Language Scales 102
Royal Berkshire Hospital 4
Russian LARSP 3

samples of language 34, 78, 86, 93, 141, 150, 168, 192–4, 206–7, 220–23, 236, 282
school vs clinic 7
screening 7–8
semantic bootstrapping 15
sentence 6–7
  vs utterance 48
shortcuts 40
sociolinguistic perspective 116
Spanish
  grammar outline 245–9
  LARSP 2, 245–81
speech acts 54–6
Stage I 17, 19
  Bengali 142–6
  Chinese 223
  Dutch 95
  French 237
  Frisian 198–9
  German 81
  Hebrew 56–8
  Irish 156
  Persian 175–6
  Spanish 251–2
  Turkish 287–90
  Welsh 117

Stage II 15–22
  Bengali 142–6
  Chinese 223–5
  Dutch 95
  French 237–40
  Frisian 199
  German 81, 85
  Hebrew 58–60
  Irish 156–9
  Persian 176–8
  Spanish 252–6
  Turkish 290–94
  Welsh 117
Stage III 15–22
  Bengali 142–6
  Chinese 225
  Dutch 95, 97
  French 237–40
  Frisian 199–201
  German 81, 85
  Hebrew 60–64
  Irish 159–60
  Persian 178–9
  Spanish 256–61
  Turkish 294–8
  Welsh 120
Stage IV
  Bengali 142–6
  Chinese 225
  Dutch 97
  French 238–40
  Frisian 201–2
  German 81, 85
  Hebrew 64–6
  Irish 160–61
  Persian 180–81
  Spanish 261–6
  Turkish 298–302
  Welsh 123
Stage V 22–5
  Chinese 225
  Dutch 98
  French 239, 243
  Frisian 202–3
  German 81, 85–6

Hebrew 67–9
Irish 161
Persian 181–3
Spanish 267–70
Turkish 302–3
Welsh 123
Stage VI 31
  Chinese 225
  Dutch 98
  French 243
  Frisian 203–4
  Hebrew 69–71
  Irish 161
  Persian 183–4
  Spanish 270–72
  Welsh 123
Stage VII
  Chinese 225
  French 243
  Frisian 204–5
  Irish 161
  Persian 184
  Spanish 272–8
  Welsh 124
statements 7, 14, 15, 19–20, 34
  Chinese 210, 215–16, 225–6
  Frisian 190, 194, 196–7, 201–2
  Hebrew 55, 57–8
  Irish 153–4, 157–8, 161
  Persian 173–80
  Spanish 252–8, 261–3, 267–8
  Turkish 289–90, 292–7, 300
  Welsh 117, 120–21, 123–5, 137
stereotypes 17, 156, 193, 198
subjectless constructions
  Bengali 140
  German 85–6, 88
  Hebrew 47, 52, 60, 65
  Persian 169
  Spanish 245
subjunctive in Spanish 79, 185, 246,
    248, 250–51, 255, 261, 275, 280
subordination *see* connectivity
Sylheti LARSP 2, 139–48
syntax vs morphology 7

TARSP 189–207
tense marking 21–2, 31
  Bengali 140–42
  Dutch 95, 97–8, 104–6
  French 231–2, 237, 241
  Frisian 190–91, 199, 202
  German 79
  Hebrew 45–7, 50, 52–5, 58–63, 66, 71, 72
  Irish 151, 156–7, 162
  Persian 171, 176–7, 185
  Spanish 260–61
  Turkish 283, 287, 290, 293
  Welsh 117, 119, 122, 125, 127
terminology
  Irish 150–51
  Welsh 116–17, 137
test vs profile 7
therapy 4–11, 29–42, 78, 89–90, 93, 102, 106–7, 128, 131, 140–41, 148, 150, 167, 175, 189, 198, 206–7, 209, 220–21, 241, 279, 283–4
time, therapeutic 6–9, 29–42, 90, 206–7, 227, 236, 241
transfer in bilingualism 115
transitivity 14–15, 17–19, 26
  Hebrew 45–6, 52–3, 62, 65, 67, 69, 72
  Irish 158
  Turkish 286
  Welsh 119
Turkish LARSP (TR-LARSP) 2, 282–305

utterance vs sentence 48

variability 12–13
valency 15, 32
verb forms and phrases 4–5, 7, 9–10, 14–24, 26, 31–3, 39
  Bengali 140–45
  Chinese 211–19, 223–5
  Dutch 95–8, 106–7
  French 230–34, 237–40
  Frisian 189–92, 198–205
  German 79–89
  Hebrew 44–72
  Irish 151–62, 164
  Persian 167, 169, 171–80, 183–6
  Spanish 245–66, 271–2. 274–5, 279–80
  Turkish 283, 286–304
  Welsh 112, 114–27, 130
verbless constructions 85–6, 176
vocabulary 5–6, 13–18, 54, 111, 113

Welsh LARSP 2, 110–38, 150, 152–3, 163, 169, 173, 175, 179, 185
word classes 72, 79, 81–2, 216
word order
  Bengali 140–41
  Chinese 225
  French 230–31
  Frisian 189–90, 198
  German 77, 80–81, 85
  Hebrew 48
  Irish 150–51, 153, 157–61
  Persian 169, 176, 184–5
  Spanish 245, 251, 256, 280
  Turkish 283–4, 292–3
  Welsh 114–15, 119–24

Author Index

Adams, C. 24
Aguado, G. 279
Aksu-Koç, A. 282, 289, 292, 296, 298, 299, 300
Albalá, M. J. 251
Andersen, R. W. 112
Ascott, F. 131
Awbery, G. M. 128

Baker, C. R. 111
Ball, M. J. 1–3, 110–38, 150, 151, 152, 153, 154, 162, 169, 173, 175, 179, 185, 223, 282–305
Bateni, M. 169, 170
Bates, E. 13
Behrenbeck, B. 90
Bellin, W. 128, 131
Bellugi, U. 176
Berman, R. A. 2, 43–76
Bertz, F. 90
Blasco-Dulbecco, M. 232
Bloom, L. 112
Boehm, J. 49, 251
Bol, G. W. 2, 92–109, 189, 230, 236
Botting, N. 222
Braine, M. 112
Brennan, S. 150
Brown, R. 5, 12, 162, 178, 184

Cameron, T. 150
Cameron-Faulkner, T. 150
Can, C. 296
Cangökçe-Yaşar, O. 282–305
Çapan, S. 289
Caselli, M. C. 112
Channell, R.W. 34
Chao, J. Z. 209
Chao, Y. R. 210, 212

Chen, Q. R. 208, 220
Cheung, H. 208
Chiat, S. 18
Chomsky, A.N. 14
Clahsen, H. 2, 77–91
Clark, E.V. 23, 112
Cobo-Lewis, A. 111
Codesidi-García, A.I. 245–81
Coloma C. J. 245–81
Cortazzi, M. 221
Cronbach, L.J. 206
Crystal, D. 1, 2, 4–11, 12, 14, 17, 18, 20, 24, 26, 29, 30, 31, 32, 34, 35, 38, 40, 43, 49, 77, 110, 120, 132–3, 151, 158, 162, 164, 175, 181, 184, 198, 220, 223, 251, 284

Dabir-Moghadam, M. 169
Dannenbauer, F. M. 89, 90
Darley, F. L. 207
De Houwer, A. 110
Deevy, P. 18
Diessel, H. 24, 25, 51
Dijkstra, J. E. 2, 189–207
Dodd, B. 110
Dorian, N. 113
Doroudian, M. 167
Dromi, E. 48
Dubois, J. 231
Dumez, M. 236, 243
Duncan, D. M. 139
Duranti, A. 221
Dykes, J. 24, 25

Eilers, R. E. 111
Eisenberg. S. 25
Ekmekci, Ö. 296
El Fenne, F. 231

Ellis Weismer, S. 18
Erbaugh, M. 208
Erguvanlı-Taylan, E. 283, 292

Farrokhpey, M. 169, 172
Fernández, M. 279
Fey, M. E. 39, 107
Flavell, J.H. 195
Fletcher, P. 1, 2, 6, 11, 12–28, 32, 110, 150, 208

Garayzábal-Heinze, E. 245–81
Garman, M. 1, 6, 43, 187
Gathercole, V. C. M. 111, 112, 163
Gavin, W. J. 2, 12–28, 279
Geerts G. 93
Genesee, F. 1153
Gladstone, M. 227
Göksel, A. 287
Goodluck, H. 150
Gorter, D. 189
Greenberg, J. 151
Greene, D. 151
Grosjean, F. 110, 111
Guo, Z. H. 209, 211, 212

Hadley, P. 18, 21, 22
Han, J. T. 209
Hansen, D. 2, 77–91
Hart, B. 13
Hayden, C. 150
Heidtmann, H. 90
Hesketh, A. 24
Hickey, T.M. 2, 150–66, 173, 185, 187
Hirsch, M. 43
Hsu, J. H. 208
Hua, Z. 110
Huang, B. R. 210, 211, 212
Huang, C J. 208
Huddleston, R. 26
Hunt, K. W. 93
Huttenlocher, J. 13
Hyams, N. 177

Jakubowicz, C. 241
Jimenez-Juliá, T. 279
Jin, L. 2, 208, 209, 221, 223
Johnson, B. W. 34
Johnson, J. S. 111
Jones, B. M. 113
Jones, G. 133
Jones, J. M. 115
Jones, R. M. 115, 119, 122, 124, 125
Jones, M. C. 113, 114
Jonkman, R.J. 189

Kail, M. 231
Kany, C. E. 261
Karimi, S. 169
Karmiloff-Smith, A. 72
Kershen, A. J. 139
Kerslake, C. 287
Ketrez, F.N. 288, 292
King, G. 18
Klee, T. 2, 12–28, 110, 279
Klooster, W. G. 93
Kornfilt, J. 292
Kuiken, F. 92, 106, 189, 230, 236

Labov, W. 223
Law, S 208

Leech, G.N. 21
Le Normand, M. T. 233, 235
Leonard, L.B. 18
Levin, B. 18, 26
Li, D. C. S. 111
Li, Y. A. 208, 210
Li, Y. M. 208, 220
Liao, X. D. 209, 211, 212
Lieven, E. 112
Locke, J. 187
Long, S.H. 2, 30–42
López Ornat, S. 252
Lu, F. B. 211
Lustigman, L. 2, 43–76

MacWhinney, B. 43, 71, 168, 233, 251

Maillart, C. 230–44, 279
Marchman, V.A. 111
Marinellie, S. 25
Marrero, V. 245–81
Mayberry, R. I. 111
McCabe, A. 222, 223
McCloskey, J. 158, 159
McKenna, A. 149
McLaughlin, B. 110, 111
McLeod, S. 110
Mendoza, E. 245–81
Mhic Mhathúna, M. 149
Miller, J.F. 38
Minami, M. 223
Mirhassani, A. 171
Moll, K.L. 207
Morris, D. 111
Motsch, H.-J. 90
Müller, N. 116, 128
Murphy, K, 4

Naigles, L. 15, 26
Nash, L. 241
Neeman, Y. 44
Newport, E. L. 111
Nicholls, L. 25

Ochs, E. 221
Ó Duibhir, P. 149
Oetting, J. 21
Oh, B.L. 208–29
Oller, D. K. 111, 112
Olswang, L.B. 18
Ó Sé, D. 151, 160, 162
Ó Siadhail., M. 156
O'Toole, C. 150
Owens, M. 149
Özcan, F. H. 289, 298, 300

Paradis, C. 231
Paradis, J. 111, 115, 243
Parisse, C. 2, 230–44
Paul, R. 38, 40

Pavez, M.M. 245–81
Perkins, M. R. 2, 167–88, 223
Peters, A. M. 57, 178
Peterson, C. 222, 223
Pine, J. 112
Pinker, S. 15
Pizzuto, E. 112
Pollmann, T. 93
Price, G. 116
Pullum, G. 26

Quirk, R. 4, 7, 11, 20, 21, 29, 169, 209

Radford, A. 289
Ramon-Blumberg, R. 71
Ravid, D. 44, 66, 71
Razak, R. A. 208–29
Rice, M. L. 18
Rimmington, D. 210, 212, 219
Risley, R. T. 13
Rojo, G. 279
Rom, A. 43, 71
Romaine, S. 110
Rothweiler, M. 90
Rubino, R. 112

Samadi, H. 2, 167–88, 223
Samiian, V. 169, 186
Schieffelin, B. B. 221
Schiemenz, S. 114
Schlichting, L. 2, 189–207
Schrey-Dern, D. 90
Schuele, C. 24, 25
Schwarzwald, O. R. 44
Shirai, Y. 112
Singleton, D. 150
Slobin, D. I. 48, 49, 150, 304
Stenson, N. 151, 158
Stokes, J. 2, 13, 139–48
Stokes, S. F. 13
Sturm, A. 93
Surridge, M. 113

Tallerman, M. 112
Tardif, T. 208
Tervoort, B.T. 92
Thomas, A. R. 119, 122, 125
Thomas, E. M. 2, 110–38, 163, 169, 173, 175, 179, 185
Thomas, P. W. 130
Thordadottir, E. 18
Tiersma, P.M. 189, 190
Tolbert, L. 25
Tomasello, M. 14, 25, 112
Tommerdahl, J. 230–44
Topbaş, S. 2, 282–305
Trask, R. 26
Turan, Ü. D. 286, 287
Tyack, D. 40

Underhill, R. 283

Van den Toorn, M.C. 93
Venable, G.P. 40
Vial, C. 236, 243

Waletzky, J. 223
Wall, E. 149
Ward, A. 151
Watkins, T. A. 113, 133
Wei, L. 110, 133
Wells, G. 95, 193
Williams, S. J. 131
Windfuhr, B. 169, 173, 176
Wong, V. 220

Xin, A. T. 220
Xin, J. 209, 212, 216

Yavaş, M. 283, 285
Yip, P. 210, 212, 219

Zhang, J. R. 208, 220
Zhou, G. G. 208
Zhou, J. 208, 220
Zhu, H. 208
Zhu, S. M. 208

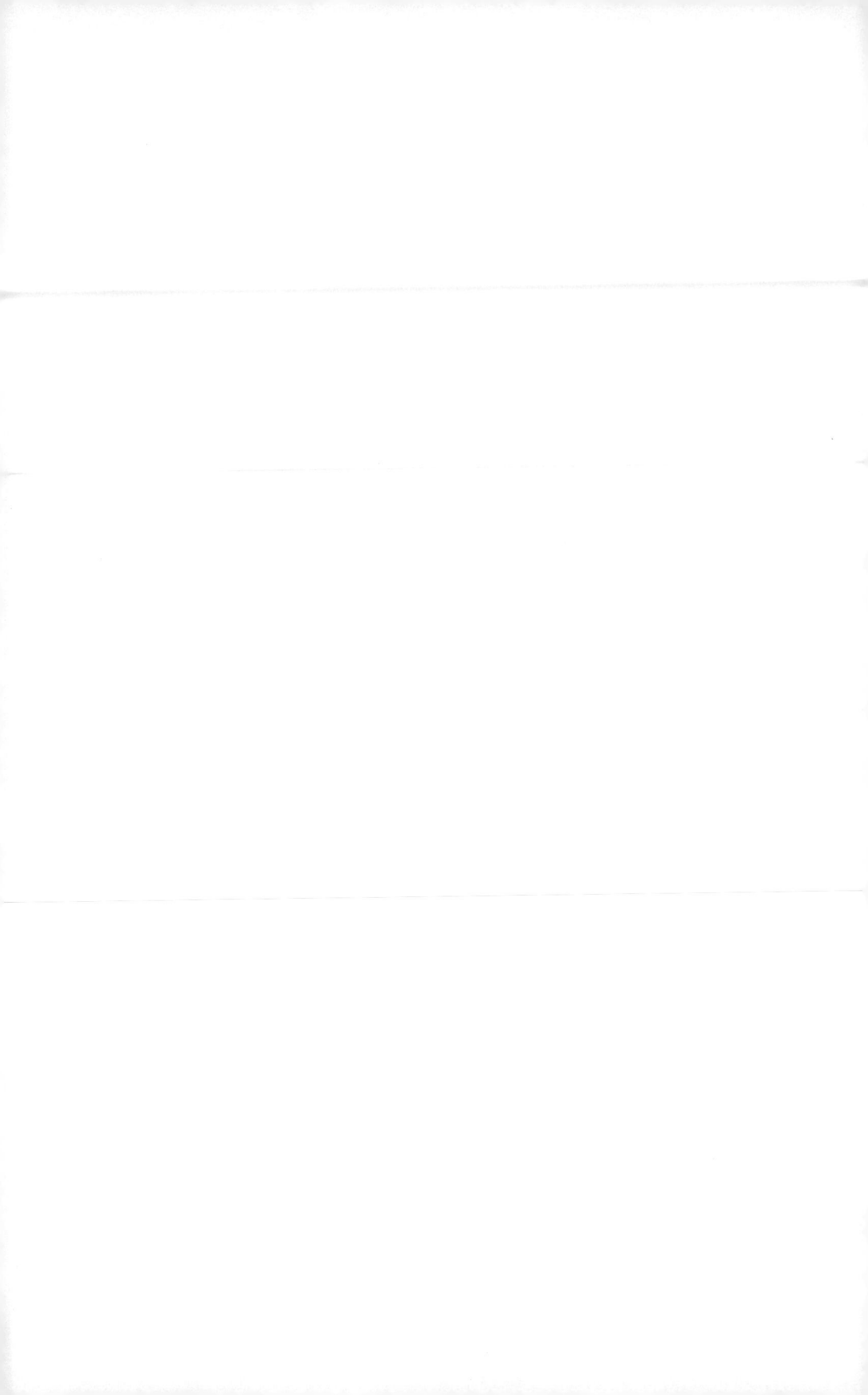